S0-BXN-362

PROGRESS IN CLINICAL AND BIOLOGICAL RESEARCH

Series Editors

Nathan Back   Vincent P. Eijsvoogel   Kurt Hirschhorn   Sidney Udenfriend
George J. Brewer   Robert Grover   Seymour S. Kety   Jonathan W. Uhr

RECENT TITLES

Vol 206: **Genetic Toxicology of the Diet,** Ib Knudsen, *Editor*

Vol 207: **Monitoring of Occupational Genotoxicants,** Marja Sorsa, Hannu Norppa, *Editors*

Vol 208: **Risk and Reason: Risk Assessment in Relation to Environmental Mutagens and Carcinogens,** Per Oftedal, Anton Brøgger, *Editors*

Vol 209: **Genetic Toxicology of Environmental Chemicals,** Claes Ramel, Bo Lambert, Jan Magnusson, *Editors.* Published in two volumes: Part A: *Basic Principles and Mechanisms of Action.* Part B: *Genetic Effects and Applied Mutagenesis*

Vol 210: **Ionic Currents in Development,** Richard Nuccitelli, *Editor*

Vol 211: **Transfusion Medicine: Recent Technological Advances,** Kris Murawski, Frans Peetoom, *Editors*

Vol 212: **Cancer Metastasis: Experimental and Clinical Strategies,** D.R. Welch, B.K. Bhuyan, L.A. Liotta, *Editors*

Vol 213: **Plant Flavonoids in Biology and Medicine: Biochemical, Pharmacological, and Structure–Activity Relationships,** Vivian Cody, Elliott Middleton, Jr., Jeffrey B. Harborne, *Editors*

Vol 214: **Ethnic Differences in Reactions to Drugs and Xenobiotics,** Werner Kalow, H. Werner Goedde, Dharam P. Agarwal, *Editors*

Vol 215: **Megakaryocyte Development and Function,** Richard F. Levine, Neil Williams, Jack Levin, Bruce L. Evatt, *Editors*

Vol 216: **Advances in Cancer Control: Health Care Financing and Research,** Lee E. Mortenson, Paul F. Engstrom, Paul N. Anderson, *Editors*

Vol 217: **Progress in Developmental Biology,** Harold C. Slavkin, *Editor.* Published in two volumes.

Vol 218: **Evolutionary Perspective and the New Genetics,** Henry Gershowitz, Donald L. Rucknagel, Richard E. Tashian, *Editors*

Vol 219: **Recent Advances in Arterial Diseases: Atherosclerosis, Hypertension, and Vasospasm,** Thomas N. Tulenko, Robert H. Cox, *Editors*

Vol 220: **Safety and Health Aspects of Organic Solvents,** Vesa Riihimäki, Ulf Ulfvarson, *Editors*

Vol 221: **Developments in Bladder Cancer,** Louis Denis, Tadao Niijima, George Prout, Jr., Fritz H. Schröder, *Editors*

Vol 222: **Dietary Fat and Cancer,** Clement Ip, Diane F. Birt, Adrianne E. Rogers, Curtis Mettlin, *Editors*

Vol 223: **Cancer Drug Resistance,** Thomas C. Hall, *Editor*

Vol 224: **Transplantation: Approaches to Graft Rejection,** Harold T. Meryman, *Editor*

Vol 225: **Gonadotropin Down-Regulation in Gynecological Practice,** Rune Rolland, Dev R. Chadha, Wim N.P. Willemsen, *Editors*

Vol 226: **Cellular Endocrinology: Hormonal Control of Embryonic and Cellular Differentiation,** Ginette Serrero, Jun Hayashi, *Editors*

Vol 227: **Advances in Chronobiology,** John E. Pauly, Lawrence E. Scheving, *Editors.* Published in two volumes.

Vol 228: **Environmental Toxicity and the Aging Processes,** Scott R. Baker, Marvin Rogul, *Editors*

Vol 229: **Animal Models: Assessing the Scope of Their Use in Biomedical Research,** Junichi Kawamata, Edward C. Melby, Jr., *Editors*

Please contact the publisher for information about previous titles in this series.

PROSTATE CANCER
Part A: Research, Endocrine Treatment, and Histopathology

PROSTATE CANCER
Part A: Research, Endocrine Treatment, and Histopathology

Proceedings of the Second International Symposium on Prostate Cancer held in Paris, France, June 16–18, 1986

Editors

Gerald P. Murphy
Department of Urology
State University of New York at Buffalo
Buffalo, New York

Saad Khoury
Clinique Urologique
Hôpital de la Pitié
Paris, France

René Küss
Clinique Urologique
Hôpital de la Pitié
Paris, France

Christian Chatelain
Clinique Urologique
Hôpital de la Pitié
Paris, France

Louis Denis
Department of Urology
A.Z. Middelheim
Antwerp, Belgium

RC280
P7
I56
v.1
1986

ALAN R. LISS, INC. • NEW YORK

Address all Inquiries to the Publisher
Alan R. Liss, Inc., 41 East 11th Street, New York, NY 10003

Copyright © 1987 Alan R. Liss, Inc.

Printed in the United States of America

Under the conditions stated below the owner of copyright for this book hereby grants permission to users to make photocopy reproductions of any part or all of its contents for personal or internal organizational use, or for personal or internal use of specific clients. This consent is given on the condition that the copier pay the stated per-copy fee through the Copyright Clearance Center, Incorporated, 27 Congress Street, Salem, MA 01970, as listed in the most current issue of "Permissions to Photocopy" (Publisher's Fee List, distributed by CCC, Inc.), for copying beyond that permitted by sections 107 or 108 of the US Copyright Law. This consent does not extend to other kinds of copying, such as copying for general distribution, for advertising or promotional purposes, for creating new collective works, or for resale.

Library of Congress Cataloging-in-Publication Data

International Symposium on Prostate Cancer (2nd :
   1986 : Paris, France)
   Prostate cancer.

   (Progress in clinical and biological research ;
v. 243)
   Contents: pt. A. Research, endocrine treatment, and
histopathology—pt. B. Imaging techniques, radiotherapy,
chemotherapy, and management issues.
   Includes bibliographies and index.
   1. Prostate gland—Cancer—Congresses. I. Murphy,
Gerald Patrick. II. Title. III. Series. [DNLM: 1. Prostatic Neoplasms—congresses. W1 PR668E v.243 /
WJ 752 I61 1986p]
RC280.P7I56   1986   616.99'463   87-3637
ISBN 0-8451-5093-6 (set)
ISBN 0-8451-0198-6 (pt. A)
ISBN 0-8451-0199-4 (pt. B)

Contents

BASIC CONSIDERATIONS

Contributors

H. Abourachid, ER 277 CNRS, IRSC Villejuif, France **[507]**

Per-Anders Abrahamsson, Department of Urology, University of Lund, Lund, Sweden **[489]**

Armand Abramovici, Laboratory of Developmental Pathology, J. Casper Institute of Pathology and Department of Urology, Beilinson Medical Center, Petah Tikva, Tel Aviv University, Sackler School of Medicine, Israel **[559]**

L. Adenis, Centre de Lutte contre le Cancer Oscar Lambert, 59000 Lille, France **[503]**

Herman Adlercreutz, Department of Clinical Chemistry, Helsinki University Central Hospital, Helsinki, Finland **[99]**

Frederick R. Ahmann, Division of Urology, University of Mississippi Medical Center, Jackson, MS 39216 **[283]**

D. Albano, S. Spirito Hospital, Casale, Italy **[251]**

E. Alcini, Surgical Department, Urological Division, Catholic University of Sacred Heart-Policlinico "A. Gemilli," 00168 Rome, Italy **[243]**

Olaf Alfthan, Second Department of Surgery/Urological Unit, Helsinki University Central Hospital, Helsinki, Finland **[99]**

L. Allen, Edgware General Hospital and Westminster Hospital, London, United Kingdom **[427]**

Jan Alumets, Malmö General Hospital, Malmö, Sweden **[489]**

L. Andersson, Departments of Urology, Cytology, and Medical Oncology, Karolinska Institute, Stockholm, Sweden **[547]**

G. Arvis, Service d'Urologie, Hôpital St. Antoine, Paris, France **[511]**

Masaharu Asano, Takasaki Radiation Chemistry Research Establishment, Japan Atomic Energy Research, Takasaki 370, Japan **[429]**

P. Attignac, Department of Urology, Hôpital Cochin, 75014 Paris, France **[539]**

J. Bara, ER 277 CNRS, IRSC, Villejuif, France **[507]**

E. Barasolo, Ospedale S. Andrea, Vercelli, Italy **[379]**

The numbers in brackets are the opening page numbers of the contributors' articles.

Evelyn R. Barrack, Department of Urology, The Johns Hopkins University School of Medicine, and The James Buchanan Brady Urological Institute, The Johns Hopkins Hospital, Baltimore, MD 21205 **[79]**

G. Bartsch, Department of Urology, Gynecology, and Pathology, University of Innsbruck, Innsbruck, Austria **[101]**

G. Béland, Hôpital Notre-Dame, Montreal, Quebec H2L 4M1, Canada **[391]**

A. Bélanger, MRC Group in Molecular Endocrinology and Medicine, Laval University Medical Center, Quebec G1V 4G2, Canada **[145]**

M. Bellina, Urologic Clinic, University of Turin, Turin, Italy **[239]**

A. Bergh, Departments of Physiology, Urology and Andrology, and Pathology, University of Umeå, S-901 Umeå, Sweden **[513]**

Christine Bertagna, Roussel-Uclaf, 75007 Paris, France **[33,351]**

D. Beurton, Clinique Urologique, Hôpital Necker, Paris, France **[369]**

Rashid Bhatti, Division of Urology, University of Illinois and Cook County Hospitals, Chicago, IL 60612 **[551]**

A. Bianco, Institute of Oncology, University of Naples, Naples, Italy **[251]**

H. Bittard, Service d'Urologie, Service de Pathologie, CHU Saint Jacques, 25000 Besancon, France **[517]**

M. Bittard, Service d'Urologie, Service de Pathologie, CHU Saint Jacques, 25000 Besancon, France **[517]**

B. Blin, Centre de Lutte contre le Cancer Oscar Lambert, 59000 Lille, France **[503]**

F. Boccardo, Istituto Nazionale per la Ricerca sul Cancro, Genova, Italy **[249]**

L. Boccon-Gibod, Clinique Urologique, Hôpital Cochin, 75014 Paris, France **[45,411,425]**

A. Bolgan, S. Giovanni e Paolo Hospital, Venice, Italy **[251]**

M. Bongini, Service de Biochimie, Laboratoire 413, CHU Pitié-Salpêtrière, 75634 Paris Cedex 13, France **[141]**

A.V. Bono, Urology Department, Regional Hospital, Varese, Italy **[251]**

H. Botto, Centre Médico-Chirurgical Foch, 92151 Suresnes, France **[199,411]**

Ch. Bouffioux, Urological Department, CHU Sart-Tilman, Liège, Belgium **[255]**

Freerk G. Bouman, Department of Plastic Surgery, Free University Hospital, Amsterdam, The Netherlands **[55]**

N. Bove, ER 277 CNRS, IRSC, Villejuif, France **[507]**

Charles B. Brendler, Department of Urology, The Johns Hopkins University School of Medicine, and The James Buchanan Brady Urological Institute, The Johns Hopkins Hospital, Baltimore, MD 21205 **[79]**

J.-M. Brisset, Centre Médico-Chirurgical de la Porte de Choisy, Paris, France **[111,411]**

Franck Bürki, Department of Medicine, Fondation Bergonié, 33076 Bordeaux Cedex, France **[569]**

J.M. Caillaud, Histo-pathologie, Institut Gustave Roussy, Villejuif, France **[477]**

B. Callet, Hôpital Göuin, Paris, France **[401]**

M. Camey, Centre Médico-Chirurgical Foch, 92151 Suresnes, France [199,411]

J.P. Carbillet, Service d'Urologie, Service de Pathologie, CHU Saint Jacques, 25000 Besancon, France [517]

G. Cariou, Hôpital Saint-Louis, Paris, France [411]

C. Carlu, Histo-pathologie, Institut Gustave Roussy, Villejuif, France [477]

A. Caty, Centre de Lutte contre le Cancer Oscar Lambret, 59000 Lille, France [503]

Louis Chedid, Immunothérapie Expérimentale, Institut Pasteur, 75015 Paris, France [267]

R. Chiche, Clinique Urologique, Hôpital Cochin, Paris, France [425]

Hubert I. Claes, Department of Urology, University Clinics St.-Pieter, Louvain, Belgium [229]

Donald S. Coffey, Department of Urology, The Johns Hopkins Hospital, Baltimore, MD 21205 [1, 21]

Jean-Michel Coindre, Department of Pathology, Fondation Bergonié, 33076 Bordeaux Cedex, France [569]

M. Colombo, Urologic Clinic, University of Turin, Turin, Italy [239]

Ana Maria Comaru-Schally, Endocrine, Polypeptide, and Cancer Institute, VA Medical Center and Tulane University School of Medicine, New Orleans, LA 70146 [173]

E.H. Cooper, The Unit for Cancer Research, University of Leeds, Leeds LS2 9NL, United Kingdom [505]

P. Costa, Centre Hospitalier Régional Universitaire de Nîmes, France [401]

G. Costantin, Centro Tumori, Servizio di Citologia II, Ospedale Civile, Padova, Italy [545]

M. Cotard, Roussel-Uclaf, 93230 Romainville, France [315]

E. David Crawford, Division of Urology, University of Mississippi Medical Center, Jackson, MS 39216 [283]

Patrick J. Creaven, Roswell Park Memorial Institute, Buffalo, NY 14263 [351]

J. Cukier, Clinique Urologique, Hôpital Necker, Paris, France [369]

A. D'Addessi, Surgical Department, Urological Division, Catholic University of Sacred Heart-Policlinico "A. Gemilli," 00168 Rome, Italy [243]

L. Daehlin, Departments of Physiology, Urology and Andrology, and Pathology, University of Umeå, S-901 Umeå, Sweden [513]

N. Daher, ER 277 CNRS, IRSC, Villejuif, France [507]

J.-E. Damber, Departments of Physiology, Urology and Andrology, and Pathology, University of Umeå, S-901 Umeå, Sweden [513]

D. Das, Departments of Urology, Cytology, and Medical Oncology, Karolinska Institute, Stockholm, Sweden [547]

M.C. Dauge, Service d'Anatomie Pathologique, Hôpital Bichat, Paris, France [529]

A. Daver, Centre Paul Papin, Angers, France [77]

C.J. Davis, Armed Forces Institute of Pathology, Washington, DC 20306 [445]

Marilyn A. Davis, Division of Urology, University of Mississippi Medical Center, Jackson, MS 39216 [283]

Ph. Davody, Clinique Urologique, Hôpital Necker, Paris, France [369]

G. Daxenbichler, Department of Urology, Gynecology, and Pathology, University of Innsbruck, Innsbruck, Austria **[101]**

B. Debré, Clinique Urologique, Hôpital Cochin, Paris, France **[425]**

Frans M.J. Debruyne, Department of Urology, St. Radboudhospital, Cath. University, 6500 HB Nijmegen, The Netherlands **[221,301]**

R. De Coster, Department of Endocrinology, Research Laboratory Janssen Pharma, Beerse, Belgium **[291]**

A. de Géry, Roussel-Uclaf, 75007 Paris, France **[33]**

J.P. Dehaut, Centre de Lutte contre le Cancer Oscar Lambert, 59000 Lille, France **[503]**

J. de Leval, Urological Department, CHU Sart-Tilman, Liège, Belgium **[255]**

V. Delmas, Service d'Urologie, Hôpital Bichat, Paris, France **[529]**

F. Demerle, Urologie, Hôpital du Kremlin-Bicêtre, Paris, France **[245]**

Louis Denis, Departments of Endocrinology and Urology, A.Z. Middelheim, Antwerp, Belgium **[221,255,291]**

M. De Pauw, EORTC Data Center, Brussels, Belgium **[379]**

S. Desligneres, Department of Urology, Hôpital Cochin, 75014 Paris, France **[539]**

J.P. Devissaguet, Institut Henri Beaufour, Le Plessis-Robinson, France **[435]**

Herman J. de Voogt, Department of Urology, Free University Hospital, Amsterdam, The Netherlands **[55, 379]**

O. Dietze, Department of Urology, Gynecology, and Pathology, 379 , University of Innsbruck, Innsbruck, Austria **[101]**

J. Dörsam, Department of Urology, Surgical Center, and Department of Pharmacology, University of Heidelberg, Federal Republic of Germany **[423]**

F. Dray, Institut Henri Beaufour, Le Plessis-Robinson, France **[435]**

K. Drieu, Institut Henri Beaufour, Le Plessis-Robinson, France **[435]**

R. Drury, Roswell Park Memorial Institute, Buffalo, NY 14263 **[61]**

R. Duboistesselin, Institut Henri Beaufour, Le Plessis-Robinson, France **[435]**

J. Ducassou, Hôtel Dieu de Marseille, France **[401]**

J.-M. Duclos, Hôpital Saint-Joseph, Paris, France **[411]**

A. Dupont, MRC Group in Molecular Endocrinology and Medicine, Laval University Medical Center, Quebec G1V 4G2, Canada **[145]**

A. Dupront, Roussel-Uclaf, 93230 Romainville, France **[341]**

F. Duval, Clinique Chirurgicale Mutualiste, Reims, France **[411]**

W. Ehrenthal, Department of Urology, Johannes Gutenberg University Medical School, D-6500 Mainz, Federal Republic of Germany **[207]**

T. Eichenberger, Division of Urology, University of Basel, Basel, Switzerland **[533]**

M. Elhilali, Royal Victoria Hospital, Montreal, Quebec H3A 1A1, Canada **[391]**

P. Esposti, Departments of Urology, Cytology, and Medical Oncology, Karolinska Institute, Stockholm, Sweden **[547]**

P. Evrard, Department of Urology, Hôpital Cochin, 75014 Paris, France **[539]**

E. Ezan, Institut Henri Beaufour, Le Plessis-Robinson, France **[435]**

Sture Falkmer, Department of Pathology, University of Uppsala, Uppsala, Sweden **[489]**

G. Fasolis, Urologic Clinic, University of Turin, Turin, Italy **[239]**

J. Fiet, Laboratoire Central de Biochimie, Hôpital Saint-Louis, 75010 Paris, France **[33]**

D. Fontana, Urologic Clinic, University of Turin, Turin, Italy **[239]**

Y. Fradet, Hôpital Hôtel-Dieu de Quebec, Quebec G1R 2J6 , Quebec, Canada **[391]**

J. Fretin, Urologie, Hôpital du Kremlin-Bicêtre, Paris, France **[245]**

A. Frugoni, Urology Department, S. Paolo Hospital, Savona, Italy **[251]**

M. Giusti, 2nd Medical Clinic, University of Turin, Turin, Italy **[239]**

Morris L. Givner, Department of Pathology, Dalhousie University, Halifax, N.S., Canada **[439]**

D. Gontiès, Clinique Chantereine, Brou-sur-Chantereine, France **[411]**

Louis J.G. Gooren, Department of Urology, Free University Hospital, Amsterdam, The Netherlands **[55]**

P. Gosselin, Centre de Lutte contre le Cancer Oscar Lambert, 59000 Lille, France **[503]**

J. Grall, Clinique Urologique, Hôpital Necker, Paris, France **[369]**

Lars Grimelius, Department of Pathology, University of Uppsala, Uppsala, Sweden **[489]**

R. Gschwind, Institute of Physical Chemistry, University of Basel, Basel, Switzerland **[533]**

D. Guiban, Département d'Hormonologie, Hôpital Cochin, 75014 Paris, France **[45]**

Patrick Guinan, Division of Urology, University of Illinois and Cook County Hospitals, Chicago, IL 60612 **[551]**

D. Haack, Department of Urology, Surgical Center and Department of Pharmacology, University of Heidelberg, Federal Republic of Germany **[423]**

Reijo Haapiainen, Second Department of Surgery/Urological Unit, Helsinki University Central Hospital, Helsinki, Finland **[99]**

J. Happ, Department of Urology, Johannes Gutenberg University Medical School, D-6500 Mainz, Federal Republic of Germany **[207]**

Svein Hassellund, Department of Surgery and Urology and Hormone Laboratory, Aker Hospital, Oslo, Norway **[299]**

P.O. Hedlund, Departments of Urology, Cytology, and Medical Oncology, Karolinska Institute, Stockholm, Sweden **[547]**

J.W. Hetherington, The Unit for Cancer Research, University of Leeds, Leeds LS2 9NL, United Kingdom **[505]**

Anne Hosmalin, Immunothérapie Expérimentale, Institut Pasteur, 75015 Paris, France **[267]**

Robert P. Huben, Roswell Park Memorial Institute, Buffalo, NY 14263 **[61,351]**

M. Hucher, Roussel-Uclaf, 75007 Paris, France **[33]**

J.M. Husson, Roussel-Uclaf, 75007 Paris, France **[33,111]**

Kyoichi Imai, Department of Urology, School of Medicine, Gunma University, Maebashi 371, Japan **[429]**

G.B. Ingargiola, Institute of Urology, University of Palermo, Palermo, Italy **[379]**

John T. Isaacs, Department of Oncology and Urology, The Johns Hopkins Hospital, Baltimore, MD 21205 **[1,21]**

G.C. Isaia, 2nd Medical Clinic, University of Turin, Turin, Italy **[239]**

G.H. Jacobi, Department of Urology, Johannes Gutenberg University Medical School, D-6500 Mainz, Federal Republic of Germany **[207]**

G. Janetschek, Department of Urology, Gynecology, and Pathology, University of Innsbruck, Innsbruck, Austria **[101]**

A. Jardin, Urologie, Hôpital du Kremlin-Bicêtre, Paris, France **[245]**

R. Jorest, Centre Hospitalier Regional, Creil, France **[411]**

Isao Kaetsu, Takasaki Radiation Chemistry Research Establishment, Japan Atomic Energy Research, Takasaki 370, Japan **[429]**

James P. Karr, Roswell Park Memorial Institute, Buffalo, NY 14263 **[61]**

F. Keuppens, Belgium **[221]**

Saad Khoury, Clinique Urologique, Hôpital de la Pitie, Paris, France **[xxxix]**

H. Krüger, Department of Urology, Surgical Center, and Department of Pharmacology, University of Heidelberg, Federal Republic of Germany **[423]**

Fernand Labrie, MRC Group in Molecular Endocrinology and Medicine, Laval University Medical Center, Quebec G1V 4G2, Canada **[77,145]**

L. Lamy, Hôpital de Juvisy, France **[411]**

M. Landström, Departments of Physiology, Urology and Andrology, and Pathology, University of Umeå, S-901 87 Umeå, Sweden **[513]**

B. Lardennois, Hôpital de la Maison Blanche, Centre Hospitalo-Universitaire de Reims, Reims, France **[379,401]**

B. Laroche, Hôpital St.-François D'Assisse, Quebec G1L 3L5, Canada **[391]**

M.H. Laudat, Département d'Hormonologie, Hôpital Cochin, 75014 Paris, France **[45]**

N. Ledenko, Service de Biochimie, Laboratoire 413, CHU Pitié-Salpêtrière, 75634 Paris Cedex 13, France **[141]**

A. Le Duc, Hôpital Saint-Louis, Paris, France **[411,485]**

J.M. Le Goff, Laboratoire de Cancérologie Expérimentale, Faculté de Medecine Nord, UA 1175 CNRS, 13326 Marseille Cedex 15, France **[111]**

J.C. Legrand, Service de Biochimie, Laboratoire 413, CHU Pitié-Salpêtrière, 75634 Paris Cedex 13, France **[141]**

M. Leroy, Service de Médecine Nucléaire, Hôpital Saint-Louis, Paris, France **[485]**

M. Levallois, Hôpital de la Durance, Avignon, France **[401]**

Yvan J. Levasseur, Division of Urology, University of Mississippi Medical Center, Jackson, MS 39216 **[283]**

J.F. Louis, Centre Hospitalier Régional Universitaire de Nîmes, France **[401]**

T. Löwhagen, Departments of Urology, Cytology, and Medical Oncology, Karolinska Institute, Stockholm Sweden **[547]**

G. Lunglmayr, Austria **[221]**

Isabel Luthy, MRC Group in Molecular Endocrinology and Medicine, Laval University Medical Center, Quebec G1V 4G2, Canada **[145]**

C. Mahler, Departments of Endocrinology and Urology, A.Z. Middelheim, Antwerp, Belgium **[221, 255, 291]**

C.F. Mann, Roswell Park Memorial Institute, Buffalo, NY 14263 **[61]**

P.M. Martin, Laboratoire de Cancérologie Expérimentale, Faculté de Médecine Nord, UA 1175 CNRS, 13326 Marseille Cedex 15, France **[111]**

Georges Mathe, Institut de Cancérologie et d'Immunogenetique, 94800 Villejuif, France **[173]**

F. Mathieu, Centre Médico-chirurgical Foch, 92151 Suresnes, France **[199]**

M.C. Mathieu, Histo-pathologie, Institut Gustave Roussy, Villejuif, France **[477]**

Louis Mauriac, Department of Medicine, Fondation Bergonié, 33076 Bordeaux Cedex, France **[569]**

C. Mestayer, Service de Biochimie, Laboratoire 413, CHU Pitié-Salpêtrière, 75634 Paris Cedex 13, France **[141]**

B.H. Meyer, Orange Free State University, 339 Bloemfontein, South Africa **[341]**

M.J. Mihatsch, Department of Scientific Photography, University of Basel, Basel, Switzerland **[533]**

G. Mikuz, Department of Urology, Gynecology, and Pathology, University of Innsbruck, Innsbruck, Austria **[101]**

Oliver H. Millard, Department of Urology, Dalhousie University, Halifax, N.S., Canada **[439]**

M. Moguilewsky, Roussel-Uclaf, 93230 Romainville, France **[315]**

K. Möhring, Department of Urology, Surgical Center and Department of Pharmacology, University of Heidelberg, Federal Republic of Germany **[423]**

A. Morelli, M. Vittoria Hospital, Turin, Italy **[251]**

André Morin, Immunothérapie Experimentale, Institut Pasteur, 75015 Paris, France **[267]**

F.K. Mostofi, Armed Forces Institute of Pathology, Washington, DC 20306 **[445]**

Michel Mouren, Roussel-Uclaf, Paris, France **[351]**

A. Mouton, Clinique de l'Archette, Olivet, France **[411]**

Gerald P. Murphy, Department of Urology, State University of New York at Buffalo, Buffalo, NY 14214 **[xxxix]**

Robin Murray, Cancer Institute, Melbourne, Australia **[275]**

Y. Najean, Service d'Médecine Nucléaire, Hôpital Saint-Louis, Paris, France **[485]**

H. Navratil, Faculty of Medicine, Montpellier-Nîmes, France **[401]**

D.W.W. Newling, Consultant Urologist, Princess Royal Hospital, Hull, United Kingdom **[221, 261]**

Nils Normann, Department of Surgery and Urology and Hormone Laboratory, Aker Hospital, Oslo, Norway **[299]**

M. Oberholzer, Departmet of Pathology, Department of Scientific Photography, University of Basel, Basel, Switzerland [533]

T. Ojasoo, Roussel-Uclaf, 75007 Paris, France [111]

H. Parmar, Edgware General Hospital and Westminster Hospital, London, United Kingdom [427]

M. Pavone-Macaluso, Institute of Urology, University of Palermo, Palermo, Italy [379]

Jose I. Paz-Bouza, Endocrine, Polypeptide, and Cancer Institute, VA Medical Center and Tulane University School of Medicine, New Orleans, LA 70146 [173]

Lakshmi Pendyala, Roswell Park Memorial Institute, Buffalo, NY 14263 [351]

M. Petit, Clinique Chirurgicale Mutualiste, Reims, France [411]

R.H. Phillips, Edgware General Hospital and Westminster Hospital, London, United Kingdom [427]

Paula Pitt, Cancer Institute, Melbourne, Australia [275]

J.E. Pontes, Cleveland Clinic Foundation, Cleveland, OH 44106 [61]

F. Pontonnier, Hopital de le Grave de Toulouse, France [401]

J. Pottier, Roussel-Uclaf, 93230 Romainville, France [341]

E. Pozzi, Urology Department, Regional Hospital, Varese, Italy [251]

A. Prawerman, Clinique Chirurgicale Mutualiste, Reims, France [411]

L. Proulx, Roussel-Uclaf, 93230 Romainville, France [315]

G. Pugeat, Centre Hospitale-Universitaire d'Arles, France [401]

B. Rabaud, Service d'Urologie, Hôpital Saint-Louis, Paris, France [485]

E.W. Ramsey, Health Sciences Center General Hospital, Winnipeg, Manitoba R3E 0Z3. Canada [391]

D.F. Randone, Urologic Clinic, University of Turin, Turin, Italy [239]

Sakari Rannikko, Second Department of Surgery/Urological Unit, Helsinki University Central Hospital, Helsinki, Finland [99]

B. Ram Rao, Departmentof Endocrinology, Free University Hospital, Amsterdam, The Netherlands [55]

Paul Ray, Division of Urology, University of Illinois and Cook County Hospitals, Chicago, IL 60612 [551]

J.P. Raynaud, Roussel-Uclaf, 75007 Paris, France [33,111,315]

Tommie W. Redding, Endocrine, Polypeptide, and Cancer Institute, VA Medical Center and Tulane University School of Medicine, New Orleans, LA 70146 [173]

F. Richard, Centre Médico-Chirurgical Foch, 92151 Suresnes, France [199,411]

B. Richards, United Kingdom [221]

M.R.G. Robinson, Pontefract General Infirmary, Pontefract, West Yorkshire WF8 1PL, England, United Kingdom [221,383]

L. Röhl, Department of Urology, Surgical Center and Departmen of Pharmacology, University of Heidelberg, Federal Republic of Germany [423]

L. Rolle, Urologic Clinic, University of Turin, Turin, Italy [239]

Marvin Rubenstein, Hektoer Institute for Medical Research, Chicago, IL 60612 [551]

G. Rutishauser, Division of Urology, University of Basel, Basel, Switzerland **[533]**

J. Saborowski, Department of Urology, University of Bochum, D-4690 Herne 1, Federal Republic of Germany **[365]**

Uriel Sandbank, Laboratory of Developmental Pathology, J. Casper Institute of Pathology and Department of Urology, Beilinson Medical Center, Petah Tikva, Tel Aviv University, Sackler School of Medicine, Israel **[559]**

A.A. Sandberg, Roswell Park Memorial Institute, Buffalo, NY 14263 **[61]**

Sten Sander, Department of Surgery and Urology and Hormone Laboratory, Aker Hospital, Oslo, Norway **[299]**

J.P. Sarramon, Centre Hospitalo-Universitaire de Rangueil, Toulouse, France **[401]**

I. Savatovsky, Hôpital R. Ballanger, Aulnay, France **[411]**

Andrew V. Schally, Endocrine, Polypeptide, and Cancer Institute, VA Medical Center and Tulane University School of Medicine, New Orleans, LA 70146 **[173]**

Harald Schulze, Department of Urology, The Johns Hopkins Hospital, Baltimore, MD 21205; present address: Marienhospital, 4690 Herne, Federal Republic of Germany **[1,21]**

Th. Senge, Department of Urology, University of Bochum, D-4690 Herne 1, Federal Republic of Germany **[365]**

G. Serment, Hotel Dieu de Marseille, France **[401]**

Ciro Servadio, Laboratory of Developmental Pathology, J. Casper Institute of Pathology and Department of Urology, Beilinson Medical Center, Petah Tikva, Tel Aviv University, Sackler School of Medicine, Israel **[559]**

I.A. Sesterhenn, Armed Forces Institute of Pathology, Washington, DC 20306 **[445]**

Josef Shmuely, Laboratory of Developmental Pathology, J. Casper Institute of Pathology and Department of Urology, Beilinson Medical Center, Petah Tikva, Tel Aviv University, Sackler School of Medicine, Israel **[559]**

J.K. Siddall, The Unit for Cancer Research, University of Leeds, Leeds LS2 9NL, United Kingdom **[505]**

Jacques Simard, MRC Group in Molecular Endocrinology and Medicine, Laval University Medical Center, Quebec G1V 4G2, Canada **[145]**

P.H. Smith, United Kingdom **[221]**

J.Y. Soret, Service d'Urologie, CHU Anger, France **[77]**

H.-W. Spindler, Department of Urology, Johannes Gutenberg University Medical School, D-6500 Mainz, Federal Republic of Germany **[207]**

A. Steg, Clinique Urologique, Hôpital Cochin, 75014 Paris, France **[45,425,539]**

R. Sylvester, EORTC Data Center, Brussels, Belgium **[379]**

P. Teillac, Service d'Urologie, Hôpital Saint-Louis, Paris, France **[485]**

H.D. Tewari, St. John Regional Hospital, St. John, N.B. E2L 4L2 Canada **[391]**

G. Tobelem, Service d'Urologie, Hôpital St. Antoine, Paris, France **[511]**

R. Tomic, Departments of Physiology, Urology and Andrology, and Pathology, University of Umeå, S-901 87 Umeå, Sweden **[513]**

C. Tournemine, Roussel-Uclaf, 93230 Romainville, France [315]

Dominique Tremblay, Roussel-Uclaf, 93290 Romainville, France [341,351]

R.R. Tubbs, Cleveland Clinic Foundation, Cleveland, OH 44106 [61]

U.W. Tunn, Department of Urology, Stadtische Kliniken, D-6050 Offenbach/Main, Federal Republic of Germany [365]

E. Usai, Institute of Urology, University of Calgari, Calgari, Italy [251]

D. Vacilotto, Surgical Department, Urological Division, Catholic University of Sacred Heart-Policlinico "A. Gemilli," 00168 Rome, Italy [243]

G. Vallancien, Centre Médico-Chirurgical de la Porte de Choisy, Paris, France [411]

Ludo Vandenbussche, Department of Urology, University Clinics St.-Pieter, Louvain, Belgium [229]

P. Vecsei, Department of Urology, Surgical Center and Department of Pharmacology, University of Heidelberg, Federal Republic of Germany [423]

Raymonde Veilleux, MRC Group in Molecular Endocrinology and Medicine, Laval University Medical Center, Quebec G1V 4G2, Canada [145]

P.M. Venner, Cross Cancer Institute, Edmonton, Alberta, T6G 1Z2, Canada [391]

Raoul L. Vereecken, Department of Urology, University Clinics St.-Pieter, Louvain, Belgium [229]

J.L. Verine, Service d'Urologie, CHU Anger, France [77]

G. Viggiano, Ospedale Civile Umberto 1, Mestre, Italy [379]

J.M. Villette, Laboratoire Central de Biochimie, Hôpital Saint-Louis, 75010 Paris, France [33]

H. v. Wallenberg, Department of Urology, Johannes Gutenberg University Medical School, D-6500 Mainz, Federal Republic of Germany [207]

Lars B. Wadström, Department of Tumour Pathology, Karolinska Hospital, Stockholm, Sweden [489]

Patrick C. Walsh, Department of Urology, The Johns Hopkins University School of Medicine, and The James Buchanan Brady Urological Institute, The Johns Hopkins Hospital, Baltimore, MD 21205 [79]

W. Weiglein, Department of Urology, Stadtische Kliniken, D-6050 Offenbach/Main, Federal Republic of Germany [365]

E.H.J. Weil, The Netherlands [221]

U.K. Wenderoth, Department of Urology, Johannes Gutenberg University Medical School, D-6500 Mainz, Federal Republic of Germany [207]

H. Wenzel, Service d'Urologie, Service de Pathologie, CHU Saint Jacques, 25000 Besancon, France [517]

P. Whelan, United Kingdom [221]

Fred A. Witjes, Department of Urology, St. Radboudhospital, Cath. University, 6500 HB Nijmegen, The Netherlands [301]

F. Wright, Service de Biochimie, Laboratoire 413, CHU Pitié-Salpêtrière, 75634 Paris Cedex 13, France [141]

Hidetoshi Yamanaka, Department of Urology, School of Medicine, Gunma University, Maebashi 371, Japan [429]

Masaru Yoshida, Takasaki Radiation Chemistry Research Establishment, Japan Atomic Energy Research, Takasaki 370, Japan **[429]**

Hisako Yuasa, Department of Urology, School of Medicine, Gunma University, Maebashi 371, Japan **[429]**

F. Zattoni, Istituto di Urologia, Università di Padova, Padova, Italy **[545]**

Contents of Part B: Imaging Techniques, Radiotherapy, Chemotherapy, and Management Issues

PROGRESS IN RADIOTHERAPY

Contributors to Part B

Neil K. Aaronson, The Netherlands Cancer Institute, Amsterdam, The Netherlands

E. Alcini, Surgical Department, Urological Division, Catholic University of Sacred Heart, Poli-clinico "A. Gemelli", Rome, Italy

O. Alfthan, Second Department of Surgery, Urological Unit, Helsinki University Central Hospital, Helsinki, Finland

Y.M. Allain, Service de Radiotherapie, Centre Paul Papin, Angers, France

Malcolm A. Bagshaw, Department of Radiology, Stanford University School of Medicine, Stanford, CA

G. Balconi, Clinica Chirurgicale, Divisione di Urologia, Instituto S. Raffaele, Milan, Italy

Philippe Ballanger, Hôpital du Tondu, Bordeaux, France

Roland Ballanger, Hôpital du Tondu, Bordeaux, France

Mostafa Batata, Brachytherapy Service of the Department of Radiation Oncology, Memorial Sloan-Kettering Cancer Center, New York, NY

Victor Benavente, Department of Urology, Instituto Nacional de Enfermedades Neoplasicas, Lima, Peru

Mitchell C. Benson, Department of Urology, Columbia University, New York, NY

P. Bernacchi, Urologic Department, Regional Hospital, Varese, Italy

M. Bernini, Department of Urology, Arcispedale S. Anna, Ferra, Italy

H. Biersack, Institute of Clinical and Experimental Nuclear Medicine, University Hospital, Venusburg, Bonn, Federal Republic of Germany

A. Bockish, Institute of Clinical and Experimental Nuclear Medicine, University Hospital, Venusburg, Bonn, Federal Republic of Germany

M. Bolla, Service de Radiotherapie, Centre Paul Papin, Angers, France

C. Bollack, Service de Chirurgie Urologique-C.H.U., Strasbourg, France

A.V. Bono, Urologic Department, Regional Hospital, Varese, Italy

B. Brandt, Service d'Urologie, C H U Reims, 51092 Reims Cedex, France

J.M. Brisset, Department of Urology, C.M.C. 15, 75015 Paris, France

J.M. Brule, Service de Radiologie, Chirurgie A - C.H.U., Strasbourg, France

D. Brune, Service de Radiotherapie, Centre Paul Papin, Angers, France

Patrick J. Bryan, Department of Radiology, Case Western Reserve University, School of Medicine, Cleveland, OH 44106

Konrad Burk, Urology Department, University of Frankfurt, Frankfurt, Federal Republic of Germany

Fernando Calais da Silva, Hospital Desterro, Lisbon, Portugal

E.W. Campbell, University of Maryland, School of Medicine, Division of Urology, Baltimore, MD 21201

C. Eugene Carlton, Jr., Department of Urology, Baylor College of Medicine, Houston, TX 77030

C. Carluccio, Department of Urology, Arcispedale S. Anna, Ferra, Italy

B. Castelain, Service de Radiotherapie, Center Paul Papin, Angers, France

P. Cellier, Service de Radiotherapie, Centre Paul Papin, Angers, France

Gilberto Chéchile, Department of Urology, Uro-Oncologic Unit, Puigvert Foundation, Barcelona, Spain

Munzer Chaban, Department of Epidemiology, University of Antwerp, Wilrijk, Belgium

Ch. Chatelain, Clinique Urologique, Hôpital de la Pitié, Paris, France

Richard Chopp, The Urologic Service, Department of Surgery, Memorial Sloan-Kettering Cancer Center, New York, NY

John W. Coleman, Department of Surgery (Urology), New York Hospital - Cornell Medical Center, New York, NY

P. Consonni, Clinica Chirurgicale, Divisione di Urologia, Instituto S. Raffaele, Milan, Italy

Alain Cornet, Department of Urology, AZ Middelheim, Antwerp, Belgium

Richard S. Cox, Department of Radiology, Stanford University School of Medicine, Stanford, CA

J.C. Cuillere, Service de Radiotherapie, Centre Paul Papin, Angers, France

G. Cunin, Département d'Anesthésie, Hôpital Lariboisière, Paris, France

A. D'Addessi, Surgical Department, Urological Division, Catholic University of Sacred Heart, Poli-clinico "A. Gemelli", Rome, Italy

C. Daniele, Department of Urology, Arcispedale S. Anna, Ferra, Italy

Jean B. deKernion, Department of Surgery/Urology, UCLA School of Medicine, Los Angeles, CA 90024

A.B. De La Grange, Service d'Urologie de C.H. de Boulogne s/mer, Boulogne, France

G. De Laroche, Radiotherapy Department, Centre Hospitalier, Lyon Sud, France

Louis Denis, Department of Urology, AZ Middelheim, Antwerp, Belgium

Hugo Denys, Department of Urology, AZ-St. Jan, Bruges, Belgium

W. de Riese, Urology Department, MHH Hannover, Hannover, Federal Republic of Germany

E. Despres, Service de Radiologie, Hôpital Saint Joseph, Paris, France

Edith De Tarragon, Department of Radiology, Hospital P. Morel, Vesoul, France

M. Devonec, Unité de Néphro-Urologie-Transplantation et Immunologie clinique, Hôpital E. Herriot, Lyon, France

Isabel Diaz, Department of Urology, Uro-Oncologic Unit, Puigvert Foundation, Barcelona, Spain

V. DI Girolamo, Clinica Chirurgicale, Divisione di Urologia, Instituto S. Raffaele, Milan, Italy

M. Dimitri, Clinica Urologica, Perugia, Perugia, Italia

J. Douchez, Service de Radiotherapie, Centre Paul Papin, Angers, France

Jean-Pierre E. Droz, Institut Gustave-Roussy, Villejuif, France

Albert Eisenscher, Department of Radiology, Hospital Hasenrain, Mulhouse, France

A. El Khansa, Service d'Urologie, C H U Reims, 51092 Reims Cedex, France

Willy Eylenbosch, Department of Urology, AZ Middelheim, Antwerp, Belgium

William Fair, Brachytherapy Service of the Department of Radiation Oncology, Memorial Sloan-Kettering Cancer Center, New York, NY

Pierre Fargeot, Institut Gustave-Roussy, Centre Leclerc, Dijon, France

C. Fava, Urologic Department, Regional Hospital, Varese, Italy

Hossein Firooznia, Department of Radiology, New York University Medical Center, New York, NY 10016

Sophie Dorothea Fosså, Department of Medical Oncology and Radiotherapy, The Norwegian Radium Hospital, Oslo, Norway

S. Gallais, Service de Neuro-Chirurgie, Hôpital de la Pitié-Salpêtriére, Paris, France

Gustavo Garrido, Department of Urology, Instituto Nacional de Enfermedades Neoplasicas, Lima, Peru

J.P. Gerard, Radiotherapy Department, Centre Hospitalier, Lyon Sud, France

J. Geslin, Service de Radiotherapie, Centre Paul Papin, Angers, France

Robert P. Gibbons, Section of Urology and Renal Transplantation, The Mason Clinic and Virginia Mason Medical Center, Seattle, WA 98111

M. Giustacchini, Surgical Department, Urological Division, Catholic University of Sacred Heart, Poli-clinico "A. Gemelli", Rome, Italy

Cornelia Golimbu, Department of Radiology, New York University Medical Center, New York, NY 10016

Mircea Golimbu, Department of Urology, New York University Medical Center, New York, NY 10016

R. Haapiainen, Second Department of Surgery, Urological Unit, Helsinki University Central Hospital, Helsinki, Finland

R.R. Hall, Department of Urology, Freeman Hospital, Newcastle Upon Tyne, England

Kamal A. Hanash, Department of Urology, Georgetown University Medical Center, McLean, VA 22102

J. Hauchecorne, Service d'Oncologie Médicale, Hôpital de la Salpétrière, Paris, France

M. Hay, Service de Radiotherapie, Centre Paul Papin, Angers, France

Per Olov Hedlund, Department of Urology, Karolinska Hospital, Stockholm, Sweden

J. Heintz, Service de Radiotherapie, Centre Paul Papin, Angers, France

Harry Herr, Brachytherapy Service of the Department of Radiation Oncology, Memorial Sloan-Kettering Cancer Center, New York, NY

Basil Hilaris, Urologic Service of the Department of Surgery, Memorial Sloan-Kettering Cancer Center, New York, NY

H.H. Holm, Departments of Ultrasound,, Urology and Oncology, Herlev Hospital, University of Copenhagen, Herlev, Denmark

B. Hunermann, Institute of Clinical and Experimental Nuclear Medicine, University Hospital, Venusburg, Bonn, Federal Republic of Germany

N. Jaeger, Department of Urology, University Hospital, Venusburg, Bonn, Federal Republic of Germany

A. Jardin, Clinique Urologique, Hôpital du Kremlin-Bicêtre, Paris, France

C. Jasmin, Service d'Hématologie et de Biologie des Tumeurs, Hôpital Paul Brousse, Villejuif, France

N. Javadpour, University of Maryland, School of Medicine, Division of Urology, Baltimore, MD 21201

N. Juul, Departments of Ultrasound, Urology and Oncology, Herlev Hospital, University of Copenhagen, Herlev, Denmark

S. Khoury, Department of Urology, Clinique Urologique, Hôpital de la Pitié, Paris, France

M. Koechlin, Service de Radiotherapie, Centre Paul Papin, Angers, France

L. Koonsilin, Radiotherapy Department, Centre Hospitalier, Lyon Sud, France

A.M. Korinek, Service d'Anesthesiologie et de Réanimation, Hôpital de la Pitié-Salpêtrière, Paris, France

Ivo Kraljić, Clinic of Urology, Clinical Hospital "Dr. M. Stojanović," Croatia, Yugoslavia

Elroy D. Kursh, Division of Urology, Case Western Reserve University, School of Medicine, Cleveland, OH 44106

J.L. La Grange, Service de Radiotherapie, Centre Paul Papin, Angers, France

I. Lambert, Lille, France

D. Langlois, Service de Radiotherapie, Centre Paul Papin, Angers, France

Philippe Laplaige, Institut Gustave-Roussy, Charleville Mézières, France

B. Lardennois, Service d'Urologie, C H U Reims, 51092 Reims Cedex, France

F. Larra, Service de Radiotherapie, Centre Paul Papin, Angers, France

H.M. Lauche, Service de Radiotherapie, Centre Paul Papin, Angers, France

F. Laursen, Departments of Ultrasound, Urology and Oncology, Herlev Hospital, University of Copenhagen, Herlev, Denmark

Pierre Léandri, Department of Urology, Clinic Saint Jean Languedoc, Toulouse, France

L. Lemaître, Lille, France

J.P. Leo, Department of Urology, C.M.C. 15, 75015 Paris, France

Herbert Lepor, Department of Urology, The Johns Hopkins University School of Medicine, Baltimore, MD 21205

M. Maffezzini, Clinica Chirurgicale, Divisione di Urologia, Instituto S. Raffaele, Milan, Italy

K. Malkani, Service de Radiotherapie, Centre Paul Papin, Angers, France

M. Marichez, Service de Radiologie, Hôpital Saint Joseph, Paris, France

Ernesto Martinez, Department of Urology, Uro-Oncologic Unit, Puigvert Foundation, Barcelona, Spain

G. Mathieu, Service de Radiotherapie, Centre Paul Papin, Angers, France

E. Mazeman, Lille, France

J.J. Mazeron, Service de Radiotherapie, Centre Paul Papin, Angers, France

John H. McGovern, Department of Surgery (Urology), New York Hospital - Cornell Medical Center, New York, NY

E. Mearini, Clinica Urologica, Perugia, Perugia, Italia

G. Menu, Service d'Urologie, C H U Reims, 51092 Reims Cedex, France

Pablo Morales, Department of Urology, New York University Medical Center, New York, NY 10016

Angel Moran-Ribon, Institut Gustave-Roussy, Villejuif, France

F. Mornex, Radiotherapy Department, Centre Hospitalier, Lyon Sud, France

Eliahu Mukamel, Department of Surgery/Urology, UCLA School of Medicine, Los Angeles, CA 90024

Gerald P. Murphy, Department of Urology, State University of New York, Buffalo, NY 14214

Jean P. Ory, Department of Medicine, Hospital P. Morel, Vesoul, France

R. Parienty, Service d'Urologie, Hôpital Foch, Suresnes, France

David F. Paulson, Division of Urologic Surgery, Duke University Medical Center, Durham, NC 27710

P. Perrin, Service d'Urologie, Hôpital de l'Antiquaille, Lyon Cedex, France

Gilles Piot, Institut Gustave-Roussy, Le Havre, France

J. Edson Pontes, Department of Urology, Section of Urologic Oncology, The Cleveland Clinic Foundation, Cleveland, OH 44106

M. Porena, Clinica Urologica, Perugia, Perugia, Italia

Julio Pow-Sang, Department of Urology, Instituto Nacional de Enfermedades Neoplasicas, Lima, Peru

Julio Pow-Sang, Jr., Department of Urology, Instituto Nacional de Enfermedades Neoplasicas, Lima, Peru

E. Pozzi, Urologic Department, Regional Hospital, Varese, Italy

J. Pradel, Service d'Urologie, Hôpital Foch, Suresnes, France

George R. Prout, Jr., Urologic Surgical Service, Massachusetts General Hospital Cancer Center, Harvard Medical School, Boston, MA

Mahvash Rafii, Department of Radiology, New York University Medical Center, New York, NY 10016

Graciela Ramirez, Department of Pathology, Instituto Nacional de Enfermedades Neoplasicas, Lima, Peru

S. Rannikko, Second Department of Surgery, Urological Unit, Helsinki University Central Hospital, Helsinki, Finland

F. Rasmussen, Departments of Ultrasound, Urology and Oncology, Herlev Hospital, University of Copenhagen, Herlev, Denmark

Gordon R. Ray, Department of Radiology, Stanford University School of Medicine, Stanford, CA

A. Reggiani, Department of Urology, Arcispedale S. Anna, Ferra, Italy

Martin I. Resnick, Division of Urology, Case Western Reserve University, School of Medicine, Cleveland, OH 44106

P. Ribaud, Service d'Hématologie et de Biologie des Tumeurs, Hôpital Paul Brousse, Villejuif, France

F. Richard, Service de Radiologie, Hôpital Saint Joseph, Paris, France

P. Richaud, Service de Radiotherapie, Centre Paul Papin, Angers, France

P. Rigatti, Clinica Chirurgicale, Divisione di Urologia, Instituto S. Raffaele, Milan, Italy

J.M. Rigot, Lille, France

A. Romano, Department of Urology, Arcispedale S. Anna, Ferra, Italy

P. Romestaing, Radiotherapy Department, Centre Hospitalier, Lyon Sud, France

F. Ronchi, Clinica Chirurgicale, Divisione di Urologia, Instituto S. Raffaele, Milan, Italy

Stuart Rosenberg, The Urologic Service, Department of Surgery, Memorial Sloan-Kettering Cancer Center, New York, NY

P. Rosi, Clinica Urologica, Perugia, Perugia, Italia

Georges Rossignol, Department of Urology, Clinic Saint Jean Languedoc, Toulouse, France

O. Rousseau, Lille, France

G. Ruffi, Clinica Chirurgicale, Divisione di Urologia, Instituto S. Raffaele, Milan, Italy

G.R. Russo, Department of Urology, Arcispedale S. Anna, Ferra, Italy

José Salvador, Department of Urology, Uro-Oncologic Unit, Puigvert Foundation, Barcelona, Spain

L. Sauvage, Lille, France

Jean L. Sauvain, Department of Radiology, Hospital P. Morel, Vesoul, France

Peter T. Scardino, Department of Urology, Baylor College of Medicine, Houston, TX 77030

F.H. Schroeder, Department of Urology, Erasmus University, Rotterdam, The Netherlands

W. Schultze-Seemann, Urology Department, University of Marburg, Marburg, Federal Republic of Germany

A. Serie, Département d'Anesthésie, Hôpital Lariboisière, Paris, France

C. Servadio, Department of Urology, Beilinson Medical Center, The Sackler School of Medicine, Tel Aviv University, Petah Tiqua, Israel

William U. Shipley, Radiation Medicine Service, Massachusetts General Hospital Cancer Center, Harvard Medical School, Boston, MA

Pramod Sogani, Urologic Service of the Department of Surgery, Memorial Sloan-Kettering Cancer Center, New York, NY

H. Sommerkamp, Department of Urology, University Hospital, Freiburg, Federal Republic of Germany

C. Sropp, Klinik Berg, Land Wuppertal, Federal Republic of Germany

Baudouin Standaert, Department of Epidemiology, University of Antwerp, Wilrijk, Belgium

Adolphe Steg, Department of Urology, Hôpital Cochin, Paris, France

A. Taieb, Service d'Urologie, Hôpital Foch, Suresnes, France

Marko Tarle, Nuclear Medicine and Oncology Clinic, Clinical Hospital "Dr. M. Stojanović," Croatia, Yugoslavia

J.B. Thiebault, Service de Neuro-Chirurgie, Hôpital H. Dunant, Paris, France

Cl. Thurel, Service de Neuro-Chirurgie, Hôpital Lariboisière, Paris, France

S. Torp-Pedersen, Departments of Ultrasound, Urology, and Oncology, Herlev Hospital, University of Copenhagen, Herlev, Denmark

D. Vacilotto, Surgical Department, Urological Division, Catholic University of Sacred Heart, Poli-clinico "A. Gemelli", Rome, Italy

W. Vahlensieck, Department of Urology, University Hospital, Venusberg, Bonn, Federal Republic of Germany

G. Vallancien, Department of Urology, C.M.C. 15, 75015 Paris, France

Jean-Claude Van der Auwera, Department of Epidemiology, University of Antwerp, Wilrijk, Belgium

Peter Van Oyen, Department of Urology, AZ-St. Jan, Bruges, Belgium

E. Darracott Vaughn, Department of Surgery (Urology), New York Hospital - Cornell Medical Center, New York, NY

Piet Vercruysse, Pain Relief Unit, AZ-St. Jan, Bruges, Belgium

Robert Vergison, Department of Urology, AZ-St. Jan, Bruges, Belgium

G. Vespasiani, Clinica Urologica, Perugia, Perugia, Italia

José Vicente, Urology Service, Fudación Puigvert, Barcelona, Spain

G. Virgili, Clinica Urologica, Perugia, Perugia, Italia

Patrick C. Walsh, Department of Urology, The Johns Hopkins University School of Medicine, Baltimore, MD 21205

M. Wannenmacher, Department of Radiotherapy, University Hospital, Freiburg, Federal Republic of Germany

J.J. Wenger, Service de Radiologie, Chirurgie A - C.H.U., Strasbourg, France

Willet F. Whitmore, Jr., Urologic Service, Department of Surgery, Memorial Sloan-Kettering Cancer Center, New York, NY

A. Wurtz, Lille, France

Phong Bui Xuan, Department of Radiology, Hospital P. Morel, Vesoul, France

J.D. Young, University of Maryland, School of Medicine, Division of Urology, Baltimore, MD 21201

Eduardo Zungri, Department of Urology, Uro-Oncologic Unit, Puigvert Foundation, Barcelona, Spain

Preface

The Second International Symposium on Prostate Cancer was held at the Hotel Intercontinental in Paris, France, June 16–18, 1986. Six years after the first Symposium held in 1980, more than 900 recognized specialists, representing 25 nations, met to discuss the management of this common tumor which is becoming increasingly common, due in part to the aging of the population.

Although this cancer occurs more frequently in elderly men (mean age: 72 years), there are no other specific known predisposing causes. For this reason, in contrast with other cancers, specific prevention cannot be proposed at the present time. Perhaps progress in this disease will have to come from treatment.

Treatment remains highly controversial, especially since the development in recent years of new forms of endocrine therapy. This symposium provided the opportunity to compare various approaches and to define the points of agreement and disagreement, which will be the subject of debate of smaller meetings to be held in the future.

Since the first symposium on prostate cancer in 1980, several new elements, especially in relation to endocrine treatment, have appeared in this field, which, if their value is confirmed, could change profoundly the future management of this tumor.

Another most significant progress in diagnosis is the more routine use of ultrasonography in the evaluaton of the extension of the disease, which can therefore be more accurately defined than by simple digital rectal examination. The role of CT scan and NMR has also been discussed extensively.

The treatment was also the focus of many communications. The discussion of the value of the new LHRH analogs and of the total androgen blockade concept was for the first time discussed on the basis of controlled scientific data rather than on passionate theoretical concepts.

The symposium also directed attention to new progress in the histochemistry and related pathologic topics of prostate cancer. Results from radiotherapy were presented, and the value of chemotherapy with and without hormone treatments was updated.

Surgical treatments of various stages of prostate cancer are reported. The nerve-sparing procedure of Patrick Walsh is included. A series of reports on aspects of treatment for each clinical stage of prostate cancer conclude this symposium. To the degree the report of this symposium is successful principally reflects the worldwide cooperation in cancer efforts between urologists and medical specialists in general.

Saad Khoury
Gerald P. Murphy
Paris, France,
June 18, 1986

Acknowledgment

The organizing and scientific committee of the Second International Symposium on Prostate Cancer wish to thank the ARC (Association pour la Recherche sur le Cancer-Villejuif) for their help in organization of the Symposium and the editing of the book.

Prostate Cancer, Part A: Research, Endocrine
Treatment, and Histopathology, pages 1–19
© 1987 Alan R. Liss, Inc.

A CRITICAL REVIEW OF THE CONCEPT OF TOTAL ANDROGEN ABLATION
IN THE TREATMENT OF PROSTATE CANCER

Harald Schulze, John T. Isaacs and
Donald S. Coffey

The Johns Hopkins Hospital, Department of
Urology, Baltimore, Maryland 21205, USA

I. INTRODUCTION

Forty-five years following the proposed treatment of
prostatic adenocarcinoma by androgen ablation (Huggins and
Hodges, 1941), we remain in a state of confusion regarding
this type of therapy. For example, how much can survival
be increased by castration? Should treatment with androgen
ablation be initiated early or late in the disease process?
Do people relapse following castration because of small
amounts of androgen remaining in the serum or tissue? Are
there clones of tumor cells within the prostate that are
androgen-insensitive? Are there any new hormonal
treatments of prostate cancer that are better than
castration for survival?

There is added confusion as LH-RH analogs join our
armamentarium of drugs to treat prostate cancer. These
exciting new drugs can achieve castration levels of serum
testosterone and are probably of therapeutic equivalence to
diethylstilbestrol (DES) or castration. What is not so
clear is whether adding flutamide or another antiandrogen
to early treatment with LH-RH analogs will produce a
remarkable increase in efficacy such as proposed by Labrie
et al. (1983). That is, can you increase the survival of a
patient treated early with LH-RH and flutamide beyond that
observed with castration alone? Why do patients die of
prostate cancer following relapse from castration? Is
relapse due to small remaining amounts of DHT residing in
the tumor tissue which might be derived from adrenal
androgens or by direct synthesis within the prostate?

We propose in this review that the scientific evidence
at the moment supports the concept that patients who die of
prostate cancer following relapse to castration do so not
from residual androgens remaining in the serum nor from
androgens residing in the prostate, but from androgen-
independent cells. This is because the tumor has reached
an androgen autonomous state which is a common process
throughout tumor biology in many forms of resistance to
drug therapy. An attempt will be made to put these issues
in proper focus from both the historical and scientific
perspective. It is possible to selectively choose papers
from the voluminous literature on this topic that will
support almost any hypothesis. We will try to focus on the
strongest studies to help the reader through this confusing
arena. Unfortunately, there are no controlled, randomized
prospective studies on LH-RH plus flutamide with a long
enough follow-up to adequately answer the question of the
efficacy of this treatment. Until these data become
available the debate will continue.

II. <u>EARLY APPROACHES TO TOTAL ANDROGEN ABLATION</u>

   a.) <u>ADRENALECTOMY</u>

   Following the classic studies of Huggins and his
associates for the use of castration or estrogen therapy to
treat prostate cancer, it became apparent that patients
subsequently failed this treatment and relapsed to what
appeared to be a hormonally insensitive state. The
question arose as to whether adrenal androgens could be the
cause of this relapse. Many studies followed in which
patients were adrenalectomized and supported with
hydrocortisone replacement. In addition, many techniques
were developed to cause "medical adrenalectomies" (Robinson
et al., 1974; Worgul et al., 1983; Ponder et al., 1984;
Murray and Pitt, 1985; Pont, 1986; DeBruyne and Witjes,
1986) . These studies showed that patients can die of
prostatic adenocarcinoma without testes and adrenals. The
absence of testes and adrenals is not sufficient to stop
the progression of prostate cancer cells. Indeed, today,
adrenalectomy and chemical control of the adrenals have not
been accepted as standard treatment for advancing prostate
cancer. Some important papers which described the
objective responses to bilateral adrenalectomy for

hormonally treated and relapsed prostate cancer patients
are summarized in Table 1.

TABLE 1. ADVANCED PROSTATE CANCER:
BILATERAL ADRENALECTOMY FOLLOWING RELAPSE TO STANDARD
HORMONAL THERAPY

AUTHORS	NO. OF PTS.	REPORTED OBJECTIVE IMPROVEMENT
Huggins & Scott (1945)	4	0
Huggins & Bergenstal (1952)	7	0
Baker (1953)	10	0
Whitmore et al. (1954)	17	2
Morales et al. (1955)	20	1
MacFarlane et al. (1960)	13	1
Bhanalaph et al. (1974)	26	1
	97	5
TOTAL EVALUABLE:	89	5 (5.6%)

b.) HYPOPHYSECTOMY

Since hypophysectomy blocks both adrenal and testicular
function by the removal of ACTH and LH, this might have
provided an effective treatment for patients who relapsed
after castration therapy for prostate cancer. In addition,
prolactin might also play a role in stimulating relapse
from prostatic adenocarcinoma. In 1948, W. W. Scott and
his colleagues at Johns Hopkins carried out the first
hypophysectomy in patients who relapsed after castration.
Several studies have subsequently pursued this approach. It
is apparent that patients died of prostatic cancer without
testes and pituitary glands. Their malignancy continued to
grow in spite of the absence of adrenal androgen serum
levels. Some hypophysectomy studies are summarized in
Table 2. Today, hypophysectomy is not considered an
effective form of therapy although it would achieve almost
total androgen ablation.

TABLE 2.   ADVANCED PROSTATE CANCER:
HYPOPHYSECTOMY FOLLOWING RELAPSE TO
STANDARD HORMONAL THERAPY

AUTHORS	NO. OF PTS.	REPORTED OBJECTIVE IMPROVEMENT
Scott & Schirmer (1962)	17	7
Fergusson & Hendry (1971)	100	0
Morales et al. (1971)	23	0
Murphy et al. (1971)	34	0
Maddy et al. (1971)	20	7
Levin et al. (1978)	10	0
Smith et al. (1984)	15	0
	219	14
TOTAL EVALUABLE:	209	14 (6.7%)

c.)   ANTIANDROGENS

New drugs that could block androgen action directly at the target tissue became available in the early 1960s. These antiandrogens blocked any androgens made by the testes and adrenals, as well as androgens synthesized within the prostate gland per se by an autocrine process. As antiandrogens, such as cyproterone acetate, medroxyprogesterone, flutamide, Anandron and others achieved widespread use, it again became apparent that patients could die of prostate cancer even in the face of castration and large amounts of antiandrogen that blocked prostatic DHT.   This indicated that androgens within the prostate itself were not sufficient to account for the continued growth of prostatic cancer following castration. Although all these antiandrogens are very effective agents in blocking androgen action, some argued that slight androgenic effects of some of these antiandrogens (i.e., cyproterone acetate) might account for the inability to completely block the growth of relapsing cancer.   However, even the pure antiandrogens flutamide and Anandron have failed to stop the continued growth of relapsed prostate cancer.   Studies with the most commonly used antiandrogens, cyproterone acetate and flutamide, are summarized in Table 3.

TABLE 3. ADVANCED PROSTATE CANCER:
ANTIANDROGENS FOLLOWING RELAPSE TO
STANDARD HORMONAL THERAPY

AUTHORS	ANTI-ANDROGEN	NO. OF PTS.	REPORTED OBJECTIVE IMPROVEMENT
Wein & Murphy (1973)	Cyp.	15	1
Smith et al. (1973)	Cyp.	28	2
Stoliar & Albert (1974)	Flu.	14	1
Sogani et al. (1975)	Flu.	26	2
MacFarlane & Tolley (1985)	Flu.	14	1
TOTAL:		97	7 (7.2%)

Cyp. = cyproterone acetate
Flu. = flutamide

III. A NEW APPROACH TO ANDROGEN ABLATION - LH-RH ANALOGS

The dramatic discovery that LH secretion was regulated by a small decapeptide, LH-RH or GnRH, resulted in a new approach to the treatment of prostate cancer. Although medical orchiectomy probably provided no additional therapeutic benefit, it might prove more acceptable because the psychological impact of orchiectomy was avoided. As these agonists were clinically tested, symptomatic flares occurred due to the outpouring of testosterone from the immediate but transient stimulation of the Leydig cells by LH. Antiandrogens were added to prevent this flare. Currently, LH-RH antagonists are being developed which should not produce such flares.

The LH-RH analogs are exciting new compounds because they reduce testosterone to approximately the same levels that can be obtained with castration or diethylstilbestrol (DES) therapy. LH-RH analog therapy circumvents the need for estrogens which have well known water retention and cardiovascular side effects. They also circumvent the psychological impact of orchiectomy. The difficulty with these compounds is that they must be administered throughout the remaining life of the patient and require strict compliance. Depot formulations may aid in compliance; however, all agents remain very expensive. In summary, these LH-RH analogs provide new options for the treatment of prostate cancer. Because of the newness of these drugs, additional mechanisms of action or toxicities cannot be excluded.

IV.   IS PROSTATE CANCER MORE SENSITIVE TO ANDROGENS THAN NORMAL PROSTATE?

    a) Measurement of Intracellular Androgen Levels

    Labrie and his colleagues (1982) have recently claimed that the combination of an LH-RH analog with an antiandrogen as early therapy might be superior to castration. This concept depends upon the theory that androgens can accumulate in the prostate from adrenal sources or from autocrine synthesis and that these steroids provide for relapse following castration. In addition, Labrie has proposed that there may be supersensitive prostatic cancer cells within the prostate that can function even with small amounts of prostatic androgens. No one has yet been able to show that adrenalectomy or LH-RH and antiandrogens reduced the baseline level of DHT that remained in prostatic tissue after castration.

    The measurement of dihydrotestosterone levels in the prostate is most difficult in the very best hands. Levels of DHT in the prostate are extremely low and therefore require many controls to distinguish from normals. Problems associated with tissue processing and of DHT recovery make interpretation and reproducibility difficult. In fact, for many years it appeared that dihydrotestosterone levels were elevated in BPH tissue. This was confirmed in many laboratories before it was proven that this was an artifact of postmortem metabolism (Walsh, Hutchins and Ewing, 1983). Potential metabolic artifacts have not been ruled out in many studies with prostate cancer. We therefore cannot make major conclusions on the therapy of human prostate cancer based upon the remaining DHT levels in the prostate until further investigation.

b) Animal Models

Labrie postulated that prostatic cancer cells are more sensitive to androgens than normal prostate based upon observations of the Shionogi tumor system (Labrie and Veilleux, 1986). The Shionogi tumor system is a mouse mammary tumor grown in cell culture. Extrapolations from this in vitro system are being made to human prostate cancer. The existence of human prostatic tumor cells that are extremely sensitive to androgens remains to be established. Indeed, Ellis and Isaacs (1985) and Trachtenberg (1985) have shown that as testosterone levels are increased in the serum of castrated animals, the Dunning H rat prostatic tumor can respond at a slightly lower testosterone concentration than can normal tissue. The minimal concentration to stimulate cancer cell growth is still, however, well above that present in the serum of the castrated host. These careful studies of Dunning rat prostatic adenocarcinoma sublines demonstrated that castrate levels of testosterone are not sufficient to support any significant growth of androgen-dependent prostatic tumor cells over the long term. Extensive investigation of this animal model indicates that, in addition to androgen-dependent cancer cells, there are androgen-independent cells residing within individual prostatic adenocarcinomas that can grow in either castrated hosts or castrated hosts treated with antiandrogens. These androgen-independent tumor cells are thus resistant to androgen ablation therapy, no matter how complete.

Prostatic cancer cells comprise three different categories of androgen sensitivity. Androgen-dependent prostatic cancer cells require androgen for their existence as do many of the normal epithelial cells of the prostate. When androgen is withdrawn, these dependent cells' growth ceases and they die. Clones of cancer cells that are androgen-sensitive survive in the absence of androgen but grow at a higher rate in the presence of androgens. Androgen-independent cancer cells are not affected by the presence or absence of androgens in any appreciable manner. Tumors are heterogeneous; all of these cell types may be present in a prostatic carcinoma. They certainly are represented in the different sublines of the Dunning rat

prostatic adenocarcinoma (Isaacs, 1985). In Fig. 1, we
have summarized the growth of the Dunning R-3327-H tumor
under different hormonal therapies. The addition of an
antiandrogen showed no further reduction in tumor weight
when compared to chemical or surgical castration alone.
There is no evidence to support the concept that serum
levels of testosterone below that of castrate are capable
of supporting any significant growth in animal models of
prostate cancer.

RAT PROSTATE CANCER
DUNNING R-3327 H

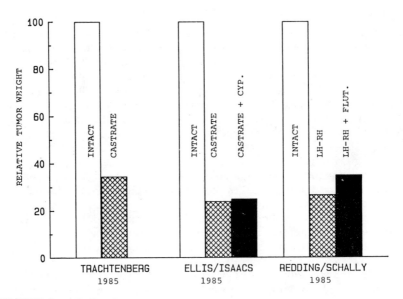

FIGURE 1. Relative tumor weight of the rat Dunning tumor
R3327H compared to the tumors grown in intact control
animals 9 weeks after the indicated treatment was started
(Cyp. = cyproterone acetate; Flu. = flutamide).

V. COMBINED THERAPY IN HUMAN PROSTATE CANCER

Labrie et al. (1984, 1985, 1986) have claimed
spectacular results following treatment of patients with
prostatic cancer using a combination of a pure antiandrogen

plus surgical or medical castration. Their results
stimulated several large prospective studies using a
combination of castration and antiandrogens. As expected
from theoretical considerations and animal studies
discussed above, early reports of prospective studies
indicate no advantage to using antiandrogens in addition to
castration or LH-RH analog treatment (Table 4).

TABLE 4. PROSPECTIVE STUDIES ON
COMPLETE ANDROGEN BLOCKADE IN PATIENTS
WITH METASTATIC PROSTATE CANCER

AUTHORS	NO. OF PTS.	RATE OF PROGRESSION AFTER 1 YEAR
ZADRA & TRACHTENBERG (1986)		
- CASTRATION	9	44%
- CASTRATION + ANANDRON	10	50%
- LH-RH + ANANDRON	11	36%
SCHROEDER ET AL. (1986)		
- LH-RH ANALOG	58	38%
- LH-RH + CYPROTERONE ACETATE	13	38%

Labrie et al. (1984, 1985, 1986) have claimed that
flutamide is a more potent antiandrogen than cyproterone
acetate. One must distinguish between potency and
efficacy. In terms of a drug dose response curve, potency
represents the dose of a drug that achieves 50% of the
maximal effect, while efficacy represents the maximal
response that can be achieved. There is absolutely no
evidence in any animal model that flutamide is more
efficacious than cyproterone acetate. For example, Neri et
al. (1972) demonstrated equivalent reduction in prostate
growth in animals treated with cyproterone acetate and
flutamide.

The studies of Labrie et al. (1984, 1985, 1986) are
difficult to interpret. In Figures 2 and 3, we summarize
their reports. Although the number of patients has

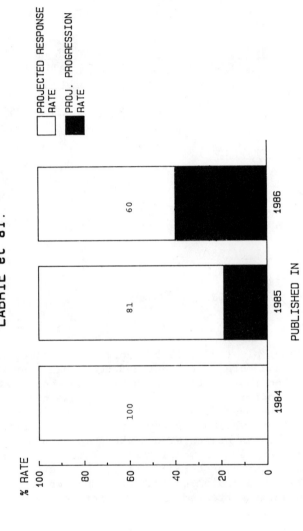

COMPLETE ANDROGEN WITHDRAWAL
PROJECTED 2 - YEAR RESPONSE RATE
LABRIE et al.

% RATE

PROJECTED RESPONSE
RATE

PROJ. PROGRESSION
RATE

100

81

60

1984   1985   1986

PUBLISHED IN

NUMBER OF PATIENTS 50 - 87 - 119
AVERAGE FOLLOW-UP (YEARS) 1.50 - 1.35 - 1.42

Fig. 2

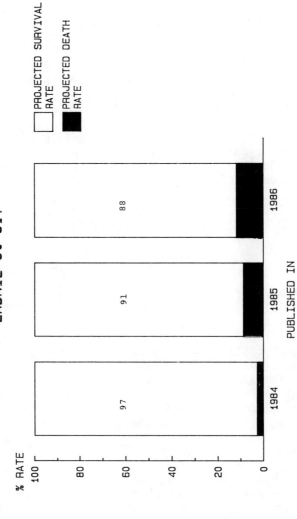

COMPLETE ANDROGEN WITHDRAWAL
PROJECTED 2 - YEAR SURVIVAL RATE
LABRIE et al.

% RATE

100
80
60
40
20
0

97   91   88

1984   1985   1986

PUBLISHED IN

☐ PROJECTED SURVIVAL RATE
■ PROJECTED DEATH RATE

NUMBER OF PATIENTS 50 - 87 - 119
AVERAGE FOLLOW-UP (YEARS) 1.50 - 1.35 - 1.42

Fig. 3

continued to increase, the average follow-up interval remains approximately 1.4 years. The _projected_ response rate at 2 years has decreased from 100% to 60% (Fig. 2). Although the projected survival rates (Fig. 3) up to now appear to have decreased only slightly, the question remains as to how much further these response and survival rates will have decreased by the time the study has been carried out for a longer period of time, so that actual rates are obtained rather than projected.

A comparison of reported response rates in several studies using different treatment modalities (Table 5) shows a wide variation of objective initial response rates (53.8-100%). A summation of the data (Table 6) shows, however, that all different hormonal treatments up to now have been equally effective. The fact that even for the same treatment a 2-fold difference in the initial response rates has been reported emphasizes the importance of performing randomized studies for evaluating the efficacy of a given treatment.

TABLE 5. REPORTED INITIAL RESPONSE RATE OF PREVIOUSLY UNTREATED PATIENTS WITH ADVANCED PROSTATE CANCER

AUTHORS	TREATMENT	NO. PTS.	RESPONSE RATE (%)
Stoliar & Albert ('74)	Flutamide	3	100
Prout et al. (1975)	Flutamide	13	53.8
Rost et al. (1978)	Cyp.Acetate	10	100
Jacobi et al (1980)	Cyp.Acetate	21	85.7
Narayama et al ('81)	Flutamide	11	100
Sogani et al. (1984)	Flutamide	72	87.5
Tunn et al (1983)	Cyp.Acetate	20	65
Murphy et al (1983)	DES/Orch.	83	80.7
Trachtenberg (1984)	Ketoconazole	13	100
Robinson et al (1974)	Aminogluteth.	6	83.3
Leuprolide Study Group (1984)	DES	94	88.9
	LH-RH	92	86
Keating et al (1986)	Flutamide	80	80
DeBruyne & Witjes ('86)	Ketoconazole	40	72.5
Wenderoth & Jacobi ('86)	LH-RH	25	84
Heybroek (1986)	LH-RH	55	78.2
Van Cangh,Opsomer ('86)	LH-RH	19	84.2

TABLE 6. SUMMARY OF INITIAL RESPONSE RATES

TREATMENT	NO. OF PATIENTS	% OBJECTIVE RESPONSE	RANGE
DES/Orchiectomy	177	83%	80.7-100
Antiandrogens			
Cyproterone acetate	51	80%	65.0-100
Flutamide	179	85%	53.8-100
Ketoconazole	53	79%	72.5-100
LH-RH Analog	191	83%	78.2- 86

Will combined therapy be more efficacious than castration or diethylstilbestrol or any other single treatment? The results may be compared with those of the National Prostatic Cancer Project Series 500 on the effect of DES or castration alone and with those of Giuliani and colleagues (1980) who had treated their patients with a combination of castration and cyproterone acetate, thus achieving a complete androgen blockade early in the treatment (Table 7). The actual two year survival rates of these 2 different treatment modalities are not different. In 1982, Labrie et al. called for a randomized prospective study. Such studies are underway and final results will reveal whether there is any advantage of combination therapy for prostate cancer.

TABLE 7. SURVIVAL RATES
METASTATIC PROSTATE CANCER

	1 YEAR	2 YEARS
Murphy et al. (1983) NPCP 500		
- DES or Orchiectomy	90%	63%
Giuliani et al. (1980)		
- Castration + Cyproterone Acetate	95%	58%

We believe that treatment with LH-RH and flutamide will be a very effective alternative to castration. Whether any therapeutic advantages will be observed beyond castration, in terms of response or survival rates, is unclear. In comparative studies, it is important that the same criteria are measured using the same types of patients, and that proper statistical analysis is performed.

The most important therapeutic need at present is a treatment for hormonally insensitive prostate cancer. We must not dilute our efforts to find these new modalities of therapy by continuing to believe that residual androgens play a role in relapsed prostate cancer. We urgently need a better understanding of the biology of prostate cancer. In the meantime, with the LH-RH analog, we have an alternative to standard hormonal therapy. Unfortunately, neither antiandrogens alone nor antiandrogens in combination with medical or surgical castration seem to provide a therapeutic advance.

REFERENCES

Bailar JC III, Byar DP (1970). Estrogen treatment for cancer of the prostate. Cancer 26:257-261.

Baker WJ (1953). Bilateral adrenalectomy for carcinoma of the prostate gland: preliminary report. J Urol 70:275-281.

Bhanalaph T, Varkarakis MJ, Murphy GP (1974). Current status of bilateral adrenalectomy or advanced prostatic carcinoma. Ann Surg 179:17-23.

Byar DP (1973). The Veterans Administration Cooperative Urological Research Group's studies of cancer of the prostate. Cancer 32:1126-1130.

DeBruyne FMS, Witjes FJ and the members of the Dutch South-East Cooperative Study group (1986). Ketoconazole high dose (H.D.) in the management of metastatic prostatic carcinoma. J Urol 135:Abstract #397.

Elder JS, Gibbons RP (1985). Results of trials of the USA National Prostatic Cancer Project. EORTC Genitourinary Group Monograph 2, Part A: Therapeutic Principles in Metastatic Prostatic Cancer, pp. 221-242, Alan R. Liss, Inc.

Ellis WJ, Isaacs JT (1985). Effectiveness of complete versus partial androgen withdrawal therapy for the treatment of prostatic cancer as studied in the Dunning

R-3327 system of rat prostatic adenocarcinomas. Cancer Res 45:6041-6050.

Fergusson JD, Hendry WF (1971). Pituitary irradiation in advanced carcinoma of the prostate: analysis of 100 cases. Br J Urol 43:514-519.

Fossa SD, Jahnsen JU, Karlsen S, Ogreid P, Haveland H, Trovag A (1985). High-dose medroxyprogesterone acetate versus prednisolone in hormone-resistant prostatic cancer. Eur Urol 11:11-16.

Giuliani L, Pescatore D, Giberti C, Martorana G, Natta G (1980). Treatment of advanced prostatic carcinoma with Cyproterone acetate and orchiectomy - 5-year follow-up. Eur Urol 6:145-148.

Harrison JH, Thorn GW, Jenkins D (1953). Total adrenalectomy for reactivated carcinoma of the prostate. N Engl J Med 248:86-92.

Heybroek RPM (1986). LHRH-depot (single and combination) therapy for advanced prostatic carcinoma. J Urol 135:Abstract #390.

Huggins C, Bergenstal D (1952). Effect of bilateral adrenalectomy on certain human tumors. Proc Nat Acad Sci 38:73-76.

Huggins C, Hodges CV (1941). Studies on prostatic cancer. I. The effect of castration, of estrogen and of androgen injection on serum phosphatases in metastatic carcinoma of the prostate. Cancer Res 1:293-297.

Huggins C, Scott WW (1945). Bilateral adrenalectomy in prostatic cancer. Clinical features and urinary excretion of 17-ketosteroids and estrogens. Ann Surg 122:1031-1041.

Isaacs JT (1985). Mechanisms for resistance of prostatic cancers to androgen ablation therapy. In: Bruchovsky N, Chapdelaine A, Neumann F, eds., Regulation of Androgen Action, pp. 71-76.

Jacobi GH, Altwein JE, Kurth KH, Basting R, Hohenfellner R (1980). Treatment of advanced prostatic cancer with parenteral Cyproterone acetate: A phase III randomised trial. Br J Urol 52:208-215.

Johansson J-E, Lingardh G (1985). High-dose medroxy-progesterone in the treatment of advanced therapy-resistant prostatic carcinoma. Eur Urol 11:9-10.

Keating MA, Griffinn PP, Schiff SF (1986). Flutamide in the treatment of advanced prostate cancer. J Urol 135:Abstract #398.

Labrie F, Belanger A, Dupont A, Emond J, Lacoursiere Y, Monfette G (1984). Combined treatment with LHRH agonist and pure antiandrogen in advanced carcinoma of the prostate. Lancet 2:1090.

Labrie F, Dupont A, Belanger A, Cusan L, Lacourciere Y, Monfette G, Laberge JG, Emond JP, Fazekas ATA, Raynaud JP, Husson JM (1982). New hormonal therapy in prostatic carcinoma: combined treatment with an LHRH agonist and an antiandrogen. Clin Invest Med 5:267-275.

Labrie F, Dupont A, Belanger A, Giguere M, Lacoursiere Y, Emond J, Monfette G, Bergeron V (1985). Combination therapy with Flutamide and castration (LHRH agonist or orchiectomy) in advanced prostate cancer: a marked improvement in response and survival. J Steroid Biochem 23:833-841.

Labrie F, Veilleux R (1986). A wide range of sensitivities to androgens develops in cloned Shionogi mouse mammary cells. The Prostate 8:293-300.

Labrie F, Dupont A, Lacourciere Y, Giguere M, Belanger A, Monfette G, Emond J (1986). Combined treatment with flutamide in association with medical or surgical castration. J Urol 135:Abstract 399.

The Leuprolide Study Group (1984). Leuprolide versus diethylstilbestrol for metastatic prostatic cancer. N Eng J Med 311:1281-1286.

Levin AB, Benson RC Jr, Katz J, Nilsson T (1978). Chemical hypophysectomy for relief of bone pain in carcinoma of the prostate. J Urol 119:517-521.

Macfarlane DA, Thomas LP, Harrison JH (1960). A survey of total adrenalectomy in cancer of the prostate. Am J Surg 99:562-572.

MacFarlane JR, Tolley DA (1985). Flutamide therapy for advanced prostatic cancer: a phase II study. Br J Urol 57:172-174.

Maddy JA, Winternitz WW, Norrell H (1971). Cryohypophysectomy in the management of advanced prostatic cancer. Cancer 28:322-328.

Morales A, Blair DW, Steyn J (1971). Yttrium[90] pituitary ablation in advanced carcinoma of the prostate. Br J Urol 43:520-522.

Morales P, Brendler H, Hotchkiss RS (1955). The role of the adrenal cortex in prostatic cancer. J Urol 73:399-409.

Murphy GP, Beckley S, Brady MF, et al. (1983). Treatment of newly diagnosed metastatic prostate cancer patients with chemotherapy agents in combination with hormones versus hormones alone. Cancer 51:1264-1272.

Murphy GP, Reynoso G, Schoonees R, Gailani S, Bourke R,
Kenny GM, Mirand KA, Schalch DS (1971). Hypophysectomy
and adrenalectomy for disseminated prostatic carcinoma.
J Urol 105:817-825.
Murray R, Pitt P (1985). Treatment of advanced prostatic
cancer, resistant to conventional therapy, with
aminoglutethimide. Eur J Cancer Clin Oncol 21:453-458.
Narayana AS, Loening SA, Culp DA (1981). Flutamide in the
treatment of metastatic carcinoma of the prostate. Br J
Urol 53:152-153.
Neri R, Florance K, Koziol P, Van Cleave S (1972). A
biological profile of a nonsteroidal antiandrogen, SCH
13521 (4'-nitro-3'-trifluoromethylisobutyranilide).
Endocrinology 91:427-437.
Ponder BAJ, Shearer RJ, Pocock RD, Miller J, Easton D,
Chilvers CED, Dowsett M, Jeffcoate SL (1984). Response
to aminoglutethimide and cortisone acetate in advanced
prostatic cancer. Br J Cancer 50:757-763.
Pont A (1986). Longterm experience with high-dose
ketoconazole therapy for prostate cancer. J Urol
135:Abstract #389.
Prout GR, Irwin RJ Jr, Kliman B, Daly JJ, Maclaughin RA,
Griffin PP (1975). Prostatic cancer and SCH-13251: II.
Histological alterations and the pituitary gonadal axis.
J Urol 113:834-840.
Redding TW, Schally AV (1985). Investigation of the
combination of the agonist D-Trp-6-LH-RH and the
antiandrogen Flutamide in the treatment of Dunning R-
3327H prostate cancer model. The Prostate 6:219-232.
Robinson MRG, Shearer RJ, Fergusson JD (1974). Adrenal
suppression in the treatment of carcinoma of the
prostate. Br J Urol 46:555-559.
Rost A, Hantelmann W, Fiedler U (1978). Cyproterone
acetate and testosterone levels in serum and first
clinical results after intramuscular application of
cyproterone acetate in the treatment of prostatic cancer.
Proceedings of the II International Symposium on the
Treatment of Carcinoma of the Prostate. Rost A and
Fiedler U, Berlin, pp. 84-88.
Schroeder FH, Klijn JG, de Jong FH (1986). Metastatic
cancer of the prostate managed by Buserelin acetatae
versus Buserelin acetate plus Cyproterone acetate. J Urol
135:Abstract #392.
Scott WW, Schirmer HKA (1962). Hypophysectomy for
disseminated prostatic cancer. In: On Cancer and

Hormones: Essays in Experimental Biology, Univ. of Chicago Press, pp. 175-204.

Smith JA JR, Eyre HJ, Roberts TS, Middleton RG (1984). Transphenoidal hypophysectomy in the management of carcinoma of the prostate. Cancer 53:2385-2387.

Smith RB, Walsh PC, Goodwin WE (1973). Cyproterone acetate in the treatment of advanced carcinoma of the prostate. J Urol 110:106-108.

Sogani PC, Ray B, Whitmore WF Jr (1975). Advanced prostatic carcinoma. Flutamide therapy after conventional endocrine treatment. Urology 6:164-166.

Sogani PC, Vagaiwala MR, Whitmore WF Jr (1984). Experience with Flutamide in patients with advanced prostatic cancer without prior endocrine therapy. Cancer 54:744-750.

Stoliar B, Albert DJ (1974). SCH 13521 in the treatment of advanced carcinoma of the prostate. J Urol 111:803-807.

Trachtenberg J, Pont A (1984). Ketoconazole therapy for advanced prostate cancer. Lancet, August 25, pp. 433-435.

Trachtenberg J (1984). Ketoconazole therapy in advanced prostatic carcinoma. J Urol 132:61-63.

Trachtenberg J (1985). Optimal testosterone concentration for the treatment of prostatic cancer. J Urol 133:888-890.

Tunn UW, Graff J, Senge Th (1983). Treatment of inoperable prostatic cancer with cyproterone acetate. In: Androgens and Anti-Androgens, Schroeder FH (ed.), Schering Nederland BV, pp. 149-160.

Van Cangh PJ, Opsomer RJ (1986). Treatment of advanced carcinoma of the prostate with a depot LHRH-analogue (ICI-118-630). J Urol 135:Abstract #395.

Walsh PC, Hutchins GM, Ewing LL (1983). Tissue content of dihydrotestosterone in human prostatic hyperplasia is not supranormal. J Clin Invest 72:1772-1777.

Wein AJ, Murphy JJ (1973). Experience in the treatment of prostatic carcinoma with cyproterone acetate. J Urol 109:68-70.

Wenderoth UK, Jacobi GH (1986). Experience with a depot-preparation of the LH-RH-analogue D-trp[6] in the treatment of 25 patients with advanced prostatic carcinoma. J Urol 135:Abstract #386.

Whitmore WF Jr, Randall HT, Pearson OH, West CD (1954). Adrenalectomy in the treatment of prostatic cancer. Geriatrics 9:62-69.

Worgul TJ, Santen RJ, Samojlik E, Veldhuis JD, Lipton A, Harvey HA, Drago JR, Rohner TJ (1983). Clinical and

biochemical effect of aminoglutethimide in the treatment
of advanced prostatic carcinoma. J Urol 129:51-55.
Zadra J, Bruce AW, Trachtenberg J (1986). Total androgen
ablation therapy in the treatment of advanced prostatic
cancer. J Urol 135:Abstract #388.

Prostate Cancer, Part A: Research, Endocrine
Treatment, and Histopathology, pages 21–31
© 1987 Alan R. Liss, Inc.

DEVELOPMENT OF ANDROGEN RESISTANCE IN PROSTATIC CANCER

John T. Isaacs, Harald Schulze and
Donald S. Coffey

The James Buchanan Brady Urological Institute, The
Johns Hopkins Hospital; Department of Urology and
The Oncology Center, The Johns Hopkins University
School of Medicine, Baltimore, Maryland 21205, USA

I. PROSTATIC CANCER AND ANDROGEN SENSITIVITY

One of the most common characteristics of cancers is
their ability to develop resistance to chemotherapy and/or
hormonal manipulation to which they were initially
responsive (Skipper et al., 1978; Goldie and Coldman, 1979;
Isaacs, 1982; Ling, 1982). For example, there is a greater
than 80% initial response rate of prostatic cancer patients
to androgen ablation, however, essentially all of these
patients eventually relapse to an androgen-independent
state in which further antiandrogen therapy is no longer
effective. Following relapse, all further attempts to
ablate the low level of nontesticular androgens remaining
following castration or estrogen therapy by means of
hypophysectomy, adrenalectomy, or administration of direct
acting antiandrogens have proven unsuccessful in stopping
the continuous tumor growth in this androgen-independent
state (Scott, Menon and Walsh, 1980; Schulze, Isaacs and
Coffey, 1986).

This nearly universal development of resistance to a
wide spectrum of therapeutic modalities by cancers is
rather unusual when one realizes that normal tissues do not
develop similar resistance to the toxic effects of these
therapies with continuous exposure. Hence the propensity
of prostatic cancers to develop resistance to androgen
ablation therapy is in direct contrast to the normal
prostate. The normal prostate chronically requires
androgen to maintain its normal function and cell number.
Following castration, the normal prostate rapidly involutes

with a more than 80% reduction in total epithelial cell
number (Lesser and Bruchovsky, 1973). The involuted normal
prostate can, however, be fully restored simply by
treatment with exogenous androgen. Once fully restored,
the prostate will re-involute if the treatment with
exogenous androgen is discontinued. By alternating
treatment of castrated hosts with exogenous androgen
followed by a period of no treatment, the normal prostate
can be made to go through a cyclic process of restoration-
involution. Even if this process of androgen treatment
followed by a period of no treatment is cyclically
continued many times, the normal prostate always responds
with restoration-involution, demonstrating that it does not
become resistant to androgens (Sandford, Searle and Kerr,
1984; Isaacs, 1986). This demonstrates that there is a
fundamental difference between the normal and malignant
prostate with regard to the ability to develop resistance
to androgen withdrawal.

When the Dunning R-3327 rat prostatic adenocarcinoma
became available, we studied the basis for the relapse
following castration with this reliable and reproducible
model (Smolev et al., 1977; Isaacs et al., 1978). Several
months after subcutaneous implantation of Dunning-H subline
cells into intact male rats, a growing tumor could be
palpated. At that time the animals were castrated and an
involution of the tumor was observed. Like human prostatic
cancer, the initial response of the H-tumor to androgen
ablation was followed by a relapse. The relapsed H-tumor
could be shown to be completely androgen-independent
(Isaacs et al., 1978; Isaacs and Coffey, 1981). This was
demonstrated by the fact that when the relapsed tumor was
transplanted into a castrated rat and subjected to high
concentrations of antiandrogens, the tumor grows at the
same rate as if it had been placed into an intact animal
with testes. Even treating animals bearing this relapsed
tumor with high doses of exogenous androgen did not
increase its growth rate.

Kinetic studies demonstrated that this relapse of the
R-3327-H tumor to castration resulted from the continuous
growth of cancer cell clones which were androgen-
independent and which already existed in the initial tumor
at the time of castration (Smolev et al., 1977; Isaacs et
al., 1978; Isaacs and Coffey, 1981). These observations
demonstrated that prostatic cancer can be heterogeneously

composed of a variety of phenotypically distinct cell clones even before hormonal therapy is begun. For example, with regard to androgen responsiveness, there are three distinct phenotypes possible for prostatic cancer cells: androgen-dependent, androgen-sensitive, or androgen-independent. Androgen-dependent cancer cells chronically require a critical level of androgenic stimulation for their continued maintenance and growth (i.e., without adequate androgenic stimulation, these cells die), and in this regard, they are very similar to the androgen-dependent non-neoplastic cells of the normal prostate. In contrast, androgen-sensitive cancer cells do not die, even if no androgen is present, however, their continuous rate of growth is decreased following androgen ablation. Androgen-independent cells neither die nor slow their continuous growth following androgen ablation, no matter how complete; these cells are completely autonomous to androgenic effects on growth. Thus, of the three phenotypes of prostatic cancer, the only one which is eliminated by androgen ablation, even if complete, is the androgen-dependent cancer cell.

In human prostatic cancer, the response following androgen ablation varies from almost complete remission to essentially no effect. The initial response of the individual prostatic cancer to androgen ablation is dependent upon the ratio of the androgen-dependent, -sensitive and -independent cells heterogeneously preexisting within the tumor before therapy. Indeed, individual metastatic lesions can be heterogeneously composed of various ratios of these three different cell types. Due to variations in the ratio of these three cell types within individual metastases, it is not uncommon to observe remission and progression at different rates in different metastases within the same patient following androgen ablation.

II. Tumor Cell Heterogeneity

Prostatic cancers are rarely phenotypically homogeneous with regard to the clones of cancer cells comprising individual tumors. For example, Kastendieck (1980) demonstrated that of 180 clinically manifest prostatic cancers removed surgically from previously hormonally untreated patients, 60% of these cancers were

already histologically heterogeneous being composed of a
mixture of several different cancer cell types of widely
varying differentiation (admixture of glandular,
cribriform, and anaplastic morphology within the same
cancer). These results clearly demonstrate that prostatic
cancer cell heterogeneity can occur early in the clinical
course of the disease and there is no requirement for any
reduction in serum androgen levels (i.e., no requirement
for hormonal therapy) in order to induce this morphological
heterogeneity. This last point is also demonstrated by the
study of Viola et al. (1986) in which immunoperoxidase
staining methods were used to examine the cellular
distribution of prostate-specific antigen, carcinoembryonic
antigen and p21 Harvey-ras oncogene protein within
individual prostatic cancers from patients with metastatic
disease and who had received no prior hormonal therapy.
This study again demonstrates that each of these phenotypic
parameters was heterogeneously distributed with multiple
foci of both nonreactive and reactive cancer cells present
within individual prostatic cancers. Similar cellular
heterogeneity within individual prostatic cancers, even
before hormonal therapy was initiated, was also
demonstrated by Mostofi et al. (1981) using
immunocytochemical localization of prostatic specific acid
phosphatase as a phenotypic marker. There is also a great
variation in the amount of androgen receptors throughout
different areas of the same prostatic cancer (Blankenstein,
Bolt-deVries and Foekens, 1982).

Based upon these morphological, biochemical, and
immunological studies, it is clear that individual
prostatic cancers are heterogeneously composed of clones of
phenotypically distinct prostatic cancer cells even before
therapy is begun. The initial response of prostatic cancer
to any therapy will therefore depend upon the
responsiveness of each of the heterogeneous cell types
existing within the tumor. It appears that this cellular
heterogeneity develops early in the life of an individual
tumor and may result from genetic instability (Nowell,
1976; Isaacs et al., 1982). The change in the state of
the genome or DNA content within the tumor cells
(aneuploidy, polyploidy, abnormal chromosomes) reflects
this genetic instability of the tumor (Nowell, 1976).

Tumor cell heterogeneity is a common denominator in
practically all cancers in humans and animals that have

been studied (Owens, Coffey and Baylin, 1982). This intratumor heterogeneity is the major cause of the rapid development of resistance of a cancer to a variety of different types of therapy. Hence the development of resistance to further antiandrogen therapy which occurs in prostatic cancer patients following relapse to castration is not a unique, but a common, feature of cancers in general. This resistant state has been called the autonomous phase of tumor growth. In fact, there are prostate cancer cells that can grow in culture in the complete absence of androgens in a synthetic medium (Chan, 1981). This indicates that these cancer cells do not require the presence of any androgens to grow. One might propose that a prostatic cancer cell might be capable of making its own androgens in an autocrine manner, similar to the situation observed for other cancers, in which the cells make their own growth factors (Sporn and Roberts, 1985). If prostate cancer cells could synthesize their own androgens, it still should be possible to block the growth of these cells by administration of antiandrogens. As antiandrogens have the ability to block the binding of androgens to the receptor within the cell, the activation of the receptor by androgen is blocked by antiandrogens regardless of the source of androgens. Since androgen-independent cells continue to grow in the absence of androgens and in the presence of antiandrogens, it appears that the growth of these cancer cells is completely independent and autonomous to androgens.

III. Future Aspects

How might the growth of prostate cancers be better controlled? A more complete androgen ablation is not the answer. Such an approach does not stop the continuous growth of either the androgen-sensitive or the androgen-independent cells present within the prostate cancer. In order to effectively manage prostatic cancer patients, what is needed is a therapy directed towards all of the phenotypically different clones of cancer cells present within the tumor. There are a variety of effective hormonal therapies for the elimination of the androgen-dependent cancer cells presently available. What is not presently available is a therapy effective against the androgen-sensitive and androgen-independent prostatic cancer cells.

Why have androgen-sensitive and androgen-independent prostate cancer cells been so refractory to control by standard cancer chemotherapeutic agents presently studies? This is probably because most of our chemotherapeutic agents are directed towards blocking DNA synthesis. Since prostate cancer grows at such a very slow rate, only very few cells are in mitosis and DNA synthesis studies show less than 0.5% of all prostate cancer cells actually in DNA synthesis at one time (Meyer, Sufrin and Martin, 1982). In contrast, bone marrow and gastrointestinal epithelial cells in normal tissue are turning over with a much higher rate of DNA synthesis than prostate cancer cells. It has been estimated that in the human approximately 40 kg of normal gastrointestinal epithelial cells, approximately 20 kg of normal bone marrow cells, and about 10 kg cells of skin and hair are made per year. Thus a normal human produces approximately his own body weight of 70 kg in new normal cells per year.

As there is nothing unique about DNA synthesis between normal and cancer cells that has yet been shown and that could be capitalized upon as a therapeutic approach, it becomes apparent that treatment of a slow growing tumor such as prostate cancer with any cytotoxic agent directed towards DNA synthesis will cause a highly toxic effect on normal cells while only a small amount of cancer cells will be affected.

This again indicates that a completely new therapeutic approach to controlling the growth of androgen-sensitive and androgen-independent prostate cancer cells is urgently needed (Isaacs, 1985). The mass of any cell population can be increased either by elevating the rate of its proliferation or by decreasing its rate of death. Thus the increase in total cellular mass of a tumor represents an imbalance between the cell proliferation and death rate. The mechanism of what controls cell death is a fruitful area to concentrate our attention upon in the future since it may be possible to therapeutically increase the rate of cell death and thus eliminate these cancer cells (Isaacs, 1985). Indeed, the involution of a prostate following withdrawal of androgens is not due to the lack of nutrients but is an active and induced process (Bruchovsky, Lesser and VanDoorn, 1975; Lee, 1981; Isaacs, 1984a; Montpetit, Lawless and Tenniswood, 1986) More information is needed on this active process of prostate cell death in the hope that it may give us some new approaches to the treatment of prostate cancer.

A major area of research is the study of the biological defense of the host against the tumor. Such studies have resulted in several new therapeutic modalities that involve the immune system of the host. Examples of these are gamma interferon (Schiller et al., 1986), interleukin II (Rosenberg et al., 1985) and tumor necrosis factor (Old, 1985). Presently, it is unclear exactly what these substances are directed toward since there is no specific tumor antigen yet shown on all of the solid tumors. Modification of the immune system is an area that will require far more research and may be an exciting approach to controlling growth of prostate cancer.

When cancer cells grow, they require the growth of a wide variety of normal cells to keep the tumor alive. This includes the endothelial cells that make up the capillaries. In fact, a 1 cc tumor has approximately 10,000 capillary branches that support the one billion cells growing within this tumor (Folkman, 1985). Blocking the growth of a tumor by blocking the angiogenesis process is another promising research field (Folkman, 1985).

Besides the growth of endothelial cells, the expansion of a tumor necessitates normal stromal elements like smooth muscle and connective tissue. Prostate epithelial cells have been shown to be exquisitely sensitive to the stroma to which they are attached (Cunha et al., 1983). Stromal-epithelial interaction is one of the most exciting areas of tumor biology. We do not yet know how the epithelial cell communicates with the basement membrane and how this interaction is directed by the stromal cells. However, there is little doubt that this interaction has been altered in the pathogenesis of cancer.

IV. Conclusion

Since 1941, most of the attention on prostatic cancer has been focused upon the role of androgens in tumor growth. It is important to realize that the approach of controlling prostatic cancer growth simply by deprivation of androgens alone will not be curative since this therapy will kill only the androgen-dependent cells. The androgen-sensitive and -independent cells also present with the

heterogeneous cancer will not be eliminated, no matter how
complete the androgen ablation (Ellis and Isaacs, 1985).
In order to increase the effectiveness of the treatment of
prostatic cancer, androgen ablation must be combined with
therapies targeted specifically at controlling the
androgen-sensitive and androgen-independent cancer cells.
Using such a combined approach, it should be possible to
affect the growth of all populations of malignant cells
within the prostatic cancer (i.e., androgen-dependent, -
sensitive, and -independent) and thus increase the
effectiveness of the combined therapy above that obtained
with hormonal therapy alone. Indeed, in animal models,
such combinational therapy early in the course of the
disease, does produce substantial increases in survival
above that produced by hormonal therapy alone (Isaacs,
1984b).

Presently, there are a large variety of effective ways
to eliminate the androgen-dependent prostatic cancer cells
within a prostatic cancer (i.e., surgical castration,
estrogens, LHRH analog plus or minus antiandrogen, etc.).
Unfortunately, there is no effective therapy for the
elimination of either the androgen-sensitive or the
androgen-independent cancer cells within a prostatic
cancer. Since it is these androgen-sensitive and androgen-
independent prostatic cancer cells which eventually lead to
the demise of the patient, future attention should focus on
finding new nonhormonal therapies to eliminate these cells.
Several new approaches to limiting the growth of these
androgen-sensitive and androgen-independent prostatic
cancer cells have been presented.

REFERENCES

Blankenstein MA, Bolt-deVries J, Foekens JA (1982).
  Nuclear androgen receptor assay in biopsy-size specimens
  of human prostatic tissue. The Prostate 3:351-359.
Bruchovsky N, Lesser B, VanDoorn E (1975). Hormonal
  effects on cell proliferation in rat prostate. Vit Horm
  33:61.
Chan SY (1981). A chemically defined medium for the
  propagation of rat prostate adenocarcinoma cells. The
  Prostate 2:291-298.
Cunha GR, Chung LWK, Shannon JM, Taguchi O, Fujii H (1983).
  Hormone-induced morphogenesis and growth: role of

mesenchymal-epithelial interactions. Recent Prog Horm Res 39:559.

Ellis W, Isaacs JT (1985). Effectiveness of complete _versus_ partial androgen withdrawal therapy for the treatment of prostatic cancer as studied in the Dunning R-3327 system of rat prostatic adenocarcinoma. Cancer Res 145:6041-6050.

Folkman J (1985). Tumor angiogenesis. Adv Cancer Res 43:175-203.

Goldie GH, Coldman AJ (1979). A mathematical model formulating the drug sensitivity of tumors to their spontaneous metastatic rate. Cancer Trt Rep 63:1727.

Isaacs JT (1982). Cellular factors in the development of resistance to hormonal therapy. In: Drug and Hormone Resistance in Neoplasia (Bruchovsky N and Goldie JH, eds.), Vol. I, 139-156, CRC Press, Boca Raton, FL.

Isaacs JT (1984a). Antagonistic effect of androgen on prostatic cell death. The Prostate 5:545-557.

Isaacs JT (1984b). The timing of androgen ablation therapy and/or chemotherapy in the treatment of prostatic cancers. The Prostate 5:1-18.

Isaacs JT (1985). New principles in the management of metastatic prostatic cancer. Prog Clin Biol Res 185A:303-405.

Isaacs JT (1986). Control of cell proliferation and cell death in the normal and neoplastic prostate: A stem cell model. In: Proceedings of the 2nd NIADDK Symposium on Benign Prostatic Hyperplasia (in press).

Isaacs JT, Coffey DS (1981). Adaptation _versus_ selection on the mechanism responsible for the relapse of prostatic cancer to androgen ablation therapy as studied in the Dunning R-3327-H adenocarcinoma. Cancer Res 41:5070-5075.

Isaacs JT, Heston WDW, Weissman RM and Coffey DS (1978). Animal models of the hormone-sensitive and -insensitive prostatic adenocarcinomas, Dunning R-3327-H, R-3327-HI, and R-3327-AT. Cancer Res 38:4353-4359.

Isaacs JT, Wake N, Coffey DS and Sandberg AA (1982). Genetic instability coupled to clonal selection as a mechanism for tumor progression in the Dunning R-3327 rat prostatic adenocarcinoma system. Cancer Res 42:2353-2361.

Kastendieck H. (1980). Correlation between atypical primary hyperplasia and carcinoma of the prostate. Histologic studies on 180 total prostatectomies due to manifest carcinoma. Pathology, Research, and Practice 169:366-387.

Lee C (1981). Physiology of castration-induced regression in rat prostate. In: Murphy GP, Sandberg AA, Karr JP (eds), The Prostate Cell: Structure and Function, Part A. New York:Alan R. Liss, Inc., p. 145.

Lesser B, Bruchovsky N. (1973). The effects of testosterone, 5α-dihydrotestosterone, and adenosine 3',5'-monophosphate on cell proliferation and differentiation in rat prostate. Biochim Biophys Acta 308:426-437.

Ling V (1982). Genetic basis of drug resistance in mammalian cells. In: Drug and Hormone Resistance in Neoplasia (Bruchovsky N, Goldie JH, eds.), Vol 1, 1-19, CRC Press, Boca Raton, FL.

Meyer JS, Sufrin G, Martin SA (1982). Proliferative activity of benign human prostate, prostatic adenocarcinoma, and seminal vesicle evaluated by thymidine labeling. J Urol 128:1353-1356.

Montpetit ML, Lawless KR, Tenniswood M (1986). Androgen-repressed messages in the rat ventral prostate. The Prostate 8:25-36.

Mostofi K, Sesterhenn J (1981). The role of prostatic acid phosphatase in histological diagnosis of carcinoma of the prostate. Proceedings of the 76th Annual Meeting of the American Urological Association, Abstract #42.

Nowell PC (1976). The clonal evolution of tumor cell populations. Science 194:23-28.

Old LJ (1985). Tumor necrosis factor (TNF). Science 230:630-632.

Owens AH, Coffey DS, Baylin SB (eds.) (1982). Tumor Cell Heterogeneity: Origins and Implications. Bristol-Myers Cancer Symposium, Vol. 4, Academic Press:New York.

Rosenberg SA, Lotze M, Maul LM, Leitman S, Change AE, Ettinghausen SE, Matory YC, Skibber JM, Shilonic E, Velto JT, Seipp CA, Simpson C, Reichert CM (1985). Observations on the systemic administration of autologous lymphokine-activated killer cells and recombinant interleukin-2 to patients with metastatic cancer. New Eng J Med 313:1485-1492.

Sandford NL, Searle JW, Kerr JFR (1984). Successive waves of apoptosis in the rat prostate after regulated withdrawal of testosterone stimulation. Pathology 16:406-410.

Schiller JH, Groveman DS, Schmid, SM, Wilson JKV, Cummings KB, Borden EC (1986). Synergistic antiproliferative

effects of human recombinant α54- or βser interferon with
γ-interferon on human cell lines of various histogenes.
Cancer Res 46:483-488.

Schulze H, Isaacs JT, Coffey DS (1986). A critical review
of the concept of total androgen ablation in the
treatment of prostate cancer. In: 2nd International
Symposium on Prostatic Cancer (Murphy G, ed.), New York,
Alan R. Liss, Inc., In press.

Scott WW, Menon M, Walsh PC (1980). Hormonal therapy of
prostatic cancer. Cancer 45:1929-1936.

Skipper HE, Schabel FM, Lloyd MM (1978). Selection and
overgrowth of specifically and permanently drug-resistant
tumor cells. Exp Ther Kinetics 15:207-217.

Smolev JK, Heston WD, Scott WW, Coffey DS (1977).
Characterization of the Dunning R-3327-H prostatic
adenocarcinoma: An appropriate animal model for prostatic
cancer. Cancer Trt Rep 61:273-287.

Sporn MB, Roberts AB (1985). Autocrine growth factors and
cancer. Nature 313:745-747.

Viola MV, Framowitz F, Oravez MS, Deb S, Finket G, Lundy G,
Harel P, Thor A, Schlom J (1986). Expression of rat
oncogene p21 in prostatic cancer. New Eng J Med 314:133-
137.

Prostate Cancer, Part A: Research, Endocrine
Treatment, and Histopathology, pages 33–44
© 1987 Alan R. Liss, Inc.

PLASMA HORMONE LEVELS BEFORE AND AFTER ORCHIECTOMY IN PROSTATE CANCER PATIENTS

J. Fiet, J.M. Villette, C. Bertagna, A. de Géry,
M. Hucher, J.M. Husson and J.P. Raynaud
Laboratoire Central de Biochimie (J.F. & J.M.V.)
Hôpital Saint-Louis, 75010 Paris, France
Roussel-Uclaf, 75007 Paris, France

INTRODUCTION

Prostatic carcinoma is considered to be an essentially androgen-dependent disease and the question thus arises to what extent classical treatment such as bilateral subcapsular orchiectomy eradicates all androgen influence on tumor growth. Castration eliminates androgens of testicular origin but may not have much effect, if any, on adrenal androgens. Studies reported in the literature suggest that the plasma levels of testosterone, of Δ_4-androstenedione and of dehydroepiandrosterone sulphate in castrate men are similar to or somewhat lower than those of post-menopausal women (Vermeulen, 1980; Crilly et al., 1980; Vermeulen et al., 1982; Horton and Lobo, 1986). However, in women, alterations in adrenal androgen secretion and distribution can result in abnormally high plasma levels of these androgens and in androgen-dependent disorders such as hirsutism. Similar variations in plasma adrenal androgens in castrate men could greatly influence an exquisitely androgen-sensitive organ, the prostate, which could convert these adrenal androgens into the biologically trophic hormones, testosterone and dihydrotestosterone, with the potential to sustain tumor growth.

In the course of multicentre clinical trials of the action of an antiandrogen, Anandron, in castrate patients (Raynaud et al., 1985; Moguilewsky et al., 1986; Brisset et al., in press, this volume; Navratil et al., this volume), the plasma concentrations of twelve hormones (testosterone (T), dihydrotestosterone (DHT), estradiol (E_2), FSH, LH, prolactin (PRL), Δ_4-androstenedione ($\Delta4$), 11β-hydroxy-Δ_4-androstenedione (11β-OH-$\Delta4$), dehydroepiandrosterone (DHEA), dehydroepiandrosterone sulphate (DHEA-S), cortisol (F) and androstanediol glucuronide (3α-diol-G)), and of the plasma protein TeBG were measured. Results for the placebo group before and after orchiectomy are reported in this chapter.

PATIENTS

Thirty-two men (46-88 yrs, median age 72 yrs) suffering from metastatic prostate adenocarcinoma (stage D2) and who had received no previous hormone treatment underwent surgical castration. Blood samples (20 ml) were drawn before castration and one month, three months, and six months after castration, quickly centrifuged and frozen, then stored at −20° until assay.

MATERIALS AND METHODS

Determination of DHT, Δ_4, DHEA and 11β-OH-Δ_4-androstenedione (11β-OH-Δ_4)

All cold **steroids** were purchased from Steraloids (California, USA). Tritiated steroids (s.a. 40 - 60 Ci/mmol) were purchased from Amersham (UK). Stock solutions (1 mCi/mmol) were kept at +4°C and were renewed every three months. Aliquots were diluted in pure ethanol (12.5 uCi/mmol). The intermediary solutions were kept at +4°C and used to prepare aqueous working solutions immediately prior to assay (20,000 dpm/0.1 ml phosphate buffer).

All **solvents** (isooctane, dichloromethane and diethylene glycol) were of spectroscopic quality and used without purification. A 0.4 M phosphate gelatin buffer (PGB) (pH 7.4) containing 0.1% gelatin (Prolabo, Paris) was prepared. **Celite** Analytical Filter Aid (Johns Manville, Touzard & Matignon, Vitry/Seine, France) was prepared as previously described (Fiet et al., 1980).

Anti-DHT, anti-DHEA, anti-Δ_4, and anti-11β-OH-Δ_4 **antisera** were induced in rabbits (Fiet et al., 1980) by intradermal injection of DHT-1-CMO/BSA, DHEA-7-CMO/BSA, Δ_4-6-CMO/BSA and 11β-OH-Δ_4-3-CMO/BSA. The cross-reactivities of anti-Δ_4, anti-DHEA and anti-11β-OH-Δ_4 have already been reported (Fiet et al., 1980). The cross-reactivity of anti-DHT was : 5% (testosterone), 0.01% (DHEA) and 0.5% (Δ_4).

Radioactive steroids (^{3}H-DHT, ^{3}H-Δ_4, ^{3}H-11β-OH-Δ_4, 6000 dpm) were added to 1 ml samples for recovery determinations. After 30 min equilibration at room temperature, plasma was extracted with ethylacetate/cyclohexane (10 ml, 1 min). The dry extracts were dissolved in 1.5 ml isooctane for celite elution chromatography.

Steroids were separated by **celite partition column chromatography** (Fiet et al., 1980) in 5 ml siliconized pipettes (Kimble, Touzard & Matignon, Paris). Each pipette was filled with 0.75 g of a mixture of celite/ethylene glycol (1 g/0.5 ml w/v). Steroids were eluted after layering 1.5 ml of isooctane-steroid solution onto the celite using isooctane/dichloromethane solvent of increasing polarity. Δ_4 was then eluted in the following 4 ml of pure isooctane, DHT and DHEA were eluted together in isooctane/dichloromethane (94/6 v/v) and 11β-OH-Δ_4 in isooctane/dichloromethane (70/30 v/v).

The elution fractions were evaporated to dryness and dissolved in PGB (2.5 ml for Δ_4, 4 ml for DHT + DHEA, 2.5 ml for 11β-OH-Δ_4). Δ_4, DHEA and 11β-OH-Δ_4 were **radioimmunoassayed** in two 0.2 ml and two 0.5 ml elution fractions and DHT in two 0.5 ml elution fractions ; 0.5 ml of each fraction was transferred to a counting vial for measurement of recovery.

Three standard curves covering a range of 0-600 pg/tube were established from standard aqueous solutions of Δ_4, DHEA, DHT and 11β-OH-Δ_4 (0.1 ml standard per tube).

Specific tracer solutions (20.000 dpm) and 0.1 ml of diluted specific antisera were added to the above elution fractions and standard solutions. The final volume of each tube was brought up to 0.7 ml by adding PGB. All tubes were vortexed and allowed to equilibrate overnight at +4°C. Bound fractions were measured in a liquid scintillation counter after separation of the free fractions by a dextran-coated charcoal suspension.

Recoveries were 75% $\pm$ 6% (SD), 70% $\pm$ 7% (SD), 70% $\pm$ 6% and 71% $\pm$ 8% (SD) respectively for Δ_4, DHEA, DHT and 11β-OH-Δ_4.

The plasma blank was undetectable. The lowest detectable doses on the standard curves were 6, 10, 2 and 15 pg
for Δ_4, DHEA, DHT and 11β-OH- Δ_4 respectively corresponding
to 40, 114, 22 and 105 pg per ml of plasma.

The **specificity** of the method depends on the cross-
reactivity of the antisera used and on the relative plasma
concentrations of the steroids eluted in the same elution
fraction during chromatography. Androstanedione, which
cross-reacts with our anti- Δ_4-androstenedione antiserum
(30%), was eluted in the first 1.5 ml of pure isooctane
elution and thus does not interfere with the assay of Δ_4.
DHT does not interfere with the assay of DHEA since cross-
reaction with anti-DHEA antiserum is low (0.35%) (Fiet et
al., 1980). In addition, the plasma concentration of DHT is
much lower than that of DHEA. Conversely, the very low
cross-reactivity (0.01%) of anti-DHT antiserum with DHEA
enables plasma DHT to be accurately assayed even though the
concentration of DHEA in the elution fraction also
containing DHT is much higher.

Testosterone assay

Plasma testosterone was performed with a radioimmunoassay kit ("SB-Testo" ORIS/CEA, Gif/Yvette, France)
using iodinated tracer and an anti-testosterone-19-
hemisuccinate/BSA serum. The specificity of the kit was
checked by comparison with classical methods, using
tritiated testosterone, extraction and a chromatographic
step. The results of this comparison were excellent
(unpublished data).

Plasma cortisol, estradiol and DHEA-S were assayed using
the following commercially available kits : cortisol gamma
coat clinical assays, estradiol ^{125}I ER 155 and DHEA-S
^{125}I ER-660 (Travenol, Maurepas, France). The analytical
performance of each of these kits was checked by comparison
with corresponding methods using tritiated isotopes. The
specificities of these methods were satisfactory.

Androstanediol glucoronide assay (3α-diol-G)

The plasma concentration of 3α-diol-G was determined as follows after extraction of free unconjugated 3α-diol from plasma by ethylacetate/cyclohexane :

1/ The 3α-diol-G was hydrolysed to free unconjugated 3α-diol using β-glucuronidase according to Horton et al. (1984). 0.5 ml plasma was adjusted to pH 6.4 (0.1 ml of 1M phosphate buffer pH 6) and left at 45° for 24 hrs in the presence of highly purified β-glucuronidase (10,000 Fishman Units, corresponding to 0.25 ml β-glucuronidase, Inst. Pasteur).

2/ Extraction of hydrolyzed plasma with cyclohexane/ ethylacetate (10 ml) followed by celite chromatography. Before extraction, 2000 dpm of tritiated 3α-diol (SA = 50 Ci/mmol) were added for recovery. The organic extract was evaporated to dryness and the residue redissolved in iso-octane (1.5 ml) for chromatography. 3α-diol was eluted with a mixture of isooctane and dichloromethane (64/35 v/v).

3/ The organic elution fraction of 3α-diol was evaporated and the dry residue was dissolved in phosphate gelatin buffer for radioimmunoassay (Fiet et al., 1982).

TeBG Assay

TeBG was assayed by a radioimmunologic competitive method (Milab Malmö Immunolaboratorium AB, Sweden ; Mallinckrodt, Evry Lisses, France).

FSH, LH, PRL Assays

All these pituitary hormones were radioimmunoassayed with ORIS/CEA kits (FSHK-PR, LHK-PR, SB-PROL).

Quality control

The reproducibility of all assays was checked by mea-suring the same control samples (one or two concentration levels) in each batch of assays. The coefficient of varia-tion did not exceed 13% for any of the assays.

Statistical methods

Comparisons between groups were made using Student's t-test. Values after castration were compared with the baseline values using Student's paired t-test. Correlations were calculated using Pearson's correlation coefficient.

RESULTS AND DISCUSSION

Plasma hormone levels before and after orchiectomy are shown in Figure 1.

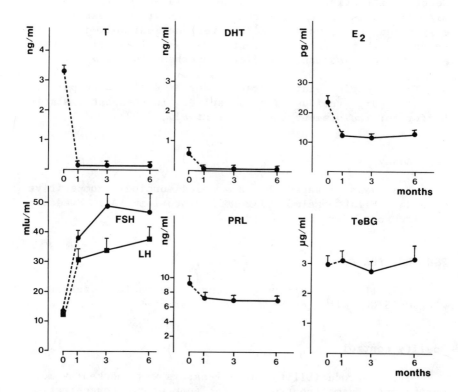

Figure 1. Plasma hormone levels before (●---) and
          after (●—) (1, 3, 6 months) orchiectomy

(Fig. 1 continued on page

As previously widely reported (Bergman et al., 1982; Varenhorst et al., 1982; Maatman et al., 1985 and others), the plasma concentrations of the biologically potent hormones T and DHT were low after bilateral subcapsular orchiectomy, i.e. 5 and 10% of the initial concentrations, respectively. Plasma levels of T were, however, three times higher than those found in prepubertal boys (Forest et al., 1974) and thus indicative of remaining functional Leydig cells and/or of an extragonadal source of T. Furthermore, the increase observed in the DHT/T ratio after castration, supporting the result of Bartsch et al. (1977), suggests that DHT could originate from precursors other than T.

FSH and LH increased until they reached 3.5 and 2.5 times the baseline levels, respectively.

Estradiol can stimulate both TeBG and prolactin secretion. TeBG might lower androgen uptake by the prostate whereas prolactin might exert a stimulatory effect on the tissue (Farnsworth, 1972; Harper et al., 1976). The literature reports a decrease in estradiol after orchiectomy, no change in TeBG and no change (Carlström et al., 1985) or distinctly elevated prolactin values in 15% of cases (Bartsch et al., 1977). In this study, estradiol levels fell by one-half after orchiectomy, TeBG did not change and prolactin levels fell slightly.

It has been suggested that adrenal androgen secretion might undergo a compensatory increase after orchiectomy (Sciarra et al., 1973) although other studies have shown decreased or little modified plasma levels (Sanford et al., 1976; Vermeulen et al., 1982; Parker et al., 1984). In our patients, the DHEA level exhibited a non-significant increase (110 to 115% of base-line levels) whereas DHEA-S fluctuated between 75 and 105% of its base-line value. The concentrations of Δ_4-androstenedione were significantly decreased, by 30 to 50% ($p < 0.006$), and highly significantly correlated ($p < 0.001$) with cortisol and testosterone levels, supporting the hypothesis that it is a key metabolite in the formation of peripheral androgens. Since its 11β-OH derivative, which is of strictly adrenal origin (Goldzieher et al., 1978; Fiet et al., 1980), does not vary significantly upon orchiectomy, the residual Δ_4 (50 to 70%) must arise from the adrenals.

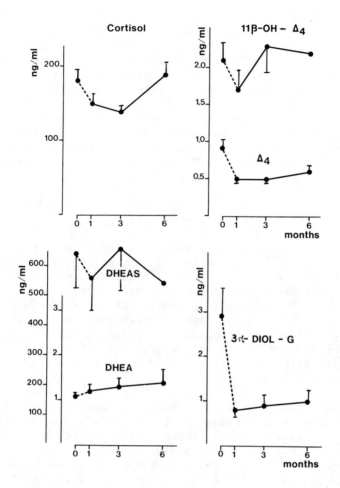

Figure 1. (contd) Plasma hormone levels before (●--) and
(●—) after (1, 3, 6 months) orchiectomy

The bioactivity of these plasma hormones on the prostate is difficult to assess. Jacobi et al (1980) concluded
that, when investigating prolactin in neoplastic prostatic
growth, it is necessary to study cellular events, i.e.
receptor-mediated tumor responsiveness and interference
with androgen-converting enzymes. Intraprostatic conversion
of adrenal androgen precursors into testosterone and DHT,
which are concentrated into target cells by high-affinity
receptors, has been put forward as a major hypothesis for

explaining sustained tumor growth (Geller, 1985; Labrie et al., 1983). An end-product of testosterone metabolism by androgen target tissues, recovered in the plasma, is thus probably the most reliable index of an androgenic environment. Several studies have suggested that the glucuronides of 5α -androstane-3α,17β -diol and of androsterone might be good markers of the peripheral formation and conversion of DHT by the prostate, skin and other androgen-receptive organs (Morimoto et al., 1981; Moghissi et al., 1984; Serafini and Lobo, 1985; Rao et al., 1986; Gompel et al., 1986; Bélanger et al., 1986 and in press; Brochu et al., 1986).

In the present study, following orchiectomy, 30% of the initial level of plasma 3α -diol-G was detected compared to only 5% of testosterone and 10% of DHT suggesting that this glucuronide might have an origin other than testicular testosterone. It could partly arise from adrenal androgen metabolism occurring in the prostate according to the following pathway : DHEA-S $\rightarrow$ DHEA $\rightarrow \Delta4 \rightarrow$ T $\rightarrow$ DHT $\rightarrow 3\alpha$-diol-G. As shown in Table 1, the levels of the adrenal androgens, of DHT and of 3α -diol-G were significantly correlated with plasma testosterone levels (Table 1).

TABLE 1. Correlations with plasma testosterone (149)
1 to 6 months after orchiectomy

Cortisol	0.02	(140)	11β-OH-Δ_4	0.52*	(57)
Estradiol	0.06	(141)	DHEA	0.53*	(139)
Prolactin	0.09	(137)	3α-diol-G	0.54*	(33)
TeBG	0.25	(37)	DHT	0.62*	(77)
DHEA-S	0.40*	(139)	Δ-4	0.66*	(136)

( ) number of assays performed in 58 castrate patients in whom testosterone was assayed at 1, 3 or 6 months.
* p <0.01. Pearson correlation coefficient r=0.40

These findings are to be correlated with the relatively high DHT content remaining in the prostate of castrated men (Geller, 1985) and underline the importance of adrenal androgens in such patients.

REFERENCES

Bartsch W, Horst HJ, Becker H, Nehse G (1977). Sex hormone binding globulin binding capacity, testosterone, 5α-dihydrotestosterone, oestradiol and prolactin in plasma of patients with prostatic carcinoma under various types of hormonal treatment. Acta Endocrinol 85: 650-664.

Bélanger A, Brochu M, Cliche J (1986): Levels of plasma steroid glucuronides in intact and castrated men with prostatic cancer. J Clin Endocrinol Metab 62: 812-815.

Bélanger A, Brochu M, Cliche J (in press): Plasma levels of steroid glucuronides in prepubertal, adult and elderly men. J steroid Biochem.

Bergman B, Damber JE, Tomic R (1982). Effects of total and subcapsular orchiectomy on serum concentrations of testosterone and pituitary hormones in patients with carcinoma of the prostate. Urol Int 37: 139-144.

Brisset JM, Bertagna C, Fiet J, de Gery A, Hucher M, Husson JM, Tremblay D, Raynaud JP (in press). Total androgen blockade versus orchiectomy in stage D prostate cancer. In :" Hormonal Manipulation of Cancer: Peptides, Growth Factors and New (Anti)steroidal Agents". New York: Raven Press.

Brochu M, Tremblay RR, Bélanger A (1986). Plasma levels of C-19 steroids and C-19 steroid glucuronides in hirsute hyperandrogenic women. 68th Ann Meet Endocr Soc, Abstract n° 350, p. 348.

Carlström K, Eriksson A, Gustafsson SA, Henriksson P, Pousette Å, Stege R, von Schoultz B (1985). Influence of orchidectomy or estrogen treatment on serum levels of pregnancy associated α2-glycoprotein and sex-hormone binding globulin in patients with prostatic cancer. Int J Androl 8: 21-27.

Crilly RG, Marshall DH, Nordin BEC (1980). Adrenal androgens in post-menopausal osteoporosis. In Genazzani AR, Thijssen JHH, Siiteri PK (eds): "Adrenal Androgens". New York, Raven Press, pp. 241-258.

Farnsworth EW (1972). Prolactin and the prostate. In Boyns AR, Griffiths K (eds): "Prolactin and Carcinogenesis". Cardiff, Alpha Omega Alpha, p. 217.

Fiet J, Gourmel B, Villette JM, Brerault JL, Julien R, Cathelineau G, Dreux C (1980). Simultaneous radioimmunoassay of androstenedione, dehydroepiandrosterone and 11β-hydroxy-androstenedione in plasma. Horm Res 13:133-149.

Fiet J, Morville R, Chemama D, Villette JM, Gourmel B, Brerault JL, Dreux C (1982). Plasma androgen and gonadotrophin levels in normal adult men after percutaneous administration of 5α-dihydrotestosterone. Int J Androl 5: 586-594.

Forest M, Sizonenko PC, Cathiard AM, Bertrand J (1974). Hypophysogonadal function in human during the first year of life. Evidence for testicular activity in early infancy. J Clin Invest 53: 819-828.

Geller J (1985). Rationale for blockade of adrenal as well as testicular androgens in the treatment of advanced prostate cancer. Seminars in Oncology, XII (suppl.1): 28-35.

Goldzieher JW, de la Pena A, Aivaliotis MV (1978). Radioimmunoassay of plasma androstenedione, testosterone and 11β-hydroxyandrostenedione after chromatography on Lipidex-5000 (hydroxyalkoxy propyl Sephadex). J steroid Biochem 9: 169-173.

Gompel A, Wright F, Kuttenn F, Mauvais-Jarvis P (1986). Contribution of plasma androstenedione to 5α-androstanediol glucuronide in women with idiopathic hirsutism. J Clin Endocrinol Metab 62: 441-444.

Harper ME, Peeling WB, Cowley T, Brownsey MG, Phillips MEA, Groom G, Fahmy DR, Griffiths K (1976). Plasma steroid and protein hormone concentrations in patients with prostatic carcinoma before and during oestrogen therapy. Acta Endocrinol (Kbh) 81: 409.

Horton R, Endres D, Galmarini M (1984). Ideal conditions for hydrolysis of androstanediol 3α, 17β-diol glucuronide in plasma. J Clin Endocrinol Metab 59: 1027.

Horton R, Lobo RA (eds) (1986). Androgen metabolism in hirsute and normal females. Clinics Endocrinol Metab 15: 213-409.

Jacobi GH, Rathgen GH, Altwein JE (1980). Serum prolactin and tumors of the prostate: unchanged basal levels and lack of correlation to serum testosterone. J Endocrinol Invest 3: 15-18.

Labrie F, Dupont A, Bélanger A, Lacoursière Y, Raynaud JP, Husson JM, Gareau J, Fazekas ATA, Sandow J, Monfette G, Girard JG, Emond J, Houle JG (1983). New approach in the treatment of prostate cancer : complete instead of partial withdrawal of androgens. The Prostate 4: 579-594.

Maatman TJ, Gupta MK, Montie JE (1985). Effectiveness of castration versus intravenous estrogen therapy in producing rapid endocrine control of metastatic cancer of the prostate. J Urol 133: 620-621.

Moghissi E, Ablan F, Horton R (1984). Origin of plasma androstanediol glucuronide in men. J Clin Endocrinol Metab 59: 417-421.

Moguilewsky M, Fiet J, Tournemine C, Raynaud JP (1986). Pharmacology of an antiandrogen, Anandron, used as an adjuvant therapy in the treatment of prostate cancer. J steroid Biochem 24: 139-146.

Morimoto I, Edmiston A, Hawks D, Horton R (1981). Studies on the origin of androstanediol and androstanediol glucuronide in young and elderly men. J Clin Endocrinol Metab 52: 772-778.

Parker L, Lai H, Wolk F, Lifrak E, Kim S, Epstein L, Hadley D, Miller J (1984). Orchiectomy does not selectively increase adrenal androgen concentration. J Clin Endocrinol Metab 59: 547-550.

Rao PN, Burdett JE Jr, Moore PH, Jr, Horton R (1986). Isolation and identification of androstanediol glucuronide from human plasma. 68th Ann Meeting Endocr Soc, Abstract n° 346, p. 117.

Raynaud JP, Moguilewsky M, Tournemine C, Pottier J, Coussedière D, Salmon J, Husson JM, Bertagna C, Tremblay D, Pendyala L, Brisset JM, Vallancien G, Serment G, Navratil H, Dupont A, Labrie F (1985): Pharmacology and clinical studies with RU 23908 (Anandron[R]). In Schröder FH, Richards B (eds): "EORTC Genitourinary Group Monograph 2, Part A. Therapeutic Principles in the Management of Metastatic Prostatic Cancer". New York, Alan Liss, pp. 99-120.

Sanford EJ, Drago JR, Rohner TJ, Santen R, Lipton A (1976). Aminoglutethimide medical adrenalectomy for advanced prostatic carcinoma. J Urol 115: 170-174.

Sciarra F, Sorcini G, di Silverio F, Gagliardi B (1973). Plasma testosterone and androstenedione after orchiectomy in prostate adenocarcinoma. Clin Endocrinol 2: 101-109.

Serafini P, Lobo RA (1985). Increased 5α-reductase activity in idiopathic hirsutism. Fertil Steril 43: 74.

Varenhorst E, Wallentin I, Carlström K (1982). The effects of orchiectomy, estrogens and cyproterone acetate on plasma testosterone, LH, and FSH concentrations in patients with carcinoma of the prostate. Scand J Urol Nephrol 16: 31-36.

Vermeulen A (1980). Adrenal androgens and aging. In Genazzani AR, Thijssen JHH, Siiteri PK (eds): "Adrenal Androgens". New-York, Raven Press, pp. 207-217.

Vermeulen A, Schelfhout W, de Sy W (1982). Plasma androgen levels after subcapsular orchiectomy or estrogen treatment for prostatic carcinoma. The Prostate 3: 115-121.

Prostate Cancer, Part A: Research, Endocrine
Treatment, and Histopathology, pages 45–53
© 1987 Alan R. Liss, Inc.

HORMONAL CONSEQUENCES OF ORCHIDECTOMY FOR CARCINOMA OF THE PROSTATE. WITH SPECIAL REFERENCE TO THE MEASUREMENT OF FREE TESTOSTERONE IN THE SALIVA

L. BOCCON-GIBOD*, M.H. LAUDAT**, D. GUIBAN**,
A. STEG*.

Clinique Urologique* et Département d'Hormonologie**- Hôpital COCHIN - 75014 PARIS - FRANCE.

Summary : 22 patients with metastatic carcinoma of the prostate were treated by subcapsular orchidectomy and followed by regular determinations of plasma T, DHT, D4A Dione, SDHEA, and TeBG as well as salivary T which measures the free Testosterone. Subcapsular orchidectomy constantly induced a dramatic and stable decrease of testicular androgens or TeBG. Free Testosterone levels vary widely for a given value of plasma T, probably due to individual variations of TeBG. Therefore salivary T should be used preferably to plasma T to monitor hormonal therapy of metastatic carcinoma of the prostate.

Introduction : Orchidectomy, suppressing the source of testicular androgens, reduces plasma Testosterone (T) to 0,5 ng/ml in a few hours. Although the long term effect of orchidectomy on plasma levels of T Dihydrotestosterone (DHT) and Adrenal androgens is well documented (2, 3, 4, 5, 8) its real impact on free Testosterone is usually deducted from calculations based on plasmatic values of T ans Testosterone Estradiol Binding Globuline (TeBG) (9, 10, 11). Free Testosterone passively diffuses in the salivary glands and therefore the salivary level of T reflects exactly the plasma level of free Testosterone (12, 13). As free T is the only active form of the hormone, its determination may be practical importance in the monitoring of patients with metastatic carcinoma of the

prostate, submitted to various forms of hormonal
manipulation.

Patients and Methods :

22 patients aged 55 - 86 (over 70) with carcinoma
of the prostate unamenable to radical treatment
because of metastatic disease or age were submitted to subcapsular orchidectomy. Plasma levels of
Testosterone (Tp), Dihydrostestosterone (DHT),
Testosterone Estradiol Binding Globuline (TeBG),
D4 Androstene Dione (D4A) and Dehydroepiandrosterone Sulfate (DHEA-S) as well as salivary Testosterone (Ts) were assayed before orchidectomy
and during follow up visits at 1 week, 1 and 12
months. Tp and DHT values were obtained by Radio-
Immunoassay using specific antibodies prepared by
Prof. J. MAHOUDEAU (6) in our laboratory, after
extraction with Ethyl Acetylate iso-octane and
separation on Celite Column, normal values are Tp:
4 - 10 ng/ml, DHT : 0,4 - 0,9 ng/ml.

Salivary Testosterone (Ts) :

Saliva was obtained from patients at 8 a.m.
After freezing   and centrifugation of the saliva
T was extracted and treated as described for plasma T. However, in castrated patients this measurement requires a more important salivary sample,
convenient dilution of specific antibodies and
standard curves of T adapted to the small quantities of salivary T.

TeBG :

Endogenous steroïds are removed from the serum
sample prior to the assay by absorption with
charcoal.
TeBG is separated from the serum by binding
to concanavaline A. TeBG binding sites are then
saturated with an excess of 3H-DHT.
After centrifugation pellet was resuspended in
scintillation fluid and counted. The results
obtainedafter calculation are considered as the
binding capacity of TeBG for DHT and expressed
in ng/ml of DHT.
Normal values are $5 \pm 2,5$ ng/ml.

D4 Androstenedione :
D4 was measured by Radio-immunoassay using a
specific antibody (Bio MERIEUX) after extraction
and isolation on celite column.
Normal values are D4 Adione : 0,8 - 2,4 ng/ml.
SDHEA : 0,8 - 3,3 mcg/ml.

DHEA S :
DHEA S was directly measured from plasma by Radio
immunoassay (Specific antibody : Bio MERIEUX).

Results :
Subcapsular orchidectomy produces a dramatic
and stable reduction in the plasma levels of T
and DHT. From a mean pre-orchidectomy level of
5,97 $\pm$ 2,22 ng/ml (extremes : 1,22 - 10,95 ng/ml)
Tp decreases to 0,16 $\pm$ 0,06 ng/ml at week 1 and
remains at 0,14 $\pm$ 0,07 NG/ml at 1 year (extremes:
0,06 - 0,34 ng/ml) (Fig. 1). Thus subcapsular
orchidectomy suppresses 97,7 % of plasma T, by the
same token plasma DHT decreases from a mean pre-
orchidectomy level of 0,58 $\pm$ 0,27 ng/ml (extremes : 0,21 - 1 ng/ml) to 0,14 $\pm$ 0,07 ng/ml at
week 1 and to 0,09 $\pm$ 0,06 ng/ml at 1 year (extremes : 0,03 - 0,17) which represents a decrease
in 85 % of plasma DHT (Fig. 2). Salivary Testosterone (Ts) which represents the free active
form of Testosterone in the plasma under-goes
the same dramatic and stable reduction, from a
mean pre-operative level of 56,6 $\pm$ 23 pg/ml (extremes : 6 - 93) it decreases to 15 $\pm$ 7 pg/ml on
week 1 and to 10 $\pm$ 5 pg/ml at 1 year (Fig. 1)
(extremes : 4 - 27 pg/ml). There is no direct
correlation between Tp and Ts levels, for a
Tp < 0,10 ng/ml Ts can vary from 4 to 15 pg/ml
and for a Tp > 15 ng/ml Ts can vary from 4 to
25 pg/ml. These variations probably reflect in
part, individual variations in TeBG concentrations (Table 1).
TeBG remained stable throughout the study : from
a mean pre-orchidectomy value of 8,85 $\pm$ 3,45 ng/
ml it decreased to 7,88 $\pm$ 2,47 ng/ml at 1 year
which is not statistically significant (p > 0,5).

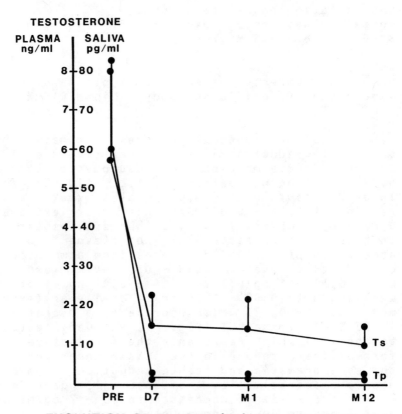

**EVOLUTION OF PLASMA (Tp) AND SALIVARY (Ts)
TESTOSTERONE AFTER ORCHIDECTOMY**

FIGURE 1.

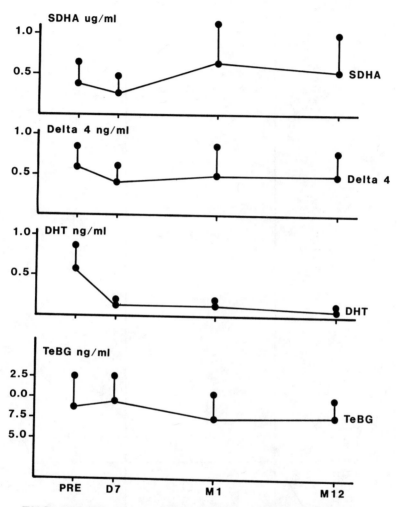

**EVOLUTION OF PLASMA TeBG, DHT, DELTA 4 A,
DHEA-S AFTER ORCHIDECTOMY**

FIGURE 2.

TL pg/mL \ Tp pg/mL	< 100	100 – 150	≥ 150
≤ 5 : 5	3		2
6 – 10 : 8	1	3	4
11 – 15 : 7	2	3	2
≥ 15 : 2		1	1
Tp	6	7	9

Tp vs Tl

TABLE 1.

There is a correlation between TeBG and Ts levels
However for a same value of TeBG, Ts can vary
widely and although the ratio $\frac{Tp - Ts}{Tp}$ tends
towards 1 when TeBG rises there are wide individual variations. Delta 4 Adione slightly decreased during the study from a mean preopera-
tive value of 0,58 ± 0,05 ng/ml to a mean value
of 0,48 ± 0,06 ng/ml at 1 year, which achieves
statistical significance (p > 0,0005).

Discussion :
After others (2, 3, 4, 5, 7, 8) this study
demonstrates that orchidectomy, be it standard
on subcapsular, produces constantly dramatic
and stable decrease in circulating androgens
down to female levels. We did not observe a single value of post-orchidectomy superior to 0,34
ng/ml as previously reported (5, 7). The same observations can be made concerning DHT which remains at its lowest values 1 year after orchidectomy eventhough there is a slight increase in
the level of plasma SDHEA. Thus it can be concluded that at 1 year there is no apparent compensatory secretion of Adrenal Androgens, nor a
rise in their peripheral conversion to Testosterone or DHT. The second observation concerns
the clinical use of the salivary Testosterone
assay. Plasma Testosterone levels only roughly
correlate with free Testosterone levels, due to
variations of TeBG concentrations which can
vary from individual to individual even in the
absence of any concommitent medications known to
increase the circulating levels of TeBG. For any
given value of plasma Testosterone, there is a
wide range of values of salivary Testosterone.
Until recently free Testosterone determinations
necessitated complex calculations based on determinations of TeBG and plasma T or a very sophisticated technique to measure free T in the plasma
(9, 10, 11, 13).

The development of the salivary assay (12, 13)
which reflects free T the only active form of
Testosterone in the plasma provides the clinician
with a simple and efficient tool to monitor
the hormonal therapy of carcinoma of the prostate. In the future, the salivary assay of free
Testosterone will allow the clinician to determine the usefulness, of any reduction of free
Testosterone levels obtained through elevation
of TeBG or inhibition of Androgen synthesis.

Bibliography :

ABRAHAM G., MANLINOS F., GARZA R.
Radio-immunoassay of Steroïds - Chapter 20 in
G.E ABRAHAM Hand-book of Radio-Immunoassay.
M. DEKKER Ed. 1977.

BRACCI U., DI SILVERIO F., SCIARRA F., SORCINI,
PIRO C., SANTORO F.
Hormonal patern in prostatic carcinoma following
orchidectomy.
Brit. J. Urol. 1977, 49, 161.

CATALONA W.J.
Prostate Cancer
Grun & Stratton Ed. Londres - New-York, 1985.

GHANADIAN R., PUAH C.M.
The clinical significance of steroïds hormone in
the management of patients with prostatic cancer.
World Journal of Urology, 1981, 1, 49.

KLUGO R.C., FARAH R.N., CERNY J.C.
Bilateral orchidectomy for carcinoma of the
prostate.
Urology, 1981, 17, 49.

MAHOUDEAU J.A., BRICAIRE H.
Dosages simultanés de la Testosterone et de la
Dihydrotestosterone par méthode Radio-Immunolo-
gique. Revue Française d'Endocrinologie Clinique,
Nutrition et Métabolisme, 1972, 13, 413.

SANFORD J., PAULSON F., ROHNERT J., DRAGO J.R.,
SANTEN R.J., BARDIN C.W.
The effects of castration on Adrenal Testoste-
rone secretions in men with prostatic carcinoma.
J. Urol. 1977, 118, 1019.

SHEARRER J., HENDRY W.F., SOMMERVILLE I.F.,
FERGUSON J.D.
Plasma Testosterone : an accurate monitor of
hormone treatment in prostatic cancer.
Brit. J. Urol. 1973, 45, 668 - 677.

TOMIC R.
Some effects of orchidectomy, oestrogens treatment and Radiation therapy in patients with
prostatic carcinoma.
Scand. J. Urol. and Nephrol. suppl. 77, 1983.

USUI T., SAGANI K., KITANO T., NIHIRA H.,
NIYACHI Y.
The changers in the binding capacity of Testosterone Oestradiol binding Globuline (TeBG) following castration and DES administration in patients with prostatic carcinoma.
Urol. Res. 1982, 10, 119.

VARENHORST E., WALLENTIN L., CARLSTROM K.
The effects of orchidectomy : oestrogens and
Cyproterone Acetate on plasma Testosterone LH
and FSH concentration in patients with carcinoma
of the prostate.
Scand. J. Urol. and Nephrol. 1982, 16, 31.

WALKER R.F., WILSON D.W., READ G.F., RIAD-FAHOU Y
Assessment of testicular function by Radio-
Immunoassay of Testosterone in saliva.

WANG C., PLEYMA T.E., NIESCHLAG E., PAULSON E.
Salivary Testosterone in men : further evidence
of a direct correlation with free serum Testosterone.
J. Clin. End. Metab. 1981, 53, 1021.

Prostate Cancer, Part A: Research, Endocrine
Treatment, and Histopathology, pages 55–60
© 1987 Alan R. Liss, Inc.

THE EFFECTS OF SUPPRESSING OF ANDROGEN ACTION ON THE
NORMAL PROSTATE

Herman J. de Voogt, B.Ram Rao, Louis J.G.Gooren and
Freerk G.Bouman

Departments of Urology, Endocrinology (Andrology) and
Plastic Surgery, Free University Hospital, Amsterdam

INTRODUCTION

Our study of agonadal men was initiated by a patient,
who was castrated for moral offense at 40 years of age and
who at the age of 80 came to our department with a poorly
differentiated prostatic carcinoma. Although his serum
testosterone (1,2 mmol/l) was below castration level (as
could be expected) he had developed a prostate cancer.
Androgen-receptor level (DHT-receptor 57 fmol/mg protein)
was measured in the tumor cytosol fraction.

A few years before in the Andrology department a study
was completed on the influence of testicular hormones on the
secretion of Luteinising Hormone (LH), Follicle Stimulating
Hormone (FSH) and Prolactin (Prl). Patients who had lost
their gonads by accident as well as those who optioned for
male-to-female transformation consented to participate in
the study.

We decided that further studies on agonadal men might
provide an insight in what happens with the normal prostate
and steroid metabolism after castration, in order to understand better the various forms of hormonal therapy which
may be effective in the management of prostatic cancer.

MATERIAL AND METHODS

The subjects studied were male-to-female transsexuals
in the age-range of 22-40 years. They were all genetically

males with 46 XY Karyotype and their basal levels of T, LH, FSH and Prl were in the normal range at the time of first examination.

After thorough information and instruction they all consented to participate in the study.

They usually were treated for periods of 18-24 months with a combination of anti-androgens and estrogens to adapt socially and psychologically to the female state before gender reassignment surgery is performed.

Seventeen of these men were treated for the first 8 weeks with a pure anti-androgen, RU 23908 (Anandron), kindly provided by Roussel-UCLAF for this purpose. At 4 and 8 weeks levels of T, LH, FSH and Prl were determined. In 6 of these men the prostate was examined by transrectal ultrasonography to assess dimensions and volume of the prostate before and after 8 weeks of anti-androgen treatment.

In 5 men, treated for 1-2 years with a combination of anti-androgens and estrogens, the prostate was measured by transrectal ultrasonography and at the time of gender reassignment surgery biopsies from the prostate were taken for histological examination. The removed testes were examined histologically as well as biochemically. Leydig cells were isolated from the testes using collagenase treatment and centrifugation procedures. In all cases vital Leydig cells could be harvested and they were investigated for T production after hCG treatment.

RESULTS

The effect of a pure anti-androgen on basal levels of T, LH, FSH and Prl is given in fig. 1 . As can be seen T-levels rose steadily to 2-3 fold the initial values during the first 4-6 weeks of Anandron administration whereafter these values reached a plateau. The same was seen to occur with LH levels. Basal FSH levels were not affected, Prolactin levels were slow to rise after 4 weeks.

All these patients clinically showed signs of feminisation such as gynaecomastia and loss of hairgrowth.

The 6 prostates studied did not change in volume or

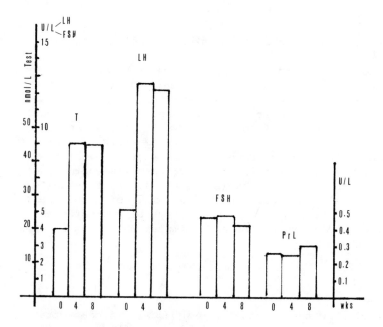

fig. 1. Effect of RU 23908 on basal levels of
Testosteron, LH, FSH and prolactine

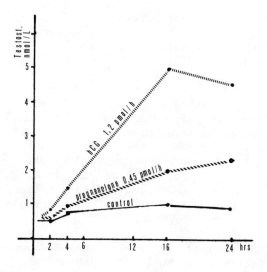

fig 2. T-synthesis of Leydig cells in culture
after pregnolone and hCG-stimulation

diameter during 8 weeks treatment with anti-androgens!

Also in patients, treated for 1 year or more with Cypro-terone acetate (CPA) and estrogens the prostates had the same volume and diameter as seen in normal men of the same age. However, histologically in all specimens an abundance of stromal tissue was found with few, if any, atrophic glandular structures, which were still positive for prostatic acid phosphatase or prostate specific antigen by histo-chemistry. As to testicular tissue, there was spermatogenic arrest and thickening of basal membranes of the seminiferous tubules as well as reduction in the number of Leydig cells. However vital Leydig cells could always be harvested and brought into culture and on hCG stimulation showed increase in T synthesis (fig 2).

DISCUSSION

Studies with eugonadal and agonadal men demonstrated that estrogens most likely inhibit LH secretion at the hypothalamic level by influencing the LH release, while FSH-secretion is inhibited by a direct action on the gonado-trophic cells of the pituitary. This latter action is proba-bly due to a synergistic effect of estrogens and inhibin. Besides it could be demonstrated that DHT in eugonadal men has no effect on gonadotrophic-secretion, but in agonadal men (in the absence of T) a suppressic effect on LH and FSH-secretion was observed (Gooren, 1981)

In the present study the use of the anti-androgen (RU 23908) in eugonadal men resulted in high serum T and LH levels and slightly elevated Prl levels, but FSH remained unaffected. Together with the clinical signs of feminisation these results indicate that RU 23908 is indeed a pure anti-androgen in that it blocks androgen action in target cells while the effective androgen receptor blocking stimulates LH secretion and subsequently T production. The fact that FSH was not affected could mean a confirmation that androgens do not influence FSH production. (Raynaud, 1984)

More important is the finding that a pure anti-androgen causes T and LH levels to rise, but that after 4-8 weeks a tendency developes for T levels to remain in general at a plateau. This could mean that RU 23908 induces a new equili-brium in the negative feedback regulation of the testis with elevated levels of LH and T in the presence of normal active gonads. Irrespective of the new hormonal equilibrium, it is evident from our studies that the androgen action in the androgen target organs is blocked. Therefore, an optimal effectiveness of nontoxic dosage may readily be achieved in the absence of gonads. However the increase in serum T and LH levels might make the pure anti_androgens less suitable for combination with LHRH-agonists, while the ratio androgens/ anti-androgens in the target organs might be such that insufficient protection against high androgen levels is reached (Habenich 1986). These considerations may have important consequences for the hormonal treatment of prostatic cancer.

From several studies in the past it is known that medical castration (by means of DES or EE) resulted in the prostate that histologically carcinomatous glandular tissue disappeared and was replaced by stroma. We observed a similar effect in normal prostates after prolonged treatment with CPA and EE; glandular structures became atrophic or disappeared while the stromal tissue increased. However the volume of the prostates remained the same. This also confirms studies that indicated an effect of steroids on stroma as well as on glands of the prostate in benign (BPH) and malignant diseases. (Bartsch, 1981)

Finally we found that prolonged androgen suppressive treatment (up to 2 years) did not destroy Leydig cell function. Although the number of Leydig cells was reduced, still vital Leydig cells were present and could be harvested as well as brought to T production in vitro.

CONCLUSIONS

After androgen deprivation by different methods the normal prostate does not change in volume but only in histologicfeatures: glandular tissue becomes atrophic and disappears while there is an increase in stromal tissue.

By administration of pure anti-androgens, although resulting in LH and T levels increase, the androgen action at the target tissue levels is effectively blocked.

Prolonged suppression of T production, other than by orchidectomy, for up to 2 years does not necessarily destroy

Leydig cells. As long as vital Leydig cells remain present
deprivation can be reversible. Orchidectomy in combination
with anti-androgens may be the choice of therapy in the
management of prostate cancer.

Castration after puberty does not preclude the development of prostate cancer. This should be kept in mind
for patients after gender reassignment procedures.

REFERENCES

Bartsch G, Rohr HP (1981). The use of anti hormones in human
    prostatic hyperplasia. In: Anti hormone ed. by Altwein,
    Bartsch und Jacobi. Zuckschwerdt Verlag München, p 21-40.
Gooren LJG (1981). Testicular hormones and the secretion
    of LH, FSH and Prolactin. Thesis, Amsterdam.
Habenich UF, Witthaus E, Neumann F (1986). Anti-androgene
    und LHRH-Agonisten: Endokrinologie in der Initialphase
    Ihrer Anwendung. Akt.Urol. 17: 10-16.
Raynaud JP et al. (1984). The pure anti-androgen RU 23908
    (Anandron), a candidate of choice for the combined anti
    hormonal treatment of prostatic cancer: A revieuw.
    The prostate 5: 299-311.

Prostate Cancer, Part A: Research, Endocrine
Treatment, and Histopathology, pages 61–76
© 1987 Alan R. Liss, Inc.

PROSTATE METABOLISM OF STEROIDS FOLLOWING CASTRATION

J.P. Karr, R. Drury, C.F. Mann,
R.P. Huben, R.R. Tubbs, J.E. Pontes,
and A.A. Sandberg

Roswell Park Memorial Institute, 666
Elm Street, Buffalo, New York 14263
(J.P.K., R.D., C.F.M., R.P.H., A.A.S)
and Cleveland Clinic Foundation,
Cleveland, Ohio 44106 (R.R.T.,
J.E.P.)

The subject of prostatic metabolism of steroids,
whether it be in tissue from normal or castrated subjects,
is one which primarily gives focus to the 5α-reduction of
testosterone to dihydrotestosterone, which in turn is further
reduced to the 3α-and 3β-androstanediols (Coffey and Isaacs,
1981; Ofner et al, 1984; Gupta 1982; Ghanadian and Smith,
1982). In addition, there has been renewed interest in the
oxidative pathways for the metabolism of testosterone
including studies recently presented at the 81st Annual
Meeting of the American Urologic Association (Mann et al.,
1986; Stone and Fishman, 1986), which point to the potential
importance of the oxidation of testosterone to androstenedione and the possible role of a prostatic aromatase system
in the synthesis of estrogens both in the normal and
neoplastic prostate (Figure 1).

Following castration, regression of the prostate is
accompanied by well-characterized cellular and biochemical
alterations with clear cut effects on enzymes involved with
prostatic metabolism of steroids. Prostatic regression in
castrated animals is an active catabolic process that is
associated with specific increases in the synthesis and
release of degradative enzymes (Lee, 1981). In addition to
the temporal decline in weight and protein content, there is
an increased acid ribonuclease activity that reaches a
maximal level approximately six days following castration and
this coincides with a rapid decline in total RNA content,
suggesting that the process of prostatic involution following
castration involves equally important roles for protein

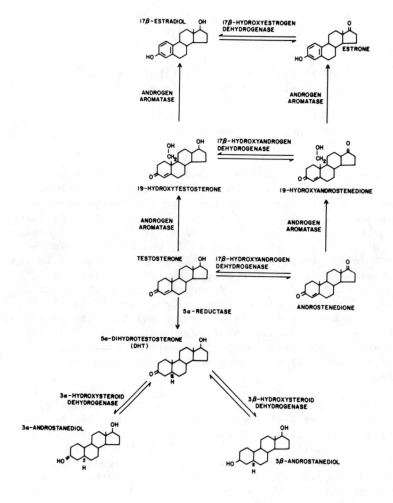

Figure 1. Reductive, oxidative and aromatic metabolism of testosterone.

degradation and synthesis (Lee, 1981; Lee and Jesik, 1983). However, mechanisms are retained in the regressed prostate through which the gland can be restored to essentially normal size and function with replacement hormonal therapy. Thus, the pronounced reduction of actual and normalized rat ventral prostate weights by day seven following castration is readily reversed with subcutaneous injections of 100 µg testosterone alone or in combination with different doses of estradiol ranging from 10 - 100 µg (Karr et al, 1974). This study also indicated that 100 µg of testosterone approaches the physiologic restorative dosage for castrated rats and that low levels of estradiol may enhance the restorative effects of testosterone on ventral prostate weights.

The concentrations of two important classes of protein that are involved with the metabolism of steroids, 5α-reductase and steroid hormone receptors, are markedly affected by castration. A recent and comprehensive review of 5α-reductase and its importance in both normal and malignant prostate tissue, (Petrow and Padilla, 1984) points out that in 1965 Shimazaki et al established that 5α-reductase activity in microsomal and mitochondrial fractions of rat ventral prostate requires NADPH as cofactor and, as an enzyme that is tightly bound to cell membranes including those of the nucleus and endoplasmic reticulum. The activity of this enzyme decreases following castration, but this can be reversed with increases to levels which exceed seven times those of normal rats upon treatment with testosterone propionate over an eight-day period (Shimazaki et al, 1969; Moore and Wilson, 1973). In castrated rats, 5α-reductase activity decreases particularly in the ventral prostate (Sandberg, 1979). That is 5α-reductase activity (expressed as nM x 10 DHT formed per 50 mg. tissue per hour) decreased from 4.5 to less than 2 in about four days, whereas about seven days were required to achieve the same percentage decrease in the dorsolateral lobe following castration. This work further compliments Yamanaka's observation in 1975 (Yamanaka, 1975) that the ventral prostate regresses more rapidly and more completely following castration than does the dorsolateral prostate. The reason for these differences is undoubtedly a reflection of the histologic, ultra-structural and biochemical differences between the lobes of the rat prostate (Sandberg et al, 1980). Similarly, the effects of medical castration on the morphology and ultrastructure of the caudal and cranial lobes of the baboon prostate differ markedly and further point to the well

documented duality of the prostate in this species as well as
that of man (Chai et al, 1981).

Studies on the effects of castration (surgical or
medical) on the different zones of the prostate, particularly
with regard to 5α-reductase, have been enhanced through the
availability of inhibitors of 5α-reductase activity which
have activity not only in vitro but in vivo as well (Petrow,
1984).

In this regard, the 4-methyl-4-aza-steroids (sodium 4-
methyl-3-oxol-4-aza-5α-pregnane-20(s)-carboxylate and 17β-N,
N-diethylcarbamoyl-4-methyl-4-aza-5α-androstan-3-one i.e.,
4-MAPC and 4-MA, respectively) are potent inhibitors of 5α-
reductase (Kadohama et al, 1984; Kadohama et al, 1985).
Studies on rats bearing the androgen responsive Noble
prostatic adenocarcinoma (2 Pr-121D) showed that both
compounds produced significant decreases in average final
tumor sizes and weights. Furthermore, analysis of tumor
growth curves showed that both drugs have a retarding effect
on tumor progression that is similar to the growth curves of
this tumor in castrated males or intact females. In prostate
glands and tumors derived from untreated and 4-MAPC-treated
rats, Kadohama et al. demonstrated that total 5α-reductase
activity, i.e. dihydrotestosterone and androstanediol reduced
from testosterone, was diminished in both the ventral and
dorsolateral prostates (Kadohama et al, 1985). The important
finding of this study, however, was that even though the
amount of DHT formed in tumor tissue from treated animals was
less than that of the controls, the overall 5α-reduced
metabolites (DHT + 3α- and 3β-diols) did not differ,
suggesting that an alternate pathway to androstanediols could
compensate for the drug effect on 5α-reduction. In organ
culture, both of these 4-methyl-4-aza steroids are potent
inhibitors of 5α-reductase in rat and human prostate tissues
(Kadohama et al, 1984). In addition, 4-MAPC, but not 4-MA,
exhibited both a strong inhibition of 5α-reduction and a
considerable stimulation of 17β-oxidation. However the
selectivity of this action by 4-MAPC was observed in the
dorsolateral lobe but not the ventral lobe of the rat
prostate. That is, 4-MAPC inhibited the reductive and to
some extent oxidative activity in ventral prostate, whereas
in the dorsolateral prostate the drug selectively inhibited
the reductive pathway by 91% and stimulated by over 6-fold
the oxidation of testosterone to Δ^4-androstenedione. In
tumor prostate cancer, similar selectivity was observed in

that both inhibitors strongly inhibited 5α-reductase, whereas only 4-MAPC produced significant enhancement of 17β-oxidation akin to that observed in the rat dorsolateral prostate. Moreover, in human BPH, the reciprocal action of 4-MAPC on oxidative and reductive pathways was also evident, but it should be noted that histologic examination of these tissues suggested that the stimulatory effect on the BPH oxidative pathway was correlated with the glandular vs the stromal content of the specimen. The importance of these and other studies on 5α-reductase inhibitors becomes apparent if one accepts the thesis that these inhibitors are more potent in castrated animals with measurable concentrations of prostatic dihydrotestosterone. That is, since the efficacy of 5α-reductase inhibitors varies inversely with testosterone concentrations, such agents presumably will have greater activity and could presumably have greater activity in castrated subjects in whom there are measurable levels of testosterone (Petrow, 1984; Petrow, 1986).

The heterogeneous nature of the prostate is demonstrated by the fact that a subset of cells which populate the normal gland are able to survive hormonal withdrawal and retain their hormonal sensitivity and respond to androgen therapy with renewed prostatic growth. Such cells are hormonally independent in the sense that they persist in the absence of testicular androgens and they are hormonally sensitive in the sense that they have preserved or retained elements which permit a stimulatory response to testosterone with subsequent restoration of prostatic weight and function. The fact that hormone action is mediated by specific receptor proteins in the prostate is well documented (Sandberg and Karr, 1987). Intracellular elements that regulate hormonal action are preserved in castrated animals, but the mechanisms involved have not been studied extensively. Some light has been shed on this subject, however, in the elegant studies reported by Hoisaeter et al., who measured cytoplasmic androgen receptor (8S in low salt buffer) in rat ventral prostate grown in organ culture for various periods of time 24 hours after castration with no hormones in the culture medium. He showed that after four hours of incubation only traces of the 8S peak could be detected and no specific 8S peak was found in explants grown in organ culture after 24 hours (Hoisaeter et al, 1981). Even in the presence of androgen no cytosolic binding of tritiated DHT in one-day castrates was noted after four hours of culture and nuclear high salt extractable receptors were

minimally detected after seven days, whereas high salt
resistant nuclear binding was maintained in the absence of
androgen after the first day of culture for up to seven days.
This work suggests that at least part of the receptor
mechanism that survives in the prostate of castrated animals
resides in the nuclear matrix. Even though neither
cytoplasmic nor nuclear receptors could be reinduced in
tissue which had been explanted for 24 hours, nuclear residue
binding i.e., the remaining radioactivity after extraction of
nuclear receptors, could be found throughout the total seven-
day culture period and this type of binding could be
reinduced after 24 hours in culture. Thus, the persistence
of androgenic effects in the explants may be related to the
persistence of high-salt-resistant nuclear binding in sites
associated with the nuclear matrix.

One of the central issues addressed in this Second
International Symposium on Prostate Cancer concerns the
source and amount of steroids available to the prostate in
both normal and castrated men. The values given in Table 1
indicate that normal serum testosterone and dihydrotestosterone can be expressed over a wide range, and that
such testosterone levels values will vary between
laboratories. Moreover, serum testosterone levels decline,
although not in physiologically significant amounts, with age
(Sandberg, 1980; Coffey and Isaacs, 1981). We and others
have previously documented serum testosterone values of
healthy men in comparison to those of untreated prostate

**Table 1. Serum Testosterone and Dihydrotestosterone
Concentrations in Healthy Men (ng/100 ml)**

T	DHT	
407–583*	66 $\pm$ 3.7*	Vermuelen '76
361 $\pm$ 145	36 $\pm$ 7.2	Jacobi et al '80
611 $\pm$ 186	56 $\pm$ 20	Coffey & Isaacs '81

* <50 years old

cancer patients (Table 2), and have further noted the marked depression of serum testosterone following castration and/or estrogen therapy (Karr et al, 1980). It should also be noted

Table 2. Mean Serum Testosterone Concentrations of Male Controls and Prostatic Cancer Patients

| | N | Testosterone (ng/100 ml) | |
		Mean ± Standard Error	Range
Controls:			
Men <50 yrs. old	10	730 ± 43	540-963
Men >65 yrs. old	4	432 ± 16	186-452
Prostatic cancer patients:			
No hormone therapy	14	493 ± 108	141-1535
Bilat. orchiectomy	28	72 ± 11	4-163
DES	22	76 ± 24	7-387
Bilat. orchiectomy and DES	28	65 ± 13	8-339

Karr et al, 1980

that in the case of estrogen therapy there is a marked elevation in serum TeBG levels which accompanies the depression of serum testosterone and this further reduces the availability of serum androgens to the prostate (Karr et al, 1980). With the ablation of testicular steroids the important question becomes whether adrenal steroids alone can affect normal and malignant prostate tissue. The hormonal regulation of the prostate has been the subject of excellent reviews (Coffey and Isaacs, 1981; Sandberg, 1981) and it is generally agreed that the testes account for over 95% of the circulating testosterone and that the adrenal contribution of relatively weak androgens to the circulation is not sufficient to restore the size of the prostate in castrated animals (rodents, dogs, non-human primates, etc.) nor in man. Nature's own experiments have further shown that the adrenal steroids alone are not sufficient to stimulate prostatic growth in patients with Kallmann's syndrome, i.e., hypogonadotrophic eunuchoidism (Kallmann et al, 1979), panhypopituitarism (Oesterling et al, 1986), prepubertal castration or in patients with 5α-reductase deficiency (Imperato-McGinley et al, 1974). In the case of rats bearing the Dunning prostatic adenocarcinoma, evidence that has been reported in the literature thus far suggests that there is no additional treatment benefit from combining the anti-androgen flutamide with medical castration using an LHRH agonist (Redding and Schally, 1985) or the anti-androgen cyproterone acetate with surgical castration (Ellis and Isaacs, 1985). The point has been made that the rat normally secretes only a marginal amount of adrenal androgens and that this is often neglected in the interpretation of experiments (Moguilewsky et al, 1986). A recent study by Foldesy et al showed the combination of an LHRH agonist and flutamide given to adrenalectomized rats produced a greater reduction in prostate weights than did either drug alone, indicating that the role of adrenal androgens in this additive effect on decreasing prostate weights is negligible. These authors suggest that the additive effects of LHRH agonist and anti-androgens in rats appear to focus on testicular rather than adrenal androgens.

In adults with intact adrenals and testes, various investigators have measured testosterone and dihydro-testosterone concentrations in prostate tissue (Table 3). As these data show, the steroid concentrations in specimens from untreated prostate cancer patients appear to fall in the range of BPH and normal prostate tissue specimens obtained at surgery. It should be noted, in particular, that Walsh et al, 1983 have reported that the tissue content of dihydrotestosterone in human BPH removed at surgery, as opposed to specimens obtained at autopsy, is not supranormal. Geller has been a leader in this field in terms of measuring DHT levels in prostate cancer tissue prior to the initiation of endocrine therapy and at the time of relapse (Geller et al, 1984a). They have shown that dihydrotestosterone levels in tumor tissue from men with advanced prostate cancer correlated with clinical response to hormonal therapy (Geller et al, 1984b). Specifically, the average disease-free interval in patients with prostatic DHT levels less than 2.0 ng per gram of tissue was significantly less than that of patients with DHT levels greater than 2.0 ng per gram. Following medical or surgical castration, DHT can still be detected in

Table 3. Human Prostate Testosterone and Dihydrotestosterone Concentrations (ng/gm tissue)*

	T	DHT
Normal	0.2 - 0.9	1.3 - 2.0
Normal	1.2 ± 0.3	5.1 ± 0.4**
Normal	0.2 ± 0.1	1.6 ± 1.0
BPH	1.8 ± 0.6	5.0 ± 0.4
BPH	0.3 ± 0.1	4.5 ± 1.4
BPH		3.9
BPH	0.3 - 0.9	4.5 - 6.0
CaP		4.0
CaP	1.2 - 1.8	3.2 - 4.2
CaP	1.2 - 0.8	3.9 ± 0.3
CaP-DES		2.4
CaP-Megace		1.1
CaP-Castrate		1.6

* These data, expressed as means or ranges, were compiled from the following reports:

Isaacs and Coffey, '79; Krieg et al, '79; Walsh, '83; Gellar '84a, b, '85;

** specimens obtained at surgery

prostatic tissues (Table 3). As many as one-tenth or more of castrated men as well as estrogen treated patients had prostatic DHT levels greater than 2.4 ng per gram in contrast to the depression of DHT levels in the majority of patients to concentrations less than 2.4 ng per gram (Geller et al, 1984a). The question is thus raised as to whether or not the adrenal androgens, androstenedione and dehydroepiandrosterone, are converted to testosterone via 17β-hydroxysteroid dehydrogenase and 3β-hydroxysteroid dehydrogenase enzyme activities, respectively, in this subset of patients. Studies in animals have shown that serum testosterone levels need not be completely eliminated to produce a maximal therapeutic response (Trachtenberg, 1985). Indeed, a threshold of serum testosterone exists for serum androgen (80ng/dl) below which the Dunning R3327H tumor is inhibited from growing, thus raising the question of whether total ablation of serum androgens is necessary for optimal treatment of prostate cancer in man. It may be important to identify subsets of patients, if such indeed exist, with unique capabilities of converting adrenal steroids to testosterone in the circulation and/or prostatic tissue.

In a collaborative study that has just begun between the Cleveland Clinic and Roswell Park Memorial Institute (Table 4), analyses of DHT concentrations in human prostate specimens obtained at surgery have revealed wide overlapping ranges in malignant, normal and BPH specimens. These determinations are based on radioimmunoassay analysis of extracted and purified steroids from whole tissue. The RIA was performed according to the methodology of Abraham using a dextran-charcoal based radioimmunoassay procedure (Abraham, 1977). The tissue was homogenized in three to five volumes of Tris buffer and an aliquot of the homogenate was mixed with known amounts of tritiated DHT and tritiated testosterone for extraction. The samples were next incubated for 30 minutes at 37°C followed by the addition of hexane:ethylacetate in a two:three ratio. The sample was frozen in liquid nitrogen thereby freezing the aqueous layer so that the upper solvent layer could be decanted and saved for purification. Chromatographic purification procedures were based on a modification of the methodology of Manlimos and Abraham (1985). The extracts were dried with nitrogen followed by the addition of 0.5 ml of iso-octane to each vial. Separation of the tissue steroids was accomplished on the basis of the variations in polarities and lipophilic strengths of the steroids. A 5.0-ml disposable serological

Table 4. **Testosterone and Dihydrotestosterone Concentrations (ng/gm tissue) in Surgical Specimens of Human Prostate**

Tissue	T	DHT	Gleason Score	Prior Treatment
CaP	.058	1.50	7	
CaP	ND	2.93	7	
CaP	ND	3.30	6	
CaP	ND	6.28	7	
CaP	.035	1.61	7	Radiation
CaP	.008	7.12	8	Radiation
CaP	.003	11.47	7	Radiation
Normal	ND	1.89		
Normal	ND	3.75		
Normal	ND	5.94		
Normal	.011	9.07		
BPH	ND	2.05		
BPH	ND	2.63		
BPH	ND	5.76		
BPH	ND	8.52		
BPH	ND	13.24		

pipette containing Celite Filter Aid and ethylene glycol was used to separate the testosterone and dihydrotestosterone from the other steroids extracted in this sample. The column was first washed with 6 ml of iso-octane that was forced through the column under nitrogen pressure (10 psi). The sample contained in 0.5 ml iso-octane was then added to the column followed by elution with iso-octane (the moving phase) under nitrogen pressure, and 1.0-ml fractions were collected. Fractions 9-13 were saved for DHT analysis. Elution was continued with 15% ethyl acetate, which is more polar than iso-octane; fractions 16-19 were saved for radioimmunoassay analysis of testosterone.

Three of the prostate cancer patients listed in Table 4 had positive biopsies two years after receiving definitive radiation to the prostate. Following salvage prostatectomy we noted that the DHT levels in two of these patients were markedly elevated. The question is raised as to whether a positive biopsy is reflective of viable or biologically aggressive tumor. These data clearly suggest that at least certain components of the intracellular mechanisms for androgen metabolism were indeed functional when these biopsies were taken. These studies are still in progress with careful patient follow-up and correlations with response to therapy to be reported later.

In summary, measurable concentrations of enzymes and mechanisms associated with receptor hormone interactions that are essential for steroid metabolism are retained in prostatic tissue following castration. Moreover, measurable concentrations of DHT can be determined in human prostate cancer following medical and surgical castration as well as definitive radiation therapy. These data have raised questions as to whether future research emphasis should be directed at defining the meaning of measurable concentrations of DHT in prostate cancer following androgen ablation or radiation therapy in terms of tumor viability and progression. Moreover, one could ask whether there is a potential therapeutic role for 5α-reductase inhibitors in patients with measurable prostatic DHT levels following reduction of serum testosterone levels to castrate levels. Answers to these and other questions, such as whether hormonal therapy accelerates the progression of prostatic tumors from hormonal dependency to autonomy, can only be answered through continued support of basic and clinical research programs.

REFERENCES

Abraham GE (1977). Clinical biochemical analysis. In "Handbook of Radio-immunoassay", Vol. 5 Marcell Dekker, pp 591-656.

Chai LS, Karr JP, Murphy GP, Sandberg AA (1981). Effects of DES on the morphology of the lobes of the baboon prostate. Invest Urol 19:202-208.

Coffey D, Isaacs J (1981). Control of prostate growth. Urology 17:17.

Ellis WJ, Isaacs JT (1985). Effectiveness of complete versus partial androgen withdrawal therapy for the treatment of prostatic cancer as studied in the Dunning R-3327 system of rat prostatic adenocarcinoma. Cancer Res 45:6041-6050.

Foldesy RG, Vanderhoof MM, Canton LE, Hahn DW (1986). Role of adrenal androgens in prostate regression in rats treated with an antiandrogen and an LHRH agonist. The Prostate. (in press).

Geller J, Albert JD, Nachtsheim DA, Loza D (1984a). Comparison of prostatic cancer tissue dihydrotestosterone levels at the time of relapse following orchiectomy or estrogen therapy. J Urol 132:693-696.

Geller J, de la Vega DJ, Albert JD, Nachtsheim DA (1984b). Tissue dihydrotestosterone levels and clinical response to hormonal therapy in patients with advanced prostate cancer. J Clin Endocrinol Metab 58:36-40.

Ghanadian R, Smith CB (1982). Metabolism of steroids in the prostate. In Ghanadian R, (ed): "Endocrinology of Prostate Tumours," Boston, MTP Press, p 113.

Gupta D (1982). Prostate Cancer: Hormone Profiles. In Jacobi GH, Hohenfellner R (eds): "Prostate Cancer," Baltimore, Williams and Wilkins, p 379.

Hoisaeter PA, Kadohama N, Corrales JJ, Karr JP Murphy GP, Sandberg AA (1981). Characterization of androgen receptor and estramustine binding protein of rat ventral prostatic tissue in organ culture. J Steroid Biochem 14:251-260.

Imperato-McGinley J, Guerro L, Gautier L, Peterson RE (1974). Steroid 5α-reductase deficiency in man: An inherited form of male pseudohermaphroditism. Science 186:1213-1215.

Isaacs JT, Coffey DS (1979). Androgenic control of
prostatic growth: regulation of steroid levels.
In Coffey D, Isaacs J (eds): "Prostate Cancer,"
Geneva, UICC pp 112-125.

Jacobi GH, Gupta D, Rathgen GH, Altwein JE (1980).
Hormone dependence of prostatic carcinoma: Serum
androgens, plasma SHBG, and prostatic
androstanediol formation in untreated patients.
In Wittliff JL, Dapunt O (eds): "Steroid
Receptors and Hormone-Dependent Neoplasia,"
USA, Masson Publishing, pp 155-160.

Kadohama N, Karr JP, Murphy GP, Sandberg AA (1984).
Selective inhibition of prostatic tumor 5α-
reductase by a 4-methyl-4-aza-steroid. Cancer
Res 44:4947-4954.

Kadohama N, Wakisaka M, Kim U, Karr JP, Murphy GP,
Sandberg AA (1985). Retardation of prostate
tumor progression in the Noble rat by 4-methyl-
4-aza-steroidal inhibitors of 5α-reductase.
J NCI 74:475-486.

Kallmann F, Schonfeld WA, et al (1944). The
genetic aspects of primary eunuchoidism.
Amer J Ment Defic 42:203.

Karr JP, Kirdani RY, Murphy GP, Sandberg AA (1974).
Effects of testosterone and estradiol on ventral
prostate and body weights of castrated rats. In
Life Sciences, Pergamon Press, 15:501-513.

Karr JP, Wajsman Z, Kirdani RY, Murphy GP,
Sandberg AA (1980). Effects of diethystil-
bestrol and estramustine phosphate on serum sex
hormone binding globulin and testosterone levels
in prostate cancer patients. J Urol 124:232-
236.

Krieg M, Bartsch W, Janssen, Voight KD (1979). A
comprehensive study of binding, metabolism and
endogenous levels of androgens in normal, hyperplastic and carcinomatous human prostate.
Coffey D, Isaacs J (eds): Prostate Cancer,"
Geneva, UICC, 93-111.

Lee C (1981). Physiology of castration-induced
regression in rat prostate. In Murphy GP,
Sandberg AA, Karr JP (eds): "The Prostatic
Cell: Structure and Function," New York,
Alan R. Liss, pp 145-159.

Lee C, Jesik C (1983). Effects of castration,

estrogen, and androgen administration. In
Hinman F, Jr (ed): "Benign Prostatic
Hypertrophy," New York, Springer-Verlag, pp
229-234.

Liu J, Geller J, Albert J, Kirshner M (1985).
Acute effects of testicular and adrenal cortical
blockade on protein synthesis and
dihydrotestosterone content of human prostate
tissue. J Clin Endo Metab 61:129-133.

Manlimos FS, Abraham GE (1975). Chromatography
purification of tritiated steroids prior to
use in radioimmunoassay. Analytical letters
8:403-410.

Mann CF, Karr JP, Kadohama N, Kim U, Drury R,
Sandberg AA (1986). Androgen metabolism and
steroid concentrations in stromal and epithelial
compartments of hyperplastic baboon prostates.
J Urol 135:110A.

Moguilewsky M, Fiett J, Tournemine C, Raynaud J-P
(1986). Pharmacology of an antiandrogen,
anandron, used as an adjuvant therapy in the
treatment of prostate cancer. J Steroid Biochem
24:139-146.

Moore RJ, Wilson JD (1973). The effect of
androgenic hormones on the reduced
nicotinamide adenine dinucleotide phosphate
Δ^4-3-ketosteroid 5α-oxidoreductase
of rat ventral prostate. Endocrinology
93:581-582.

Oesterling JE, Epstein JI, Walsh PC (1986). The
inability of adrenal androgens to stimulate the
adult human prostate - An autopsy evaluation of
men with hypogonadotrophic hypogonadism and
panhypopituitarism. J Urol (in press).

Ofner P, Terracio L, Vena RL (1984). Androgen
metabolism in cultured prostatic cells. In
Kimball FA, Buhl AE, Carter DB (eds); "Progress
in Clinical and Biological Research: New
Approaches to the Study of Benign Prostatic
Hyperplasia," New York, Alan R. Liss, pp 363-
380.

Petrow V (1986. The dihydrotestosterone (DHT)
hypothesis of prostate cancer: Role of
5α-reductase. The Prostate (in press).

Petrow V, Padilla G (1984). 5α-reductase: A target
enzyme for prostatic cancer. In "Novel

Approaches to Cancer Chemotherpy," Academic Press, pp 269-305.

Redding TW, Schally AV (1985). Investigation of the combination of the agonist D-Trp-6-LH-RH and the antiandrogen Flutamide in the treatment of Dunning R-3327-H prostatic cancer model. The Prostate 6:219-232.

Sandberg AA (1979). Regulation of prostate growth in organ culture. In Coffey D, Isaacs J (eds): "Prostate Cancer," Geneva, UICC, pp 165-194.

Sandberg AA (1980). Endocrine control and physiology of the prostate. The Prostate 1:169-184.

Sandberg AA, Karr JP (1987). Hormone and receptor assays in the management of prostatic cancer. Reviews Endocrine-Related Cancer. (in press).

Sandberg AA, Karr JP, Muntzing J (1980). The prostates of dog, baboon and rat. In Spring-Mills E, Hafez ESE (eds): "Male Accessory Sex Glands," Elsevier/North-Holland Biomedical Press p 565.

Shimazaki J, Kurihara H, Ito Y, Shida K (1965). Metabolism of testosterone in prostate. (1st Report and 2nd Report). Separation of prostatic 17β-ol-dehydrogenase and 5α-reductase. Gunma J Med Sci 14:313-325 and 326-333.

Shimazaki J, Matsushita I, Furuya N, Yamanaka H, Shida K (1969). Reduction of 5α-position of testosterone in the Rat ventral prostate. Endocrinol Jpn 16:453-458.

Stone NN, Fishman J (1986). Estrogen formation in the human prostate. J Urol 135:108A.

Trachtenberg J (1985). Optimal testosterone concentration for the treatment of prostatic cancer, J Urol 133:888-890.

Vermeulen A (1975). Testicular hormonal secretion and aging in males. In Grayhack JT, Wilson JD, Scherbenske MJ (eds): "Benign Prostatic Hyperplasia," DHEW, NIH pp 177- 182.

Walsh PC, Hutchins GM, Ewing LL (1983). Tissue content of dihydrotestosterone in human prostatic hyperplasia is not supranormal. J Clin Invest 72:1772-1777.

Yamanaka H, Shimazaki J, Kyoichi I, Sugiyama Y, Shidak K (1975). Effect of estrogen administration on activities of testosterone, 5α-reductase, alkaline phosphatase and arginase in the ventral and dorsolateral prostates of rats. Endocrinol Jpn 22:297-302.

Prostate Cancer, Part A: Research, Endocrine
Treatment, and Histopathology, page 77
© 1987 Alan R. Liss, Inc.

COMPARATIVE RESULTS OF THE VARIATIONS IN INTRA-PROSTATIC ANDROGEN LEVELS AND ANDROGEN RECEPTORS FOLLOWING PULPECTOMY WITH OR WITHOUT AN ANTI-ANDROGEN (FLUTAMIDE) IN THE TREATMENT OF ADVANCED PROSTATIC CANCER

Soret* J.Y., Verine* J.L., Daver** A.,
Labrie***F.
*Service d'Urologie, CHU Anger (France)
** Centre Paul Papin, Angers (France)
*** Université de Laval (Québec)

The aim of this study was to demonstrate the effect of complete androgen suppression induced by a combination of pulpectomy and an anti-androgen in the treatment of advanced prostatic cancer.

A series of 16 patients with untreated stage D2 prostatic cancer was divided into two groups. One group (11 patients) was treated by pulpectomy associated with the administration of a pure anti-androgen (Flutamide 750 mg/day). The second group (5 patients) was treated by pulpectomy alone. The short term therapeutic response was evaluated by assaying the intra-prostatic androgens (testosterone and Delta 5 diol) and the total intra-prostatic androgen receptors before and after 8 weeks of treatment.

The mean level of androgen receptors decreased by 74% after 8 weeks of complete androgen blockade and by only 20% after orchiectomy alone.

The mean level of intra-prostatic testosterone fell by 63% after complete androgen blockade and increased by a factor of 4 after orchiectomy alone.

These preliminary results confirm the biochemical efficacy of Flutamide combined with orchiectomy in the treatment of advanced prostatic cancer.

Prostate Cancer, Part A: Research, Endocrine
Treatment, and Histopathology, pages 79–97
© 1987 Alan R. Liss, Inc.

STEROID RECEPTOR AND BIOCHEMICAL PROFILES IN PROSTATIC
CANCER: CORRELATION WITH RESPONSE TO HORMONAL TREATMENT

Evelyn R. Barrack, Charles B. Brendler, and
Patrick C. Walsh

The Department of Urology, The Johns Hopkins
University School of Medicine, and The James
Buchanan Brady Urological Institute, The Johns
Hopkins Hospital, Baltimore, Maryland 21205.

INTRODUCTION

It is estimated that 50-80% of prostatic cancer
patients first present with evidence of metastasis (stage
D). Since Huggins and Hodges (1941) demonstrated that
prostatic cancer is dependent upon androgen, androgen
ablative therapy (castration or estrogen treatment) has
been the treatment of choice for patients with stage D
disease. While most of these patients respond to androgen
ablation, the degree and duration of response are
unpredictable and highly variable (10% live <6 months, 50%
live <3 years, and 10% live >10 years) (Blackard et al.,
1973), and their prostatic cancer eventually relapses to an
androgen-independent state (Coffey and Isaacs, 1981). In
the future, hormonal therapy will be used most effectively
when poorly responsive patients can be identified at an
earlier time in their disease and treated with alternative
forms of therapy (e.g., chemotherapy) when they would be
more able to tolerate and thus possibly more likely to
respond to this therapy. Therefore, there is a great need
to predict the quality and duration of response to
endocrine manipulation.

In our ongoing efforts to devise and evaluate methods
to predict the hormonal responsiveness of human metastatic
prostatic cancer, we have been investigating two types of
approaches: biochemistry and morphology. Measurement of
any one biochemical variable alone appears to be inadequate
to discriminate completely between a good response vs. a

poor response to androgen withdrawal. However, measurement of multiple biochemical parameters (androgen receptors and selected enzyme activities) in prostatic cancer appears to enhance significantly our ability to discriminate between good responders and poor responders to androgen withdrawal therapy (Brendler et al., 1984). Recognizing that prostatic tumors may exhibit varying degrees of heterogeneity, we therefore also evaluated morphological approaches to prostatic cancer. We have developed a combined biochemical and morphological technique to overcome the problems of tumor heterogeneity. A brief summary of these studies follows.

STEROID RECEPTOR PROFILES

Based on the androgen-dependent nature of prostatic cancer and recognition that the effects of androgen are mediated via androgen receptors, it was proposed (Walsh, 1975) that measurement of androgen receptor content in the tumor might provide a method to predict which patients will respond to endocrine therapy. The hypothesis is that androgen-independent cells have few or no androgen receptors, and that cells that contain androgen receptors are androgen-sensitive. Optimism for this approach was bolstered by the numerous reports of a correlation between estrogen receptor content in breast cancer and response to endocrine manipulation (DeSombre et al., 1979; Byar et al., 1979; Alanko et al., 1985).

Although numerous methodological obstacles were initially associated with prostatic androgen receptor assays, these difficulties were overcome when we developed reliable and specific microassay methods for measuring androgen receptors in needle biopsy specimens of prostatic cancer (Hicks and Walsh, 1979; Trachtenberg et al., 1981; Ekman et al., 1982; Barrack et al., 1983; Buttyan and Olsson, 1984). While numerous investigators have measured androgen receptors in prostatic cancer, only very few attempts have been made to correlate receptor levels with response to hormonal therapy (Trachtenberg and Walsh, 1982; Ekman et al., 1981; Concolino et al., 1982; Brendler et al., 1984; Gonor et al., 1984; Fentie et al., 1986). Most studies have simply classified specimens as either androgen receptor-negative or androgen receptor-positive, and patients as nonresponders or responders. On the other hand, (a) since most patients respond to some extent to hormonal therapy, (b) since virtually all prostatic cancer specimens contain some receptors, and (c) since the duration of response is highly variable, we have therefore attempted to correlate quantitative aspects of receptor content (fmol/mg DNA) with quantitative aspects of response to androgen ablation (duration of response and duration of survival).

In our first series of 23 patients we found that those who experienced a prolonged remission (>29.9 ± 5.3 months) following androgen ablative therapy had a significantly higher level of prostatic nuclear androgen receptor than patients who had a poor response (6.7 ± 0.9 months) (Table 1). There was, however, some overlap of nuclear receptor levels in the 2 groups (Fig. 1). In contrast, average levels of cytosol androgen receptor were not significantly different for these 2 groups of patients (Table 1), and showed almost complete overlap (Fig. 2). The ratio of nuclear androgen receptor level to cytosol androgen receptor level was significantly different in the 2 groups; the nuclear/cytosol receptor ratio was almost 2 times higher in the good responders than in the poor responders (Table 1).

TABLE 1. RELATIONSHIP BETWEEN ANDROGEN RECEPTOR LEVELS
IN PROSTATIC CANCER (STAGE D2) AND
DURATION OF RESPONSE FOLLOWING CASTRATION*

Response Duration (months)	No. Pts.	Androgen Receptors (fmol/mg DNA)		
		Nuclear	Cytosol	Nucl/Cyt.
Poor (6.7 ± 0.9)	12	151 ± 39	166 ± 49	1.2 ± 0.3
Good (>29.9 ± 5.3)	11	268 ± 56	137 ± 32	2.3 ± 0.3
(p value)		(<0.05)	(N.S.)	(<0.05)

*Nuclear and cytosol androgen receptor content in stage D2 prostatic cancer biopsies taken just prior to androgen ablation therapy. Duration of response is measured from the time of therapy to the time of relapse, and classified as good (>13 months duration; mean, >29.9 ± 5.3 months) or poor (<13 months; mean 6.7 ± 0.9 months). Based on data taken from Trachtenberg and Walsh (1982).

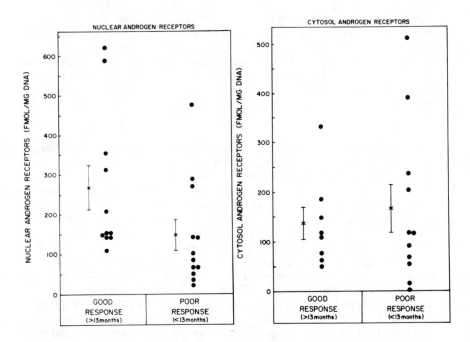

Figure 1 (left) and Figure 2 (right). Nuclear androgen receptor content (Fig. 1) and cytosol androgen receptor content (Fig. 2) in stage D2 prostatic cancer patients described in Table 1.

When patients were classified as nuclear receptor-rich or -poor (>110 vs. <110 fmol/mg DNA), Chi Square analysis indicated a significant association (p <0.01) between nuclear androgen receptor level and duration of response (>13 vs. <13 months) (Table 2). Kaplan-Meier plots (Fig. 3) show a median response duration of 8 months for receptor-poor patients and 18 months for receptor-rich patients. Table 2 shows that everyone with a nuclear receptor level below 110 fmol/mg DNA had a poor response. However, not everyone with a high nuclear receptor level (>110 fmol/mg DNA) had a prolonged response.

TABLE 2. ABILITY OF NUCLEAR RECEPTOR LEVEL
          TO IDENTIFY RESPONSE GROUP

Response	Nuclear Androgen Receptor Level	
	<110 fmol/mg DNA (n = 7 pts.)	>110 fmol/mg DNA (n = 16 pts.)
Poor (<13 months) (n = 12 pts.)	7	5
Good (>13 months) (n = 11 pts.)	0	11

Chi square test with Yates' correction for continuity,
p <0.01. Based on data in Fig. 1.

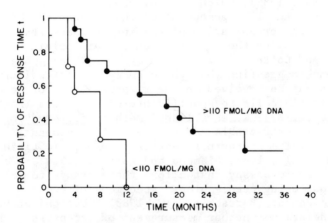

Figure 3. Kaplan-Meier plots of response of stage D2
prostatic cancer to androgen ablation in patients with high
vs. low nuclear androgen receptor content (>110 fmol
receptor/mg DNA vs. <110 fmol/mg DNA, respectively).

Thus we recognized the importance of developing a method that would allow us to further stratify patients with high nuclear receptor levels as those who do well vs. those who do poorly following androgen withdrawal. Although this type of analysis reveals the difficulty in attempting to predict the hormonal response of stage D2 prostatic cancer based on nuclear androgen receptor content alone, it appears that cytosol androgen receptor levels have no predictive value (Table 1, Fig. 2). A lack of predictive value of cytosol receptor measurements has been confirmed by other investigators (Ekman et al., 1981; Gonor et al., 1984). These data indicate the importance of measuring androgen receptors in the appropriate subcellular compartment in order to obtain accurate insight into biological behavior.

This laboratory has demonstrated that in a variety of sex hormone target tissues a significant percentage (50-90%) of the nuclear steroid receptors are associated with the nuclear matrix (Barrack et al., 1983; Barrack and Coffey, 1980, 1982), which is a discrete salt-resistant dynamic structural subcomponent of the nucleus that directs the functional organization of DNA into domains and provides sites for the specific control of nucleic acids (Barrack and Coffey, 1982; Nelson et al., 1986). Because of evidence suggesting that these nuclear salt-resistant receptors may be involved in the responsiveness of normal and neoplastic cells to specific steroid hormones (Barrack and Coffey, 1982), we established methods for studying both nuclear salt-extractable and nuclear salt-resistant (nuclear matrix) androgen receptors in prostatic tissue (Barrack et al., 1983; Diamond and Barrack, 1984). We also developed a microassay that allows these assays to be carried out using needle biopsy specimens of human prostatic cancer (Barrack et al., 1983). Our objective has been to determine whether measurement of receptors in both subnuclear compartments might more accurately reflect the androgen responsiveness of prostatic cancer following androgen withdrawal.

We have tested this hypothesis in well-defined animal models of prostatic cancer. Four different sublines of rat prostatic adenocarcinoma that differ in their response to androgen ablation were studied (Diamond and Barrack, 1984). There is no apparent quantitative relationship between androgen receptor content and tumor growth rates. There is, however, a qualitative relationship between nuclear matrix androgen receptor content and androgen responsiveness: higher levels of nuclear receptor in the R3327-H and R3327-G tumor sublines are associated with responsiveness to androgen ablation (cessation or slowing of growth, respectively), whereas lower levels of receptor in the R3327-HI and R3327-AT-2 tumor sublines are associated with androgen insensitivity (Diamond and Barrack, 1984). The data obtained using these animal tumors have important implications for human prostatic cancers (see Diamond and Barrack, 1984).

Because androgen receptors are assayed in terms of their steroid binding activity, and not in terms of a biological activity, we reasoned that an androgen-independent prostatic cancer (which would yield a poor response to androgen withdrawal) might still contain a high level of biologically inactive androgen receptors. We therefore feel it is important to identify biochemical correlates of hormone action in order to enable the classification of receptor-rich tumors into multiple subgroups. The following sections summarize some of our approaches to evaluate more accurately the degree of androgen responsiveness of prostatic cancer.

TISSUE STEROID CONTENT

Dihydrotestosterone (DHT) is the major active intracellular androgen responsible for androgenic effects in the prostate (Bruchovsky and Wilson, 1968; Anderson and Liao, 1968). Thus, there has been much interest to determine whether tissue levels of DHT might reflect various physiological or pathological states. For example, numerous investigators have reported an elevation of prostatic DHT levels in BPH compared to normal prostatic tissue and this finding has been widely accepted as a major factor in the etiology of BPH (reviewed in Walsh et al., 1983). In addition, Geller et al. (1978) and Belis and Tarry (1981) noted that DHT levels <2 ng/g of prostatic cancer were associated with failure to respond to androgen ablation therapy. Based on measurements made by Geller (1985) of prostatic DHT levels post castration (approx. 1.5 ng/g), Labrie et al. (1985) concluded that this residual tissue DHT resulted from adrenal androgen production and was biologically significant.

In order to test the hypothesis that prostatic DHT content reflects the biological potential of the tissue, we have performed 3 types of studies which we believe have important implications for future work on DHT measurements in prostatic tissue. We measured DHT content in needle biopsy specimens of stage D2 prostatic cancer taken just prior to initiation of androgen ablative therapy, and correlated these levels with duration of response to treatment (Brendler et al., 1984). There was no significant difference in the prostatic DHT content of those patients who responded poorly (7.7 $\pm$ 1.5 months; 2.9 $\pm$ 0.3 ng DHT/g tissue) vs. those who had a good response (>18.6 $\pm$ 1.6 months; 2.6 $\pm$ 0.5 ng DHT/g tissue) (Fig. 4).

In another study (Walsh et al., 1983) we discovered that prostatic DHT content in fact is not elevated in BPH (5.0 $\pm$ 0.4 ng DHT/g tissue) compared to normal prostate removed surgically (5.1 $\pm$ 0.4 ng DHT/g tissue); these findings fail to confirm the widespread belief that DHT content is elevated in BPH. This difference between our own and earlier studies was resolved by experiments performed on cadavers, which were the source of normal prostatic tissue used by other investigators; the DHT content of prostatic tissue removed at autopsy is factitiously low (0.7 - 1.0 ng DHT/g tissue). In addition, incubation of fresh prostatic tissue in vitro at 37°C for 2 hr results in similarly low DHT levels (1 ng/g). These results indicate that when prostatic tissue is harvested appropriately, DHT content of normal and hyperplastic prostatic tissue is the same (for further details see Walsh et al., 1983).

In another series of experiments we measured DHT levels in prostatic tissue obtained from men who had been castrated previously for stage D2 prostatic cancer and who were undergoing prostatectomy to relieve urinary obstructive symptoms. The prostatic DHT content of these castrated men averaged approximately 1 ng DHT/g tissue, a level essentially identical to that previously reported for nonandrogen target tissues (Geller, 1985), and similar to the level in autopsy tissue (Walsh et al., 1983). These findings fail to support the concept that adrenal androgens are an important source for DHT production in the prostates of castrated men.

BIOCHEMICAL INDEX AND CLINICAL CORRELATIONS

In order to characterize the biological potential of an individual tumor and to predict its response to endocrine manipulation prior to initiating therapy, we recognized that it may be necessary to measure multiple biochemical parameters. An example of this approach is the measurement of both progesterone receptors and estrogen receptors in breast cancer to increase the accuracy of predicting response to endocrine therapy (Alanko et al., 1985; McGuire, 1980; Siebert and Lippman, 1982). Optimism for this approach is also based on previous success in animal model studies that used multiple biochemical parameters to distinguish between histologically identical sublines of Dunning R3327 rat prostatic adenocarcinomas which differ in their androgen sensitivity (Isaacs et al., 1979), and between sublines of this rat prostatic adenocarcinoma which differ in their metastatic ability (Lowe and Isaacs, 1984). In those animal model studies in which multiple enzymatic activities were measured, no single activity could distinguish all sublines from each other. However, a ratio was derived empirically, based on the relative activities of 6 enzymes (expressed relative to the enzymatic activities in normal rat prostatic tissue); the values calculated for this relative enzymatic index were different for each of the tumor sublines, and there was no overlap among the groups (Isaacs et al., 1979).

We therefore set out to test this approach in human prostatic cancer (Brendler et al., 1984). We measured 6 enzyme activities which we believed might reflect androgen sensitivity; 3 of these enzymes are involved in androgen metabolism [5α-reductase, 17β-hydroxysteroid oxidoreductase, $3\alpha(\beta)$-hydroxysteroid oxidoreductase] and 3 are hydrolytic enzymes frequently measured in tumors (acid phosphatase, alkaline phosphatase, lactate dehydrogenase). In addition, we quantitated androgen receptor levels in 3 subcellular compartments (cytosol, nuclear salt extract, and salt-resistant nuclear matrix fractions), and tissue levels of testosterone and dihydrotestosterone. The Gleason grade of the tumor was also evaluated. All of these variables were measured in prostatic needle biopsies (total tissue 100-200 mg) obtained from 16 patients with stage D2 prostatic cancer immediately before androgen ablation (castration or estrogen therapy). These patients

were followed prospectively and the response of each
patient to hormonal therapy was assessed clinically.

Two groups of patients were again identified: a group
of poor responders (all <13 months duration; mean, 7.7 ±
1.5 months, n=7) and a group of good responders (all >13
months duration; mean, >18.6 ± 1.6 months, n=9). These 2
groups were statistically different from each other in
terms of duration of response, but they could not be
distinguished by Gleason grade, single enzymatic
activities, cytosol androgen receptor content, nuclear
matrix androgen receptor level, or tissue androgen content
(Fig. 4). In contrast, nuclear salt-extractable androgen
receptor levels were significantly different in the 2
groups (p <0.05); these data confirmed our earlier study on
23 patients (Table 1). Although mean values separated the
2 groups, there was considerable overlap of individual
nuclear androgen receptor levels between the 2 groups (Fig.
4), as we had observed in our first study (Fig. 1).

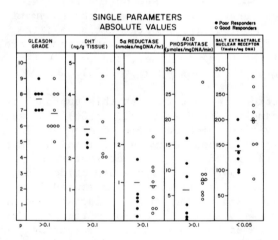

Figure 4. Single parameter measurements in stage D2
prostatic cancer biopsies of patients who had a poor
response (<13 months duration; closed circles) vs. a good
response (>13 months duration; open circles) to androgen
ablation therapy. (From Brendler et al., 1984).

An index based on multiple relative enzymatic activities was derived empirically which separated the 2 groups of patients better than any single variable alone and with less overlap (Brendler et al., 1984). When nuclear androgen receptor content was included in this multiple variable index, the 2 groups were separated with even less overlap (Fig. 5). Cancer tissue measurements were expressed relative to those in normal peripheral prostatic tissue. The index was expressed as the following ratio of relative values of $3\alpha(\beta)$-hydroxysteroid oxidoreductase activity [$3\alpha(\beta)$HSOR], 17β-hydroxysteroid oxidoreductase activity (17β HSOR), acid phosphatase activity (AP), salt-extractable nuclear androgen receptor content (SENR), and 5α-reductase activity:

$$\frac{3\alpha(\beta)\text{HSOR} \cdot 17\beta\text{HSOR} \cdot \text{AP} \cdot \text{SENR}}{5\alpha\text{-reductase}}$$

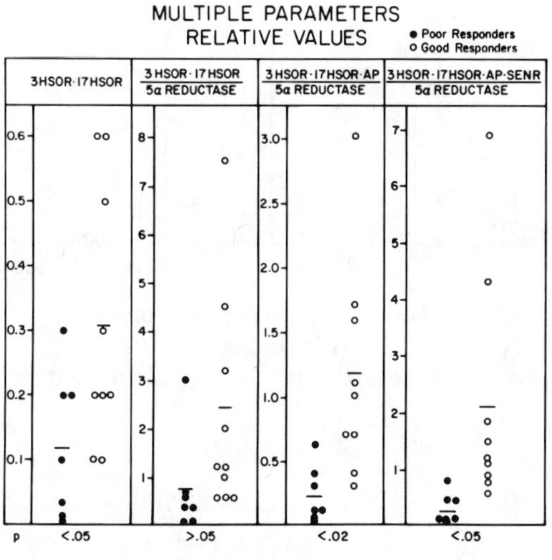

MULTIPLE PARAMETERS
RELATIVE VALUES

• Poor Responders
o Good Responders

Figure 5. Use of multiple parameters to develop index that predicts hormonal response in the patients shown in Fig. 4. All values are relative to normal prostate. 3HSOR, $3\alpha(\beta)$hydroxysteroid oxidoreductase activity. 17HSOR, 17β-hydroxysteroid oxidoreductase activity; AP, tissue acid phosphatase activity; SENR, salt extractable nuclear androgen receptor content. (From Brendler et al., 1984.)

This preliminary study suggests that the measurement of
multiple biochemical variables may indeed be useful in
predicting hormonal response (Brendler et al., 1984).
When this original biochemical index was tested on a larger
group of 24 patients (Brendler et al., 1985), the poor and
good response groups could again be distinguished by this
same index (Fig. 6).

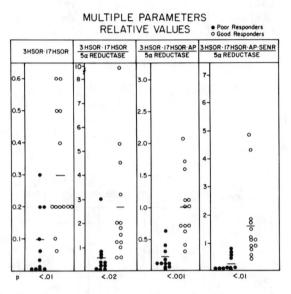

Figure 6. Test of index of multiple parameters to classify
the hormonal response of 24 patients with stage D2
prostatic cancer as described in Figs. 4 and 5.

NEED FOR A COMBINED BIOCHEMICAL-MORPHOLOGICAL APPROACH

In spite of these encouraging advances, such techniques
are not yet used clinically to predict response of
prostatic cancer to hormonal therapy. Remaining obstacles
include the limited availability of needle biopsy tissue
for analysis (approx. 30 mg/core), tumor cell
heterogeneity, and contamination of tumor biopsies with
nonmalignant prostatic tissue. Until now, all of our
steroid receptor measurements (as well as enzymatic

profiles) have been carried out using subcellular fractions of homogenized tissue; the values obtained therefore represent an average of all cells. Thus, for example, by homogenizing the biopsy tissue prior to analysis, it is not possible to assess the extent to which androgen receptor content of noncancer cells [e.g., normal and BPH cells] may contribute to the overall receptor content of the specimen. Since normal prostate and BPH are both androgen receptor-rich, contamination of the tumor biopsy with these tissue components will result in a misleading "tumor" androgen receptor content. Using homogenized tissue, it is also not possible to assess whether receptors are distributed uniformly in all tumor cells; thus prostatic cancer in different patients may contain various proportions of androgen-sensitive and androgen-insensitive cells. There is already evidence for tumor cell heterogeneity within human prostatic cancers with regard to immunocytochemical staining of prostate-specific acid phosphatase (Epstein and Eggleston, 1984), prostate-specific antigen (Epstein and Eggleston, 1984; Purnell et al., 1984), keratin (Brawer et al., 1985; Molinolo et al., 1985), carcinoembryonic antigen (Purnell et al., 1984), and ras p21 oncogene product (Viola et al., 1986).

Thus, contamination by nonmalignant prostatic tissue and tumor cell heterogeneity may account, at least in part, for androgen receptor-rich prostatic cancer biopsies of patients who experience a very poor response to androgen withdrawal therapy. Given such heterogeneity, one may not be surprised at the difficulties thus far encountered in using homogenate-based receptor assays to predict duration of response of prostatic cancer to endocrine manipulation. It also becomes apparent that the use of multiple biochemical parameters may not be sufficient to circumvent these problems of heterogeneity. Multiple biochemical parameters might, nevertheless, be useful to distinguish between cells that contain functional or non-functional receptors. We believe that further progress in developing methods to accurately predict the hormonal responsiveness of prostatic cancer in individual patients must take this heterogeneity into account.

^{3}H-STEROID AUTORADIOGRAPHY OF ANDROGEN RECEPTORS

It is apparent that in order to rigorously test whether the concentration of receptor in the cancer reflects the degree of androgen responsiveness, morphological methods are needed by which receptor content of the tumor cells themselves can be evaluated. Therefore, we have developed a new method for ^{3}H-steroid autoradiographic localization of androgen receptors in prostatic tissue which meets this need and which can be applied to needle biopsy sized specimens (Peters and Barrack, 1985, 1986). This new technique is based on a method which is now widely accepted as the method of choice for localizing neurotransmitter receptors (Kuhar, 1985). Receptors are labeled by incubating slide-mounted frozen tissue sections (10 μm thickness) under appropriate conditions in vitro with radiolabeled ligand, followed by apposition of the labeled tissue to dry emulsion-coated coverslips. Labeling receptors in slide-mounted tissue sections has the advantages both of a histological method (anatomic resolution, amenable to subsequent quantitative autoradiography, large area cross-sections of tissue can be labeled without penetration artifacts, multiple receptor classes can be examined in serial sections), and of a biochemical method (applicable to human tissue, use of frozen tissue, less expensive than in vivo methods of labeling receptors, and ability to confirm that binding of ^{3}H-steroid is to receptors of the appropriate affinity, number and steroid specificity) (Table 3).

Using human BPH and rat prostate tissues, we have recently validated this method for the labeling and autoradiographic localization of androgen receptors (Peters and Barrack, 1985, 1986). We have demonstrated that sections assayed in this way contain high affinity (K_d = 1 nM), steroid specific androgen receptors at levels comparable to the sum of those found in subcellular fractions of homogenized tissue (Peters and Barrack, 1986). It appears that all the androgen receptors in the tissue are retained in the slide-mounted tissue sections and are not eluted into the incubation medium. Extensive preliminary studies have been carried out to establish appropriate fixation conditions, incubation buffers, requirement for protease inhibitors, conditions for handling sections (storage time and temperature) prior to fixation, optimal time and temperature for efficient labeling of receptors, and washing conditions to minimize nonspecific binding (Peters and Barrack, 1986).

Using this new procedure for ^{3}H-steroid receptor autoradiography, Peters and Barrack (1985, 1986) have shown that in rat ventral prostate and human glandular BPH, androgen receptor localization is almost exclusively in the epithelial nuclei, with little or none in the stroma. Fibromuscular BPH, in contrast, contains androgen receptors both in stromal and epithelial nuclei (Peters and Barrack, 1986). This heterogeneous distribution of receptor among cell types of the prostate illustrates the improved resolution of this technique over that using homogenates of whole tissue.

TABLE 3. ADVANTAGES OF ^{3}H-STEROID AUTORADIOGRAPHY OF RECEPTORS LABELED IN SLIDE-MOUNTED TISSUE SECTIONS

1. Anatomic and cellular resolution of receptor location.
2. Tissue sections are mounted onto slides in the light.
3. No penetration artifacts in labeling sections of 10 μm thickness.
4. Less expensive than in vivo labeling.
5. Applicable to human tissue.
6. Emulsion can be protected from histochemical stains which may alter or ablate silver grains.
7. Total binding and nonspecific binding are assessed in serial sections.
8. Affinity (K_d), total receptor content (B_{max}), and kinetics of ^{3}H-steroid binding can be assessed.
9. Steroid specificity of binding can be validated.
10. Androgen, estrogen, and progesterone receptors can be measured in serial sections.
11. Regional distribution of receptors within tissue can be studied.
12. Amenable to quantitation.
13. Frozen tissue can be used.

(For details see Peters and Barrack, 1985, 1986.)

We anticipate that data obtained using this new method of steroid receptor autoradiography may provide much needed insight into the mechanism of hormonal regulation of the prostate. We believe that the data we have obtained thus far demonstrate the feasibility and appropriateness of this new approach for renewed efforts to resolve many of the issues that have hampered the study of androgen receptors in prostatic cancer and their relationship to prognosis of endocrine responsiveness.

ACKNOWLEDGMENTS

Work summarized in this report was supported by NCI Grant CA16924, and NIADDK Grant AM 19300.

REFERENCES

Alanko A, Heinonen E, Scheinin T, Tolppanen E-M, Vihko R (1985). Significance of estrogen and progesterone receptors, disease-free interval, and site of first metastasis on survival of breast cancer patients. Cancer 56:1696-1700.

Anderson KM, Liao S (1968). Selective retention of dihydrotestosterone by prostatic nuclei. Nature 219:277-279.

Barrack ER, Coffey DS (1980). The specific binding of estrogens and androgens to the nuclear matrix of sex hormone responsive tissues. J Biol Chem 255:7265-7275.

Barrack ER, Coffey DS (1982). Biological properties of the nuclear matrix: Steroid hormone binding. Recent Prog Hormone Res 38:133-195.

Barrack ER, Bujnovszky P, Walsh PC (1983). Subcellular distribution of androgen receptors in human normal, benign hyperplastic, and malignant prostatic tissues: Characterization of nuclear salt-resistant receptors. Cancer Res 43:1107-1116.

Belis JA, Tarry WF (1981). Radioimmunoassay of tissue steroids in adenocarcinoma of the prostate. Cancer 48:2416-2419.

Blackard CE, Byar DP, Jordan WP, Jr, Veterans Administration Cooperative Urological Research Group (1973). Orchiectomy for advanced prostatic carcinoma: A reevaluation. Urology 1:553-560.

Brawer MK, Peehl DM, Stamey TA, Bostwick DG (1985).
Keratin immunoreactivity in the benign and neoplastic
human prostate. Cancer Res 45:3663-3667.

Brendler CB, Isaacs JT, Follansbee AL, Walsh PC (1984).
The use of multiple variables to predict response to
endocrine therapy in carcinoma of the prostate: A
preliminary report. J Urol 131:694-700.

Brendler CB, Isaacs JT, Walsh PC (1985). An update on the
use of multiple variables to predict response to
endocrine therapy in carcinoma of the prostate.
Proceedings of the Annual Meeting of the American
Urological Association, p. 368A.

Bruchovsky N, Wilson JD (1968). The conversion of
testosterone to 5α-androstane-17β-ol-3-one by rat
prostate in vivo and in vitro. J Biol Chem 243:2012-
2021.

Buttyan R, Olsson CA (1984). Androgen receptor assays in
advanced prostatic cancer. Urologic Clinics North
America 11:311-317.

Byar DP, Sears ME, McGuire WL (1979). Relationship between
estrogen receptor values and clinical data in predicting
the response to endocrine therapy for patients with
advanced breast cancer. Eur J Cancer 15:299-310.

Coffey DS, Isaacs JT (1981). Prostate tumor biology and
cell kinetics - Theory. Urology Suppl 17:40-53.

Concolino G, Marocchi A, Margiotta G, Conti C, Di Silverio
F,Tenaglia R, Ferraro F, Bracci U (1982). Steroid
receptors and hormone responsiveness of human prostatic
carcinoma. Prostate 3:475-482.

DeSombre ER, Carbone PP, Jensen EV, McGuire WL, Wells SA
Jr, Wittliff JL, Lipsett MB (1979). Steroid receptors in
breast cancer. New Eng J Med 301:1011-1012.

Diamond DA, Barrack ER (1984). The relationship of
androgen receptor levels to androgen responsiveness in
the Dunning R3327 rat prostate tumor sublines. J Urol
132:821-827.

Ekman P, Svennerus K, Zetterberg A, Gustafsson J-A (1981).
Cytophotometric DNA analyses and steroid receptor content
in human prostatic carcinoma. Scand J Urol Nephrol
60:85-88.

Ekman P, Barrack ER, Walsh PC (1982). Simultaneous
measurement of progesterone and androgen receptors in
human prostate: A microassay. J Clin Endocrinol Metab
55:1089-1099.

Epstein JI, Eggleston JC (1984). Immunohistochemical
localization of prostate-specific acid phosphatase and

prostate-specific antigen in stage A_2 adenocarcinoma of the prostate: Prognostic implications. Human Pathol 15:853-859.

Fentie DD, Lakey WH, McBlain WA (1986). Applicability of nuclear androgen receptor quantification to human prostatic adenocarcinoma. J Urol 135:167-173.

Geller J (1985). Rationale for blockade of adrenal as well as testicular androgens in the treatment of advanced prostate cancer. Seminars Oncology 12 Suppl 1:28-35.

Geller J, Albert J, de la Vega D, Loza D, Stoeltzing W (1978). Dihydrotestosterone concentration in prostate cancer tissue as a predictor of tumor differentiation and hormonal dependency. Cancer Res 38:4349-4352.

Gonor SE, Lakey WH, McBlain WA (1984). Relationship between concentrations of extractable and matrix-bound nuclear androgen receptor and clinical response to endocrine therapy for prostatic adenocarcinoma. J Urol 131:1196-1201.

Hicks LL, Walsh PC (1979). A microassay for the measurement of androgen receptors in human prostatic tissue. Steroids 33:389-406.

Huggins C, Hodges CF (1941). Studies on prostatic cancer. I. The effect of castration, of estrogen and of androgen injection on serum phosphatases in metastatic carcinoma of the prostate. Cancer Res 1:293-297.

Isaacs JT, Isaacs WB, Coffey DS (1979). Models for development of nonreceptor methods for distinguishing androgen-sensitive and -insensitive prostatic tumors. Cancer Res 39:2652-2659.

Kuhar MJ (1985). Receptor localization with the microscope. In: Neurotransmitter Receptor Binding, 2nd ed. (Yamamura HI, Enna SJ, Kuhar MJ, Eds.), Raven Press, 153-176.

Labrie F, Dupont A, Belanger A (1985). Complete androgen blockage for the treatment of prostate cancer. In: Important Advances in Oncology (DeVita VT, Jr, Hellman S, Rosenberg SA, Eds.), JB Lippincott Company, Philadelphia, 193-217.

Lowe FC, Isaacs JT (1984). Biochemical methods for predicting metastatic ability of prostatic cancer utilizing the Dunning R-3327 rat prostatic adenocarcinoma system as a model. Cancer Res 44:744-752.

McGuire WL (1980). Steroid hormone receptors in breast cancer treatment strategy. Recent Prog Hormone Res 36:135-156.

Molinolo AA, Meiss RP, Leo P, Sens AI (1985). Demonstration of cytokeratins by immunoperoxidase staining in prostatic tissue. J Urol 134:1037-1040.

Nelson WG, Pienta KJ, Barrack ER, Coffey DS (1986). The role of the nuclear matrix in the organization and function of DNA. Ann Rev Biophys Biophys Chem 15 (In press).

Peters CA, Barrack ER (1985). Morphologic localization of androgen receptors in human prostate: A new method of steroid receptor autoradiography. Endocrinology 116 Suppl:108.

Peters CA, Barrack ER (1986). Androgen receptor localization in the prostate using a new method of steroid receptor autoradiography. 2nd NIADDK Symposium on Benign Prostatic Hyperplasia, US Govt Printing Office, Washington, DC, In press.

Purnell DM, Heatfield BM, Trump BF (1984). Immunocytochemical evaluation of human prostatic carcinomas for carcinoembryonic antigen, nonspecific cross-reacting antigen, β-chorionic gonadotrophin, and prostate-specific antigen. Cancer Res 44:285-292.

Seibert K, Lippman M (1982). Hormone receptors in breast cancer. Clinics Oncology 1:735-794.

Trachtenberg J, Hicks LL, Walsh PC (1981). Methods for the determination of androgen receptor content in human prostatic tissue. Invest Urol 18:349-354.

Trachtenberg J, Walsh PC (1982). Correlation of prostatic nuclear androgen receptor content with duration of response and survival following hormonal therapy in advanced prostatic cancer. J Urol 127:466-471.

Viola MV, Fromowitz F, Oravez S, Deb W, Finkel G, Lundy J, Hand P, Thor A, Schlom J (1986). New Eng J Med 314:133-137.

Walsh PC (1975). Physiologic basis for hormonal therapy in carcinoma of the prostate. Urologic Clinics North America 2:125-140.

Walsh PC, Hutchins GM, Ewing LL (1983). Tissue content of dihydrotestosterone in human prostatic hyperplasia is not supranormal. J Clin Invest 72:1772-1777.

Prostate Cancer, Part A: Research, Endocrine
Treatment, and Histopathology, page 99
© 1987 Alan R. Liss, Inc.

PRETREATMENT PLASMA LEVELS OF ESTRADIOL CORRELATED TO THE
CLINICAL STAGE AND SURVIVAL OF PROSTATIC CANCER PATIENTS.

Reijo Haapiainen, Sakari Rannikko, Olaf Alfthan
and Herman Adlercreutz*
Second Department of Surgery/Urological Unit and
*Department of Clinical Chemistry, Helsinki
University Central Hospital, Helsinki, Finland.

Pretreatment plasma concentration of estradiol and SHBG
were measured in 116 patients categorized into two groups
(TO-2, T3-4) according to the UICC classification. Statistically significant (p<0.05) higher estradiol (E2) values
were observed in the TO-2 than in the T3-4 category. The
mean plasma concentration of E2 was also significantly
higher (p<0.05) in the MO than in the M1 category. According to the grade of malignancy there was a tendency towards
poorer differentiation of the tumour in patients with low
E2 levels.

The patients were randomized to two therapy groups:
orchiectomy or estrogen therapy (polyestradiolphosphate 80
mg/month combined with ethinylestradiol 150 mg daily). The
mean follow-up time is now 42 months.

Analysis of survival in relation to the pretreatment
plasma levels of total E2 showed that the prognosis was
significantly better (p<0.05) in subjects with high levels
of plasma E2. The lower the E2 concentration, the poorer the
prognosis was in the estrogen and in the orchiectomy groups.
Survival was particularly poor in orchiectomized patients
with low E2 levels.

It is concluded that high endogenous plasma estrogen
level may be protective during the promotion stage of carcinogenesis and that estrogen treatment may be the treatment of
choice for patients with low pretreatment E2 levels. For
those with medium or high levels orchiectomy seems to be of
equal value as estrogen treatment.

Prostate Cancer, Part A: Research, Endocrine
Treatment, and Histopathology, pages 101–110
© 1987 Alan R. Liss, Inc.

PUNCH BIOPSY TISSUE : ENZYME AND RECEPTOR ANALYSES AS CRITERIA FOR HORMONE RESPONSIVENESS IN THE TREATMENT OF PROSTATIC CANCER - LIMITATIONS.

**Bartsch G., Janetschek G., Daxenbichler G.,
Dietze O., Mikuz G.**
Department of Urology, Gynecology and Pathology.
University of Innsbruck - Austria.

Significant quantitative differences have been demonstrated between normal prostatic and carcinomatous tissue in regard to androgen binding capacity, metabolism and endogenous androgen concentrations. It is attractive to speculate that this acquired error in androgen metabolism could play an important role in the hormone responsiveness of prostatic carcinoma. Some correlative studies in regard to this altered endocrine metabolism and prostatic cancer pathology were performed to answer the following most relevant clinical questions :
- can any conclusion regarding hormone responsiveness or resistance respectively be drawn from enzyme assays,
- are there any metabolic parameters for which the changes indicate success or failure of hormonal treatment,
- is it possible to obtain objective values indicating response or resistance to hormonal therapy by means of these biochemical investigations.

The tumor grade is believed to be a potential indicator of hormone responsiveness. However, as was shown by Dhom in 1976, carcinomas of uniform architecture account for some 45% of all cases (Dhom, 1976). About 55% show a pluriform picture with a wide variety of tumor cell grading. Areas of anaplastic, undifferentiated cells may reside within the areas of well differentiated tumor cells. This pluriform architecture also poses the question as to how grading of biopsy material is indicative of grading of the whole tumor and therefore relevant regarding the prediction of hormonal responsiveness.

5 α – reductase and 3 α- hydroxysteroid oxidoreductase activities have been shown to be metabolic parameters for which variations indicate success or failure of hormonal treatment in prostatic cancer. Testosterone uptake, 5 α-dihydrotestosterone and 5 α-androstane - 3 α - 17 β -diol formation were investigated in treated and untreated local tumors and metastases by Prout et al. (1976). These authors found a significantly decreased or absent 5 α-reductase enzyme activity in primary hormone-insensitive and hormone-resistant prostatic carcinoma. They stated that 5 α -reductase should serve as a parameter for the individual hormone responsiveness of prostatic cancer. Morfin as well as Jacobi and their co-workers showed a diminished 3 α-hydroxysteroid oxidoreductase activity in poorly differentiated prostatic carcinomas (Morfin et al., 1977, Jacobi and Altwein, 1980). In undifferentiated prostatic carcinoma testosterone is metabolized to androstenedion by the oxidative pathway instead of being metabolized to 5 α-dihydrotestosterone and 5α-androstane-3 α-17 β-diol by the reductive pathway. The interpretation of these biochemical results is difficult, since the quantitative distribution of the different tissue components (prostatic carcinoma, stromal tissue, unchanged BPH, or normal glandular cells) is unknown in these studies.

Based on the assumption that target organ responsiveness and resistance may be explained by the receptor binding capacity, receptor studies should be helpful in predicting hormonal responsiveness. Several investigators have examined the relationship between intracellular dihydrotestosterone receptor content of prostatic cancer tissue and the response of endocrine therapy. The clinical value of these endocrinologic parameters, such as enzyme levels, endogenous steroid concentration and receptor content, for predicting the response to endocrine manipulation is still highly controversial, especially because of the heterogeneity of prostatic biopsy specimens and prostatic carcinoma cells.

There is strong evidence that at the time of diagnosis prostatic cancer is not homogeneous but heteregeneous. These heterogeneous cell populations differ in growth rate, morphology, karyotype, immunogeneticity, sensitivity to hormones and radiation, invasiveness and metastatic ability. This heterogeneity of the tumor cells makes successful therapy difficult and is at present the major problem in the treatment of metastasizing prostatic cancer (Coffey and Isaacs, 1979). It is well known, that the range of the relative amounts of prostatic cancer, glandular and stromal cells varies from biopsy to biopsy from only a few per cent. A morphometric analysis of the biopsy specimens of 50 patients with prostatic carcinoma shows cancer cells in 23%,

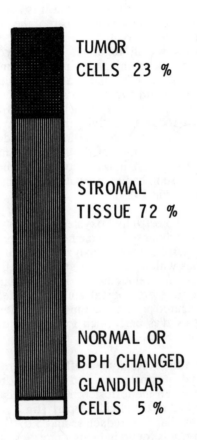

Fig 1 : Heterogeneity of punch biopsy tissue :
morphometric analysis of punch biopsy tissue specimens.

stromal tissue in 72% and normal or BPH-changed glandular cells in 4% of all biopsy specimens (fig 1); this morphometric analysis shows the heterogeneity of prostatic biopsy specimens. The stromal tissue of the elderly male is highly activated and sensitive to androgens and estrogens (Bartsch et al, 1979, Rohr and Bartsch, 1980).

At present there are strong indications that it is above all androgens which control the function of the stromal part of the human prostate. In 1977 Cowan and co-workers for the first time reported that 5 α-reductase activity, which regulates 5 α-dihydrotestosterone formation, was found predominantly in the stromal tissue of the prostate (Cowan et al, 1977). Using a mechanical technique for separating the glandular and stromal parts Krieg (Krieg et al., 1981), Romijn (Romijn et al., 1980) and Bruchovsky (Bruchovsky et al., 1980) found that 5 α-reductase activity in the stromal fraction of the prostate was considerably higher than in the glandular fraction; by comparing the stromal fractions of the normal human prostate and benign prostatic hyperplasia it was shown that the mean specific activity of 5 α-reductase in benign prostatic hyperplasia is three times greater (Bruchovsky et al., 1980).

The 5 α-reductase and 3 α (β) hydroxysteroid oxidoreductase activity of the stromal and glandular parts in the normal human prostate and in benign prostatic hyperplasia were analyzed without the use of these separation techniques which possibly destroy the cell architecture and the stromal/glandular interrelationships. In a correlative biochemical and light microscopic stereological study testosterone metabolite formation was measured in small biopsy specimens; afterwards a stereological analysis was performed to determine the amounts of glandular and stromal (Schweikert et al., 1983).

As can be seen from the correlation coefficient there is no difference between 5 α-dihydrotestosterone and 5 α-androstane 3 α (β) 17β-diol formation when the testosterone metabolism of the stromal part is compared to that of the glandular part (fig 2 and 3). These data on intact tissue show that 5 α−reductase and 3 α-(β) hydroxysteroid oxidoreductase activity is found in benign prostatic hyperplasia in the stromal part as well as in the glandular part.

Consequently enzyme and receptor assays of biopsy specimens have to be interpreted very cautiously, since androgen metabolism and binding may result not only from cancer cells but also from the stromal tissue, which is the case in a high percentage of patients. Therefore these biochemical assays should be confirmed by quantitative morphology of the tissue distribution in future; otherwise the prognostic value of these endocrinologic investigations might be compromized.

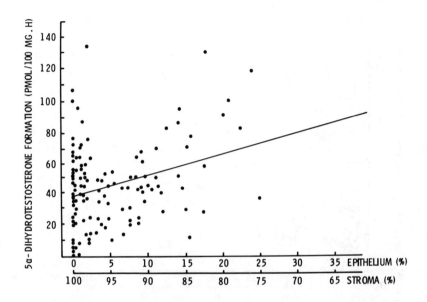

Fig 2 : Correlative biochemical and morphometric
study on human biopsy speciemns. 5 α
reductase activity is correlated to the
amount of stromal and glandular tissue of
biopsy specimens (= 100 %).

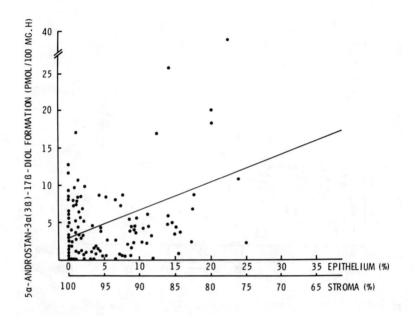

Fig 3 : Correlative biochemical and morphometric
study on human biopsy specimens.
3ɑ-hydroxysteroid-oxido-reductase
activity is correlated to the amount of
stromal and glandular tissue of the
biopsie specimen (= 100 %)

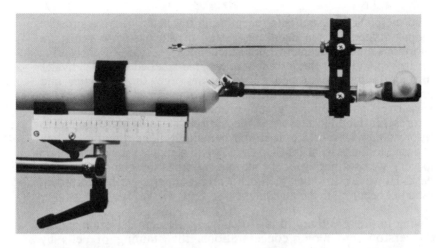

Fig 4 : By means of three pilot tubes a ultrasonically guided perineal punch biopsy can be made.

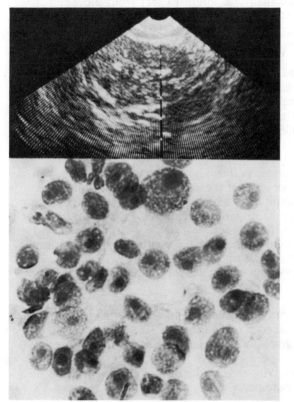

Fig 5 : In using aspiration biopsy with the help of rectal ultrasound poor cancer cells without stromal tissue can be obtained

Two methods of visualizing receptors in the heterogeneous prostate biopsy material have been suggested. In the past few years, an enormous amount of interest in histochemical methods for measuring the incorporation of fluorescence- or enzyme-labelled steroid derivates into cells has developed. Three years ago the estrogen and progesterone receptivity of the different compartments of the prostate was investigated by our group by measuring the incorporation of fluorescein-labelled steroids. The various steroids were bound to fluorescein via succinic acid and hexamethyllene-diamine. When exposed to fluorescent-labelled estradiol all samples showed moderate to very weak straining of the stroma, whereas the glands remained dark. However, in other sections a bright staining with fluorescent estradiol occurred in the glandular cells.

Owing to the sensitivity of microscopic fluorescein detection and its conversion into molar concentrations, the staining of cells by fluorescent steroid derivatives amounts to about 10^{-5} M, which corresponds to over 10 million binding sites in these cells; this is about one hundred times more than one might expect from biochemical findings. None of the methods presently used can inhibit fluorescence incorporation with the appropriate amount of the competitor (10^{-7}M). Thus it seems clear that we cannot visualize receptor sites and therefore we must not assume that hormone-sensitive cells can be localized with the help of this method. Therefore, for the time being, so-called histochemical receptor assays cannot be accepted as an alternative to traditional receptor analyses, especially in cases where clinical decisions have to be made. A second method of visualizing receptors is autoradiography, by means of which it is possible to take the heterogeneity of the biopsy specimens into account.

By using ultrasonically guided perineal punch biopsy tumor tissue can be obtained from echo poor areas of prostatic cancer; by means of three pilot tubes a punch or aspiration biopsy of the cancer tissue can be made (fig. 4). In a total of 36 patients with T1, T2 and T3 lesion, ultrasonically guided perineal punch biopsies were made; with the exception of one patient who had a false positive value all other patients had positive histological findings.
By using aspiration biopsy poor cancer cells without stromal tissue can be obtained (fig. 5).

Visualization of receptors by means of autoradiography in those aspirated cancer cells is intended to aid in :
- assessing the percentage of hormone-sensitive and insensitive tumor cells,
- assessing hormone sensitivity and cellular differentiation by means of simultaneous DNA measurements.

These tests might be helpful in identifying the 20-30% of patients who will not respond to hormonal therapy; today chemotherapy is mostly used in patients with so-called hormone-resistant tumors with a great tumor volume already; when using these tests possibly chemotherapy could be started at an earlier stage.

LITERATURE

Bartsch G., Frick J., Rüegg I., Bucher M., Holliger O., Oberholzer M., Rohr H.P.- 1979. Electron microscopic stereological analysis of the normal human prostate and of benign prostate hyperplasia.- J. Urol., 122 : 481-486

Bartsch G., Müller H.R., Oberholzer M., Rohr H.P. - 1979. Light microscopic stereological analysis of the normal prostate and of benign prostate hyperplasia. - J. Urol., 122 : 487-491

Bruchovsky N., Callaway T., Lieskovsky G., Rennie P.S. - 1980. Markers of androgen action in human prostate : potential use in the clinical assessment of prostatic carcinoma. In : Steroid receptors and hormone dependent neoplasia. Edited by Witcliff J.L. and Dapunt.O. Masson, USA p. 121-132.

Coffey D.S., Isaacs J.T.- 1979. Experimental concepts in the design of new treatments for human prostatic cancer. In : Prostate cancer Edit.Coffey D.S. and Isaacs J.T., UICC, p. 233-259.

Cowan R.A., Cowan S.K., Grant J.K., Elder H.Y. - 1977. Biochemical investigations of separated epithelium and stroma from benign prostatic hyperplastic tissue. - J. Endocr., 74 : 111-116

Dhom G. - 1976. Pathology and classification of prostatic carcinoma. In Prostatic disease. Edit. by Marberger H., Haschek H., Schirmer H.K.A., Colston J.A.C., Witkin E., Alan R., Liss inc., New-York, p.111

Jacobi G.H., Altwein J.E. - 1980. Androgenstoffwechsel im Prostatakarzinom : 3-hydroxysteroid-Dehydrogenase-Aktivität in Abhängigkeit vom Tumor-Differenzierungsgrad. - Urol.Intern., 35 : 194

Krieg M., Klötzl G., Kaufmann J., Voigt K.D. - 1981. Stroma of human benign prostatic hyperplasia : preferential tissue for androgen metabolism and estrogen binding.- Acta Endocr. Copenh. 96 :422-432

Morfin R.F., Leav I., Chavles J.F., Cavazos L.F., Ofner P., Floch H.H. - 1977. Correlative study of the morphology and C_{19}-steroid metabolism of benign and cancerous human prostatic tissue. - Cancer, 39 1517

Prout G.R. Jr., Kliman B., Daly J.J., Mac Laughlin R.A., Griffin P.D.- 1976. In vitro uptake of ^3H testosterone and its conversion to dihydrotestosterone by prostatic carcinoma and other tissues. - J. Urol., 116 : 60

Rohr H.P., Bartsch G. - 1980. Human benign prostatic hyperplasia : a stromal disease. - Urology, 625-633

Romijn J.C., Oishi K., Belt de Vriess J., Schweikert U., Mulder E., Schröder F.H. - 1980. Androgen metabolism and androgen receptors in separated epithelium and stroma of the human prostate. On steroid receptors, metabolism and prostatic cancer. Edited by Schröder F.H., de Voogt H.J.- Excerpta Medica Amsterdam, 134-139

Schweikert H.U., Bartsch G., Totzauer P., Rohr H.P. - 1983. Testosterone metabolism in the epithelium and stroma of normal human prostate in benign prostatic hyperplasia. In press.

Prostate Cancer, Part A: Research, Endocrine
Treatment, and Histopathology, pages 111–140
© 1987 Alan R. Liss, Inc.

USES AND LIMITATIONS OF HORMONE, RECEPTOR AND ENZYME ASSAYS IN PROSTATE CANCER

P.M. Martin, J.M. Le Goff, J.M. Brisset, T. Ojasoo,
J.M. Husson and J.P. Raynaud

Laboratoire de Cancérologie Expérimentale, Faculté de
Médecine Nord, UA 1175 CNRS, 13326 Marseille Cedex 15,
France (PMM, JMLG). Centre Médico-Chirurgical de la Porte
de Choisy, 75634 Paris Cedex 13, France (JMB). Roussel-
Uclaf, 75007 Paris, France (TO, JMH, JPR)

INTRODUCTION

Neoplastic transformation of endocrine target organs is
a major cause of death both in men and women. As for most
cancers, treatment is handicapped by the long latency
period before the appearance of the first symptoms and also
by the delay that often occurs between the time these symptoms appear and the moment the disease is diagnosed
(Robinson, 1984). During all this time heterogeneous cell
populations may develop in situ and be disseminated by
metastasis, two processes which limit the chances of response to therapy. There is therefore a definite need to be
able to stage the disease early and also to determine a
prognostic index for a favourable response to endocrine
therapy.

In the case of breast cancer, in spite of a few reports
to the contrary, there is a general concensus in the literature regarding the relevance of steroid hormone receptor
assays for the selection of patients liable to respond
favourably to endocrine therapy (NIH Concensus, 1986). The
presence of high levels of estrogen and progestin receptors
is considered a valuable prognostic index (Heuson et al.,
1975 ; Byar et al., 1979 ; Martin, 1985 ; McGuire et al.,
1986). Furthermore, the assay of certain enzymes such as
17β-dehydrogenase has provided proof of the functionality
of these receptors (Lübbert and Pollow, 1978 ; Fournier et
al., 1985).

In the case of prostate cancer, histochemical analysis provides an estimate of the grade of the cancer (Gleason and Mellinger, 1974) but is an inadequate prognostic index for evaluating potential response to endocrine therapy. However, as for breast cancer, the more highly differentiated the tumour, the more hormone dependent it may be. Poorly differentiated tumors may represent advanced stages of malignancy where the original make-up, including hormone dependence, of the gland has been lost. The biochemical parameters of hormone dependence (i.e. intratissular free hormone, receptor and/or enzyme levels) have consequently also been measured in prostate cancer samples in order to select those patients liable to respond. It is not yet proven that there is a clear correlation between the histological grade of a prostatic tumour and its receptor content (Pertschuk et al., 1982 ; Concolino et al., 1982) nor is there any general agreement in the literature on the value of receptor assays as response indicators (Shain and Boesel, 1978 ; de Voogt and Dingjan, 1978 ; Ekman et al., 1979 ; Ghanadian, 1983 ; Mobbs et al., 1979 ; Martelli et al., 1980 ; Concolino et al., 1982 ; Trachtenberg and Walsh, 1982 ; de Voogt and Rao, 1983 ; van Aubel et al., 1986 ; Habib et al., 1986).

The question thus arises whether the differences in prostate androgen receptor (AR) content and enzyme activity that have been observed by several teams are due to inherent properties of the prostate cells within their environment (heterogeneity, phenotype) or to technological variations in tissue sampling and assay methods. Or, in cruder terms, have these teams evaluated the relevance of AR or of their technique to measure AR ? Only rarely have optimal conditions for simple and reliable receptor and enzyme assays been determined for prostate tissue. The development of standard assays and quality control programs as for breast cancer might help to elucidate the reasons for many present controversies.

USES AND LIMITATIONS OF INTRAPROSTATIC HORMONE ASSAYS

According to anatomopathological and histological data, prostate tissue is very heterogeneous with cells ranging from totally undifferentiated to highly differentiated (Rohr, 1979 ; McNeal, 1979, 1981 ; Garnick et al., 1982 ; Poste, 1983 ; Heppner, 1984 ; Catalona, 1984 ; Ghanadian and Puah, 1983). These various cell populations may have different affinities for steroid hormones, especially androgens, and consequently different degrees of hormone sensitivity, i.e. different response thresholds to active circulating and tissue hormones (Isaacs and Coffey, 1979 ; Krieg et al., 1979 ; Vermeulen et al., 1979 ; Isaacs, 1982).

In man, besides testosterone and its metabolite dihydrotestosterone (DHT), weak androgens of adrenal origin are present in plasma (Coffey, 1979 ; Genazzani et al., 1980) which can be converted to more active androgens (i.e. DHT) by intraprostatic enzymes (Harper et al., 1984 ; Geller, 1985). Discrete levels of intraprostatic DHT have been recorded after orchiectomy or estrogen treatment (Geller et al., 1984a,b) which could possess significant stimulatory activity on the growth of prostate cancer.

Although only measurements of hormone levels **within** the prostate tissue in association with the nuclear androgen receptor content could possess any prognostic value (Krieg et al., 1979 ; Morioka et al., 1982 ; Walsh et al., 1983 ; Geller et al., 1984 a,b ; Bélanger et al., 1986), presently only total (bound + free) plasma hormone levels are measured on a routine basis (eg. on saliva). The preferential accumulation of free hormone in target cells obtained by biopsy is more difficult to ascertain since it requires a separation step by chromatography prior to RIA. Furthermore, contamination of tissue samples by plasma hormones and possible differences in the metabolic activity of the tissue over time have to be considered before interpreting the significance of the tissue hormone level in terms of the relative densities of the different populations of hormone-sensitive cells.

In the absence of an immunocytochemical analysis, a hormonal response parameter needs to be taken as reference, e.g. the activity of a prostatic secretory protein (prostatic acid phosphatase (PAP) (Lillehoj et al., 1982), of hydrolytic or proteolytic enzymes implicated in cell growth (Isaacs et al., 1979 ; Dubé et al., 1985) or of a cell proliferation-associated nuclear antigen (PaNA). The synthesis of PAP remains hormone dependent during the earlier stages of neoplastic transformation as has been demonstrated in vitro on the human prostatic cancer cell line LNCaP (Schulz et al., 1985) but the polarity of its secretion

changes (Bentz et al., 1982). The Ki-67 monoclonal antibody
to PaNA provides a reliable method for estimation of the
proliferative fraction of hormone-responsive cancer tissue
(van Steenbrugge et al., 1986). In our opinion, therefore,
intratissular androgen levels are of value only when considered in terms of their potential activity, i.e., as a
necessary parameter in a multifactorial analysis involving
receptor, enzyme and response measurements.

USES AND LIMITATIONS OF RECEPTOR ASSAYS

Several classes of steroid hormone receptor (androgen,
progestin, glucocorticoid and estrogen) have been detected
in primary prostatic carcinoma and prostatic cancer metastases (Shain and Boesel, 1978 ; Asselin et al., 1979 ; Raynaud
et al., 1980 ; Ekman, 1980) and the subject has been amply
reviewed (Trachtenberg, 1982 ; Sandberg and Karr, 1983 ;
Ghanadian and Auf, 1983 ; Buttyan and Olsson, 1984). Although higher than in normal prostate, the levels of androgen
receptor (AR) (cytosol and/or nuclear) in prostate cancer
are generally considered low. This constitutes a severe
limitation to the development of microassays for the simultaneous measurement of all steroid hormone receptors (Hicks
and Walsh, 1979 ; Martin et al., 1982) when one considers
the size of prostate punch needle biopsies (less than 0.1 g)
which may contain variable proportions of cancer cells. The
low levels of AR could be partially explained by the heat
denaturation that occurs during resection but also by the
instability of AR in the presence of high levels of proteases (Christman and Silverstein, 1973 ; Hynes et al., 1975 ;
Magnusson et al., 1975 ; Ossowski et al., 1975 ; Mullins and
Rohrlich, 1983). Surprisingly high levels of progestin
receptor (PR) can however be detected, often in the absence
of estrogen receptor, implying that the normal PR induction
mechanism may not operate. An analogous situation has been
noted in brain tumors (meningioma) where, in our experience,
ER is virtually undetectable and AR concentrations are
correlated to PR (Pertuiset et al., 1984).

In order to ascertain the value of the androgen receptor
assay as a prognostic factor -a point that is still hotly
debated- it is essential that the receptor assay technology
be fully validated. Published experiments have emphasized
the importance of the following technological features : The
use of 0.6 M KCl is recommended for optimal receptor extrac-

tion since about 80 % of the androgen binding sites in human carcinoma would appear to be occupied and located in the nucleus (Mobbs et al., 1981 ; Robel et al., 1983 ; Smith et al., 1983b). In the presence of dithiothreitol (DTT) (Barrack et al., 1983) or of NaSCN (Bresciani et al., 1980), both salt-extractable and salt-resistant nuclear receptors are measured. A phosphate buffer containing heparin and DTT has been reported to improve extraction compared to 0.4 M KCl (Foekens et al., 1981). The addition of sodium molybdate (usually 10 mM) to the incubation medium helps to stabilize the receptor (Gaubert et al., 1980 ; Krieg et al., 1981a) and protease inhibitors such as phenylmethylsulfonyl fluoride and Trasylol (Prins and Lee, 1982) minimize degradation.

The use of natural ligands such as testosterone and DHT is not recommended because of their rapid metabolism even at low temperatures and/or their binding to contaminating specific plasma proteins (i.e. sex-steroid binding protein (SBP)) (Raynaud et al., 1979). This metabolism can be prevented by pre-incubation with NAD^+-nucleosidase (Moeller et al., 1983) or by removing the SBP by absorption with Conconavalin A (Wilbert et al., 1983). But, in most studies, the natural steroid has been replaced by radiolabelled synthetic steroids, in particular by R 1881 (methyltrienolone, metribolone). Methyltrienolone binds to AR with higher affinity than DHT, is resistant to metabolic conversion during incubation, and binds only very weakly to SBP (Bonne and Raynaud, 1976 ; Ojasoo and Raynaud, 1978 ; Raynaud et al., 1979). However it lacks specificity and, like a more recently available radioligand mibolerone (Bailey et al., 1985 ; Traish et al., 1986a), binds to the progestin receptor. This binding can be selectively blocked by adding a large excess of triamcinolone acetonide (TA) to the incubation medium (Asselin et al., 1979 ; Zava et al., 1979). More recently, a hybrid ligand method using methyltrienolone as the high specific activity labelled tracer that binds only weakly to SBP and DHT as the unlabelled competitor that binds weakly to PR has been proposed (Stebbings et al., 1985).

To determine the exact concentration of receptor, the endogenously bound steroids must be removed, thereby necessitating the use of an exchange assay. The time required to exchange endogenous androgens by a radiolabelled marker such as methyltrienolone at low temperature (4°C) is in the region of 72 h compared to only 24 h for the assay of progesterone receptor. The dissociation of bound steroid can be accelerated at low temperature by adding mersalyl acid or 0.4 M NaSCN (Norris and Smith, 1983 ; Traish et al., 1981, 1986b) but many assays are still performed at higher temperatures in spite of the problems of receptor stability (Shain et al., 1982).

We are presently performing systematic steroid receptor assays using conditions described in the literature (Robel, 1984 ; Robel et al., 1985) to evaluate the variations in receptor density within benign hyperplastic and malignant prostates. Preliminary receptor assays on the left and right lobes of 51 hyperplastic prostates gave the results illustrated in Figure 1.

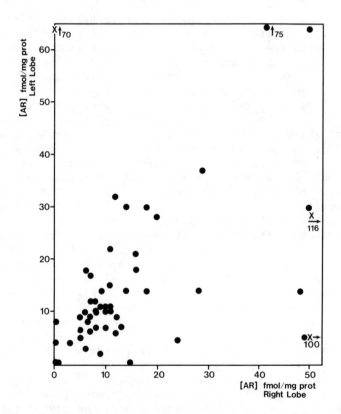

Figure 1. Plot of the androgen receptor (AR) levels in the left versus right lobes of 51 hyperplastic prostates (●) and in 3 malignant prostates (X). (The tumor was located either in the left or right lobe).(r= 0.599)

The receptor concentrations in these BPH samples tended to be low (less than 30 fmol/mg protein). A wide scatter of points is observed.

Hyperplasia and neoplasia of ageing tissues often develop simultaneously (Catalona, 1984 ; McNeal, 1979, 1981) but tend to originate from different regions of the prostate gland. The incidence of periurethral cancer is estimated as 2-3 % (Dube et al., 1973). Three of the prostates examined had malignant foci and are indicated by the sign X in Figure 1. Further details on their AR content are given in Table 1.

TABLE 1. Malignant foci in the BPH samples of Figure 1.

| Region | Androgen receptor | |
	fmol/mg prot	fmol/mg DNA
left lobe (fibrous)	0	0
right lobe (malignant)	70	340
ganglion (metastasis)	204	364
left lobe (malignant)	28	97
right lobe (malignant)	116	216
median	79	205
left lobe	5	190
right lobe	56	222
right lobe (malignant)	100	338
ganglion (metastasis)	190	250

In confirmation of data reported in the literature, the malignant foci tended to have a higher AR content than BPH but differences were minimised when results were expressed using mg DNA as a reference parameter. On a much larger published series of cancer specimens, a mean value of about 500 fmol/mg DNA has been reported and a cut-off-level of 110 fmol/mg DNA suggested for survival.

The most highly-positive BPH sample (75 fmol/mg prot) in our series gave a virtually negligible receptor content after electroresection. The heat-denaturing effect of

electroresection was confirmed on a further series of 11
BPH patients from whom 16 surgical biopsies and 11 resected
specimens were obtained. Mean AR concentrations ($\pm$ sd) of
13.67 $\pm$ 14.47 (n=16) and 4.46 $\pm$ 5.78 (n=11) were recorded
respectively. The influence of resection on androgen receptor content was therefore studied in greater detail. A
single prostate adenoma obtained by retropubic prostatectomy was divided into four segments, A to D. Within each
segment, three samples were assayed : an inner periurethral
sample A_1, an peripheral sample A_2 also cut with a
surgical knife, and a middle resected sample RA (Table 2).

TABLE 2. Influence of electroresection on androgen receptor
(AR) content in a prostate adenoma

	AR fmol/mg DNA		AR fmol/mg DNA
A_1	55	C_1	196
RA	19	RC	11.2
A_2	57	C_2	100
B_1	195	D_1	50
RB	11.2	RD	19
B_2	172	D_2	129

The results clearly indicate a decrease in receptor
content on electroresection in confirmation of earlier observations by others (Snochowski et al., 1977 ; Ghanadian
and Auf, 1983 ; Nozumi et al., 1981) but in contradistinc-
tion to some more recent reports (Smith et al., 1983b ;
Bowman et al., 1985). Furthermore, the inability to draw
Scatchard plots for certain resected specimens (even though
a single-point exchange assay gave an apparently valid result) suggests that not only could there be a loss in the
number of sites but that the protein may be denatured in
some way (unpublished data).

The above receptor determinations were performed on
samples which had all been stripped with fairly drastic
conditions of dextran-coated charcoal DCC to remove endogenous free steroids (i.e. testosterone and DHT). The impor-

tance of this DCC-treatment is shown by the results in
Table 3 for a pool of two prostate adenomas from patients
with circulating plasma testosterone levels in the range of
5000 pg/ml.

TABLE 3. Influence of the removal of endogenous steroids by
DCC-treatment on AR values (fmol/mg tissue)

	4 h incubation		20 h incubation	
	Untreated	Stripped	Untreated	Stripped
2°C	50	431	236	1030
10°C	90	545	375	1040
15°C	143	455	240	792

Systematically higher AR values were recorded after
DCC-stripping. The optimum conditions defined in this experiment were 20 h at 10°C but are being confirmed in more
extensive kinetic studies.

Apart from the difficulties associated with receptor
assay technology, one of the most acute problems in the
determination of steroid receptors in the prostate is the
heterogeneity of the gland. In order to gain some insight
into the importance of this factor in routine assays
(Bowman et al., 1986), we calculated several correlation
coefficients. AR values for 26 samples taken from the periurethral (n=13) and peripheral (n=13) regions of a single
BPH were not well correlated (r=0.22). When considering
data for 5 prostates, the correlation coefficient increased
from r=0.22 to only r=0.38. On the other hand, when the
samples were taken from the same region (periurethral or
peripheral, less than 500 mg between two samples), the
correlation coefficient for 16 pairs of values was r=0.82
(when results were expressed in fmol/mg prot) and r=0.84
(fmol/mg DNA). Increasing the number of biopsies also
increased the correlation coefficient. A single-point analysis on needle biopsy specimens before surgery was not
well correlated (r=0.26) with the value obtained with full-
multiple-point assays on tissue obtained at surgery (Benson
et al., 1985), whereas three pooled biopsies gave a correlation coefficient of 0.78. Multiple biopsies are thus

required to obtain a proper estimate of the true AR content of the tissue (Blankenstein et al., 1982).

Although the concentration of AR has been found to be greater in stromal than in epithelial nuclei (Lahtonen et al., 1983), the use of whole tissue homogenates is considered valid since the parenchymal and stromal percentages of BPH tissue have not been found to correlate with AR values (Kliman et al., 1982). However, a cytochemical method for AR (Lämmel et al., 1983 ; Pertschuk et al., 1984) would be extremely valuable as there is a tendency to use aspiration cytology more and more for diagnosis as well as follow-up of prostatic cancer.

USES AND LIMITATIONS OF ENZYME MEASUREMENTS

Considering the above limitations of intraprostatic hormone and receptor assays, the ability to measure the enzyme activities involved in the hormonal regulation of the growth and secretory activity of the prostate represents an interesting counterpart (Krieg et al., 1978, 1981b ; Bruchovsky et al., 1981 ; Habib et al., 1983 ; Hudson et al., 1983 ; Ghanadian and Smith, 1983). Certain enzymes can constitute a measure of the functionality of the receptor machinery. On the other hand, the conversion of testosterone (T) into its active metabolite DHT by a 5α-reductase is an important step, maybe even a prerequisite, preceeding the activation of the androgen receptor. The accurate in vitro assay of 5α-reductase activity could give a valuable indirect estimation of the intraprostatic presence of T and DHT since this activity, like that of any enzyme, is greatly influenced by substrate (T) and product (DHT) concentrations. Changes in affinity might be observed reflecting the variations in circulating testosterone concentration that can occur in different pathologies and between normal and castrated cancer patients who have or have not undergone endocrine therapy. Such an assay may also be an indirect way of approaching the question whether low levels of testosterone, or of other precursors such as adrenal androgens (Fiet et al., this volume), might not be converted by high enzymic activity into significant concentrations of DHT.

We have therefore tried to develop a 5α-reductase assay applicable to specimens from all sources. To establish whether any variation in activity between two tissues represents a change in enzyme concentration or a change in its affinity (or both), we calculated the classical parameters derived from a Lineweaver-Burk plot : V_{max} representative of enzyme concentration and K_m representative of enzyme affinity.

Published K_m values for 5α-reductase differ widely (Table 4). Although these differences could be attributed to species characteristics, the range of K_m values recorded by different teams for a single tissue, human BPH, is also very wide. Most investigators do not state whether they have optimised their assay conditions. Incubations are usually for half-an-hour at near neutral pH. and the stability of the cofactor is not checked. We therefore decided to determine optimal conditions for our assay which were as follows :

Whole prostate adenomas from 10 patients (60-75 yrs old) undergoing retropubic adenomectomy were cut into slices perpendicular to the urethra. Every other slice was sent for histologic examination. The remaining slices were immediately frozen in liquid nitrogen. The tissues were weighed, powdered and pooled in a high-pressure pulverizer and aliquots of about 1 g of this powder were stored in liquid nitrogen until use.

At analysis, aliquots were weighed and homogenized in three volumes of 5 mM Tris-HCl pH 7 buffer containing 50 μM of the cofactor NADPH. Great care was taken to prevent any rise in temperature by cooling the tubes in ice for 1 min between each burst. The homogenate was centrifuged at 105,000 g for 60 min at 4°C to obtain the microsomal pellet which was homogenised in 5 volumes of buffer.

Incubations were initiated by transferring 50 μl of microsomal preparation (about 0.3 mg protein) to preheated incubation tubes containing buffer (20 mM sodium acetate pH 5.5 ; NaCl to constant ionic strength of 0.2I ; 0.5 mM NADPH added less than 1 min before starting the reaction). Standard incubations contained 10^6 dpm ^{3}H-testosterone (s.a. 99 Ci/mmol) and were made up to the final concentration of substrate (0.1 μM to 20 μM) with cold testosterone. In some experiments the substrate was added in 30 μl of incubation buffer, NADPH in 30 μl of 5 mM Tris HCl pH 7, the microsomal preparation in 40 μl buffer in this order. The reaction was stopped by freezing the incubation tubes

TABLE 4. K_M values for prostatic 5α-reductase affinity according to the literature

Tissue	Incubation conditions			K_M (nM)	Reference
	Time (min)	Conc. range (μM)	pH		
RAT microsomes	10	2 – 4	6.9	2300 ± 1500	Roy, 1971
RAT DOG microsomes	30	0.5 – 5	6.5	2400 ± 1200 2200	Liang et al., 1985
DOG epithelium	45	0.01– 10	7.4	3000	McKercher et al, 1984
BPH nuclear extract	60	0.035– 0.74	6.5	600	Frederiksen and Wilson, 1971
BPH stroma epithelium	30	0.05– 2	7.4	90/120	Habib et al., 1981
BPH stroma epithelium	30	0.0025– 0.075	7.0	195 ± 44 21 ± 4	Bruchovsky et et al., 1981
BPH stroma epithelium	30	0.005– 0.125		68	Rennie et al., 1983
BPH stroma epithelium	15	0.1 – 0.33	7.4	180/250	Krieg et al., 1985
BPH microsomes	30	0.5 – 5	5.0 6.5	3300 ± 800 15200	Liang et al., 1985

in liquid nitrogen. Proteins were denatured in 10 % TCA and radioactivity was extracted by ether. Less than 1 % of the total radioactivity remains in the tubes. Incubation tubes with no microsomal preparation added were taken as controls of the spontaneous radiolysis of ^{3}H-testosterone and used to calculate non specific metabolisation in the DHT zone. Spontaneous radiolysis was less than 1 % of total and was never found to affect the DHT zone. The separation of testosterone from DHT was performed on a C18 reverse phase column. The mobile phase was a mixture of methanol : tetrahydrofuran : water (40 : 13 : 47).

With this procedure, we confirmed Liang et al.'s observation that 5α-reductase activity in human BPH is optimal at acid pH (about pH 5) (Figure 2). The pH in our incubations was thus fixed at 5.5 which provided a nearly tenfold increase in metabolic activity compared to pH 7 and enabled us to work on small quantities of material, i.e. biopsy material. Furthermore, 17β-dehydrogenase and 3-oxoreductase, two enzymes that can interfere with the transformation reaction of testosterone (T) into DHT by the homogenates, are virtually inactive at this pH. Since at optimal pH the variation in the dissociation constant of DHT from the 5α-reductase-NADPH complex is minimal, V_{max} is directly proportional to the enzyme concentration E_0.

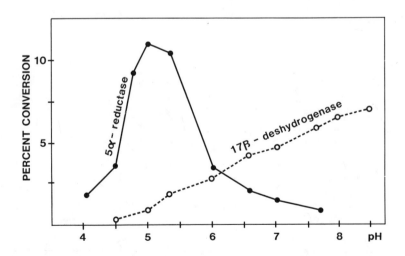

Figure 2. Optimum pH of 5α-reductase activity in human BPH

We then investigated the spontaneous disappearance of the cofactor (NADPH) as a function of pH and incubation time (Table 5). The cofactor consumption was linear from 0 to 10 minutes incubation and at quasi-optimum pH (5.5) did not exceed 10 %. Since we operated in our standard experiments at saturating (0.5 mM) NaDPH concentrations, the spontaneous disappearance largely exceeded the consumption due to the reaction.

TABLE 5. Cofactor (NADPH) requirements

pH	% consumed
6.5	1.9
6	5.7
5.5	10.5
5	21.0

The limitation of a 10 % maximum conversion, whether of cofactor or substrate, is an essential requirement for a valid Lineweaver–Burk plot which represents the **true initial rate** of product formation as a function of the reciprocal of the initial substrate concentration (Figure 3).

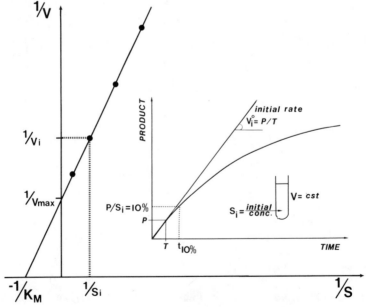

Figure 3. Requirements for a valid Lineweaver–Burk plot

Only then can the true initial rate be calculated from the quantity of DHT formed during a fixed incubation time. Since, in a given incubation volume, the rate of transformation is for ever decreasing as the substrate disappears, it is necessary to adapt the incubation time to obtain between 1 and 10 % transformation of the incubated T and less than 10 % consumption of cofactor. The lowest concentration is the fastest metabolized and the first to attain 10 % of transformation. It fixes the shortest incubation time (1 min). On increasing concentration, less and less transformation occurs during this time until the technological limitations in the sensitivity of detection of the DHT formed (1 %) due to its dilution in the untransformed testosterone pool are attained. It then becomes necessary to choose longer incubation times (4 and 15 min) for higher T concentration ranges.

Although we used a **single** microsomal preparation we obtained surprising results. For each range of testosterone concentrations [T] incubated for a fixed time (t), we obtained an excellent linear regression (r = 0.99) for the Lineweaver-Burk plot enabling classical estimations of V_{max} and K_m. However, on increasing the concentration ranges, and consequently the incubation times adapted to these ranges, we found three different K_m values. V_{max} was not significantly different (Figure 4).

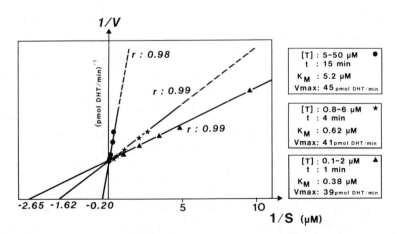

Figure 4. Lineweaver-Burk plots for a single microsomal BPH preparation incubated under conditions (●,*,▲) ensuring less than 10 % conversion of substrate and cofactor

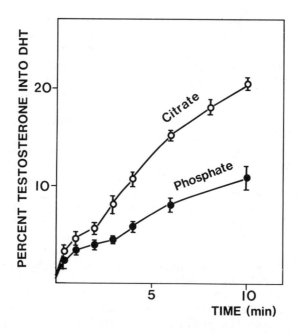

Figure 5. Time-course of metabolism of testosterone into DHT in prostatic tissue (BPH) microsomes prepared in citrate or phosphate buffer.

Finding two or more initial rates of transformation for the same testosterone concentration demonstrated that, in spite of excellent linear regressions, the Lineweaver–Burk method cannot be used to analyse data obtained by incubation of a wide range of T concentrations for a fixed time since it is based on classical first-order Michaelis–Menten kinetics for a single initial rate of transformation. This is reflected in the non-linear curves obtained in the initial phases of time-course experiments (Figure 5). It is therefore likely that 5α–reductase activity in BPH does not follow Michaelian kinetics. The change in affinity observed for this enzyme could be compared to the behavior of hysteretic enzymes (Neet and Ainslie, 1980) that conserve the memory of a previous conformation prior to in vitro manipulation.

DISCUSSION

Several problems remain outstanding in the development of a routine steroid receptor assay for human prostate tissue. The main difficulty resides in performing a low-temperance exchange over a relatively short-period of time, in obtaining multiple exploratory biopsy specimens ($\sim$ 80 mg) from a single zone and in establishing adequate quality control criteria. Furthermore, the results of such an assay should probably not be considered in isolation but should include the parallel determination of intraprostatic hormone levels and of metabolic and hormone responses for multi-parametric analysis.

In the present paper, we have made several confirmatory observations. We have established the importance of tissue sampling on androgen receptor (AR) values ; a drastic decrease in receptor content was noted in electroresected specimens. Although higher AR values were recorded in malignant tissue than in BPH specimens, this difference was greatly minimized by expressing results per mg DNA rather than per mg protein. The removal of endogenous steroids by DCC-treatment led to higher AR values. We have also performed preliminary unpublished investigations on the variations in receptor levels recorded in 12 different samples from a single hyperplastic prostate and observed marked heterogeneity and a decreased content after artificial resection. Presently, fuller investigations are underway on the heterogeneity of malignant and normal prostate by multiparametric analysis.

We have investigated the optimal conditions for an enzyme (5α-reductase) assay. In so doing, we have noted that, although good linear regressions have been observed in most of the published Lineweaver-Burk plots, the reaction may nevertheless not follow the first-order Michaelis-Menten kinetics expected at saturating cofactor levels. When investigating a wide range of testosterone concentrations, as found in prostate cancer patients (normal or castrate), at different incubation times to comply with the need to remain within a 10 % substrate consumption limit, the same V_{max} was recorded for each testosterone concentration range, but the Kms differed. This suggests that 5α-reductase activity displays variations in affinity at the beginning of incubation. Such an absence of instantaneous adaptation of an enzyme to its in vitro environment is observed with hysteretic enzymes that conserve a memory of a previous in vivo state.

This chapter has so far laid most emphasis on the choice of appropriate conditions for valid steroid receptor and enzyme assays on prostate tissue. The underlying assumption that these assays will be of use in discriminating between hormone sensitive and insensitive tissues in order that endocrine therapy be prescribed only to those patients liable to respond, and under conditions where they shall respond best, has not been addressed but deserves special attention. Besides, it is well known that, although hormone therapy has beneficial effects in a large proportion of patients, all these patients will at one stage become refractory to this treatment, show metastases, and relapse.

Therefore what is the physiological significance of the parameters involved in establishing the hormone dependence of prostate tissue ? At the **molecular level**, the presence of receptor is generally considered a sine qua non condition for an androgenic response. Decreased receptor content or an impaired receptor (Pinsky et al., 1985) could explain, and constitute a criterion for, hormone insensitivity. However, a knowledge of receptor content needs to be complemented by an appreciation of receptor functionality. At the **cellular level** the metabolism of endogenous hormones, i.e. enzyme activity (see above assay), governs the most efficient use of the receptor system. High hormone sensitivity would correspond to the effective integration of the metabolic interactions between different cell populations, whereas hormone insensitivity might be due to a loss in producer/secretory cells or an adaptation of the metabolic activity of the cells to new environmental conditions by, for instance, synthesising uncharacteristic growth factors (e.g. oncogene products). At the **tissue level**, the prime consideration is the organisational network, "ecosystem", within which hormone sensitivity can best be expressed. More than 95 % of prostate cancers are adenocarcinomas arising from the hormone-dependent epithelium of the prostatic acini usually in the periphery of the prostate gland (Catalona, 1984). But the prostate is constituted of a great diversity of cellular subpopulations (epithelial cells, stromal cells, basal cells). Cell-to-cell interactions partake in the control of the stimulatory action of plasma hormones on the growth and differentiation of the gland (Müntzing, 1980 ; Ghanadian and Puah, 1983). Both the tumoral process and hormone deprivation (e.g. castration) may dramatically modify these interactions. For instance, in tumors, the basal cells between stroma and epithelium are absent and the polarity of PAP secretion is reversed (Bentz et al., 1982). Perturbed interactions between stroma and epithelium may also end up by inducing changes in gene regulation which allow permissive coexpression of DNA areas coding for the synthesis of autonomous growth factors involved in the anarchic development of prostate epithelium (Vande Woude et al., 1984 ; Feramisco et al., 1985 ; Kris et al., 1985 ; Spandidos, 1985 ; Goustin et al., 1986 ; Stoscheck and King, 1986). Furthermore, metastatic cells originating from the primary tumor, even if they conserve their hormone machinery, may home in on cellular environments where this hormone dependence can no longer be expressed (Heppner et al., 1983 ; Poste, 1983 ; Nicolson, 1983 ; Levine et al., 1984 ; Poste et al., 1984 ; Weiss, 1985).

Conservation of the hormone sensitive phenotype and impeding the development of metastatic proclivity and autonomy (Talmadge, 1983 ; Griswold et al., 1984) are essential for successful hormone therapy. The probability of the appearance of an autonomous system independent of hormone regulation increases with time but the probability of the existence of a totally autonomous system from the birth of the first cancer clone is low since the target epithelial cells tend to be hormone-dependent. Prostate cancer cells may however lose the hormone sensitive phenotype by adapting continuously until they become totally insensitive and provoke relapse. Any endocrine treatment should therefore be administered **as early as possible** on the basis of a knowledge of the hormone sensitivity of the tumor cells. That is why valid receptor and enzyme assays are vital.

REFERENCES

Asselin J, Mélançon R, Gourdeau Y, Labrie F, Bonne C, Raynaud JP (1979). Specific binding of [^{3}H]-methyltrienolone to both progestin and androgen binding components in human benign prostatic hypertrophy (BPH). J steroid Biochem 10:483-486.

Bailey M, Carilla E, Fabre M (1985). Comparative binding studies with [^{3}H]-methyltrienolone and [^{3}H]-mibolerone, two synthetic ligands for the androgen receptor. Br J Pharmacol suppl. 54:127P.

Barrack ER, Bujnovszky P, Walsh PC (1983). Subcellular distribution of androgen receptors in human normal, benign hyperplastic, and malignant prostatic tissues : Characterisation of nuclear salt-resistant receptors. Cancer Res. 43:1107-1116.

Bélanger A, Labrie F, Dupont A (1986). Androgen levels in prostatic tissue of patients with carcinoma of the prostate treated with the combined therapy using an LHRH agonist and a pure antiandrogen. Eur J Cancer Clin Oncol 22:6.

Benson RC Jr, Utz DC, Holicky E, Veneziale CM (1985). Androgen binding activity in human prostate cancer. Cancer 55: 382-388.

Bentz MS, Cohen C, Demers LM, Budgeon LR (1982). Immuno-histochemical acid phosphatase level and tumor grade in prostatic carcinoma. Arch Pathol Lab Med 106:476-480.

Blankenstein MA, Bolt de Vries J, Foekens JA (1982). Nuclear androgen receptor assay in biopsy-size specimens of human prostatic tissue. Prostate 3:351-359.

Bonne C, Raynaud JP (1976). Assay of androgen binding sites by exchange with methyltrienolone (R 1881). Steroids 27: 497-507.

Bowman SP, Barnes DM, Blacklock NJ (1985). A minicolumn method for routine measurement of human prostatic androgen receptors. J steroid Biochem 23:421-430.

Bowman SP, Barnes DM, Blacklock NJ, Sullivan PJ (1986). Regional variations of cytosol androgen receptors throughout the diseased human prostate gland. Prostate 8:167-180.

Bresciani F, Sica V, Weizs A, Buonaguro FM, Bova R, Puca GA, Molinari AM, Endrenyi L (1980). Effect of NaSCN on receptor-estradiol interaction and application to assay total receptor ("filled" and "unfilled" sites) in tissues and tissue fractions, including nuclei, by exchange at low temperature with 17 -estradiol-^{3}H. In Bresciani F (ed): "Perspectives in Steroid Receptor Research". New York: Raven Press pp. 273-297.

Bruchovsky N, McLoughlin MG, Rennie PS, To MP (1981). Partial characterization of stromal and epithelial forms of 5 -reductase in human prostate. In Murphy GP, Sandberg AA, Karr JP (eds): "The Prostatic Cell: Structure and Function. Part A". Progr Clin Biol Res, Vol 75A. New York: Alan R Liss, pp. 161-175.

Buttyan R, Olsson CA (1984). Androgen receptor assays in advanced prostatic cancer. Urol Clinics Nth Amer 11:311-317.

Byar DP, Sears ME, McGuire WL (1979). Relationship between estrogen receptor values and clinical data in predicting the response to endocrine therapy for patients with advanced breast cancer. Eur J Cancer 15:299-310.

Catalona WJ Jr (1984). "Pathology in Prostate Cancer". New York: Grune & Stratton Inc, pp. 15-32.

Christman JK, Silverstein SC (1973). In RW Ruddon Jr (ed): "Proteinases in Membranes, Cells and Tissues". New York: Elsevier, North Holland.

Coffey DS (1979). Physiological control of prostatic growth: an overview. In Coffey DS, Isaacs JT (eds): "Prostate Cancer". Geneva: UICC Technical Report Series, Vol 48, pp.4-23.

Concolino G, Marocchi A, Margiotta G et al. (1982). Steroid receptors and hormone responsiveness of human prostatic carcinoma. Prostate 3:475-482.

Dube VE, Farrow GM, Greene LF (1973). Prostatic carcinoma of ductal origin. Cancer 32:402.

Dubé JY, Frenette G, Chapdelaine P, Paquin R, Tremblay RR (1985). Biochemical characteristics of the proteins secreted by dog prostate, a review. Exp Biol 43:145-159.

Ekman P (1980). Clinical significance of steroid receptor assay in the human prostate. In Schroeder FH, de Voogt HJ (eds): "Steroid Receptors, Metabolism and Prostatic Cancer". Amsterdam: Excerpta Medica pp. 208-224.

Ekman P, Snochowski M, Zetterberg A, Högberg B, Gustafsson JA (1979). Steroid receptor content in human prostatic carcinoma and response to endocrine therapy. Cancer 44: 1173-1181.

Feramisco J, Ozanne B, Stiles C (eds) (1985). Growth Factors and Transformation. In "Cancer Cells", Cold Spring Harbor Laboratory.

Foekens JA, Bolt-de Vries J, Mulder E, Blankenstein MA, Schröder FH, van der Molen HJ (1981). Nuclear androgen receptors in human prostatic tissue. Extraction with heparin and estimation of the number of binding sites with different methods. Clin Chim Acta 109:91-102.

Fournier S, Brihmat F, Durand JC, Sterkers N, Martin PM, Kuttenn F, Mauvais-Jarvis P (1985). Estradiol 17β-hydroxysteroid dehydrogenase, a marker of breast cancer hormone dependency. Cancer Res 45:2895-2899.

Frederiksen DW, Wilson JD (1971). Partial characterization of the nuclear reduced nicotinamide adenine dinucleotide phosphate: Δ^4-3-ketosteroid 5α-oxidoreductase of rat prostate. J Biol Chem 246:2584-2593.

Garnick MB, Prout GR Jr, Canellos GP (1982). Cancer of the prostate. In Holland JF, Frei E III (eds): "Cancer Medicine". Philadelphia: Lea & Febiger pp. 1912-1934.

Gaubert CM, Tremblay RR, Dubé JY (1980). Effect of sodium molybdate on cytosolic androgen receptors. J steroid Biochem 13:931-937.

Geller J (1985). Rationale for blockade of adrenal as well as testicular androgens in the treatment of advanced prostate cancer. Sem Oncol XII: 28-35.

Geller J, Albert JD, Nachtsheim DA, Loza D (1984a). Comparison of prostatic cancer tissue dihydrotestosterone levels at the time of relapse following orchiectomy or estrogen therapy. J Urol 132:693-696.

Geller J, de la Vega DJ, Albert JD, Nachtsheim DA (1984b). Tissue dihydrotestosterone levels and clinical response to hormonal therapy in patients with advanced prostate cancer. J Clin Endocrinol Metab 58:36-40.

Genazzani AR, Thijssen JHH, Siiteri PK (eds) (1980). Adrenal androgens. New York: Raven Press.

Ghanadian R (1983). Predictive role of steroid receptors in evaluating the response to endocrine therapy. In Ghanadian R (ed): "The Endocrinology of Prostate Tumours". Lancaster: MTP Press pp. 221-239.

Ghanadian R, Auf G (1983). Analysis of steroid receptors in the prostate. In Ghanadian R (ed): "The Endocrinology of Prostate Tumours". Lancaster: MTP Press pp. 171-219.

Ghanadian R, Puah CM (1983). Biochemical and morphometric evaluations of prostatic epithelial and stromal cells. In Ghanadian R (ed): "The Endocrinology of Prostate Tumours". Lancaster: MTP Press pp. 87-111.

Ghanadian R, Smith CB (1983). Metabolism of steroids in the prostate. In Ghanadian R (ed): "The Endocrinology of Prostate Tumours". Lancaster: MTP Press pp. 113-135.

Gleason DF, Mellinger GT (1974). Prediction of prognosis for prostatic adenocarcinoma by combined histological grading and clinical staging. J Urol 111:58-64.

Goustin AS, Leof EB, Shipley GD, Moses HL (1986). Growth factors and cancer. Cancer Res 46:1015-1029.

Griswold DP Jr, Schabel FM Jr, Dykes DJ, Trader MW, Laster WR Jr (1984). Concepts for the treatment of tumor metastasis. In Nicolson G, Milas L (eds): "Cancer Invasion and Metastasis: Biologic and Therapeutic Aspects". New York: Raven Press, pp.389-396.

Habib FK, Tesdale AL, Chisholm GD, Busuttil A (1981). Androgen metabolism in the epithelial and stromal components of the human hyperplastic prostate. J Endocr 91:23-32.

Habib FK, Beynon L, Chisholm GD, Busuttil A (1983). The distribution of 5ɑ-reductase and 3ɑ(β)-hydroxysteroid dehydrogenase activities in the hyperplastic human prostate gland. Steroids 41:41-53.

Habib FK, Odoma S, Busuttil A, Chisholm GD (1986). Androgen receptor status in cancer of the prostate : The impact of the stage and grade of the tumour on receptor content. Urol Res 14: n°13, 158.

Harper ME, Pike A, Peeling WB, Griffiths K (1984). Steroids of adrenal origin metabolized by human prostatic tissue both in vivo and in vitro. J Endocrinol 60:117-125.

Heppner GH (1984). Tumor heterogeneity. Cancer Res 44: 2259-2265.

Heppner GH, Miller BE, Miller FR (1983). Tumor subpopulation interactions in neoplasms. Biophys Biochim Acta 695: 215-226.

Heuson JC, Mattheiem WH, Longeval E, Deboel MC, Leclerq G (1975). Clinical significance of the quantitative assessment of estrogen receptors in breast cancer. In "Hormones and Breast Cancer". Editions de l'INSERM, Vol 55, pp.57-70.

Hicks LL, Walsh PC (1979). A microassay for the measurement of androgen receptors. Steroids 33:389-406.

Hudson RW, Moffitt PM, Owens WA (1983). Studies of the nuclear 5ɑ-reductase of human prostatic tissue: comparison of enzyme activities in hyperplastic, malignant, and normal tissues. Can J Biochem Cell Biol 61:750-755.

Hynes RO, Wyke JA, Bye JM, Humphryes KC, Pearlstein ES (1975). In Reich E, Rifkin PB, Shaw E (eds): "Proteases and Biological Control". New York: Cold Spring Harbor Laboratory pp:931-940.

Isaacs J (1982). Mechanisms for and implications of the development of heterogeneity of androgen sensitivity in prostatic cancer. In Owens AH Jr, Coffey DH, Baylin SB (eds) "Tumor Cell Heterogeneity : Origins and Implications", vol. 4, New York: Academic Press pp. 99-111.

Isaacs JT, Coffey DS (1979). Androgenic control of prostatic growth: regulation of steroid levels. In Coffey DS, Isaacs JT (eds): "Prostate Cancer". Geneva: UICC Technical Report Series, Vol 48, pp.112-125.

Isaacs JT, Isaacs WB, Coffey DS (1979). Models for development of nonreceptor methods for distinguishing androgen-sensitive and -insensitive prostatic tumors. Cancer Res 39:2652-2659.

Kliman B, Daly JJ, MacLaughlin RA, Eddleston MT, Prout GR
Jr (1982). Androgen receptors in relation to parenchymal
and stromal components of human benign prostatic hyperplasia. Surg Forum 33:627-629.
Krieg M, Grobe I, Voigt KD, Altenähr E, Klosterhalfen H
(1978). Human prostatic carcinoma: Significant differences in its androgen binding and metabolism compared to the
human benign prostatic hypertrophy. Acta Endocrinol 88:
397-407.
Krieg M, Bartsch W, Janssen W, Voigt KD (1979). A comparative study of binding, metabolism and endogenous levels of
androgens in normal, hyperplastic, and carcinomatous human
prostate. J steroid Biochem 11:615-624.
Krieg M, Braun BE, Lämmel A, Smith K (1981a). Androgen
receptor quantification with and without molybdate. Acta
Endocrinol 97: n°164, 243.
Krieg M, Klötzl G, Kaufmann Voigt KD (1981b). Stroma of
human benign prostatic hyperplasia: Preferable tissue for
androgen metabolism and oestrogen binding. Acta Endocrinol
96:422-432.
Krieg M, Schlenker A, Voigt KD (1985). Inhibition of androgen metabolism in stroma and epithelium of the human
benign prostatic hyperplasia by progesterone, estrone, and
estradiol. Prostate 6:233-240.
Kris RM, Libermann TA, Avivi A, Schlessinger J (1985).
Growth factors, growth-factor receptors and oncogenes.
Biotechnology 3:135-140.
Lahtonen R, Bolton NJ, Kontturi M, Vihko R (1983). Nuclear
androgen receptors in the epithelium and stroma of human
benign prostatic hypertrophic glands. Prostate 4:129-139.
Lämmel A, Krieg M, Klötz G (1983). Are fluorescein-conjuga-
ted androgens appropriate for a histochemical detection of
prostatic androgen receptors ? Prostate 4:271-282.
Levine AJ, Vande Woude GF, Topp WC, Watson JD (eds) (1984).
The Transformed Phenotype. In "Cancer Cells". Cold Spring
Harbor Laboratory.
Liang T, Cascieri MA, Cheung AH, Reynolds GF, Rasmusson GH
(1985). Species differences in prostatic steroid 5α-
reductases of rat, dog and human. Endocrinology 117:571-
579.
Lillehoj HS, Choe BK, Rose NR (1982). Monoclonal antibodies
to human prostatic acid phosphatase. Probes for antigenic
study. Proc Nat Acad Sci, USA, 79:5061-5065.

Lübbert H, Pollow K (1978). Correlation between the 17β-hydroxysteroid dehydrogenase activity and the estradiol and progesterone receptor concentration of normal and neoplastic mammary tissue. J Mol Med 3:175-183.

Magnusson S, Petersen TE, Sottrua-Jensen L, Claeys H (1975). In Reich E, Rifkin DB, Shaw E (eds): "Proteases and Biological Controls", Cold Spring Harbor Laboratory, pp. 123-131.

Martelli A, Soli M, Bercovich E, Prodi G, Grilli S, DeGiovanni C, Galli MC (1980). Correlation between clinical response to antiandrogenic therapy and occurrence of receptors in human prostatic cancer. Urology 16:245-249.

Martin PM (1985). Bases physiopathologiques de l'hormonothérapie dans le cancer du sein. In "Actualités Cancérologiques". Paris: Expansion Scientifique Française pp. 213-214.

Martin PM, Magdelenat H, Kelly P (1982). Simultaneous determination of estrogen, progestin and androgen receptors on small amounts of breast tumor cytosol. In F Cavalli et al. (eds): "International Symposium on Medroxyprogesterone Acetate". Geneva: Excerpta Medica pp. 544-588.

McGuire WL, Clark GM, Dressler LG, Owens MA (1986). Role of steroid hormone receptors as prognostic factors in primary breast cancer. In Lippman ME (ed) "NIH Concensus Development Conference on Adjuvant Chemotherapy and Endocrine Therapy for Breast Cancer", NCI Monographs n°1 pp. 19-23.

McKercher G, Chevalier S, Roberts KD, Blean G, Chapdelaine A (1984). 5α-reductase and 3β-hydroxysteroid dehydrogenase activities in isolated canine prostatic epithelial cells. J steroid Biochem 21:549-554.

McNeal JE (1979). New morphologic findings relevant to the origin and evolution of carcinoma of the prostate and BPH. In Coffey DS, Isaacs JT (eds): "Prostate Cancer". Geneva: UICC Technical Report Series, Vol 48 pp. 24-37.

McNeal JE (1981). Normal and pathologic anatomy of prostate. Urology (suppl), XVII:11-16.

Mobbs BG, Johnson IE, Connolly JG (1979). Protamins sulfate precipitation of androgen receptors in cytosols of human benign and malignant prostatic tumors. In Murphy GP, Sandberg AA (eds): "Prostate Cancer and Hormone Receptors". New York: Alan R. Liss pp. 13-32.

Mobbs BG, Johnson JE, Connolly JG (1981). Role of cytosol androgen receptor in determining androgen binding by prostatic nuclei. In Abstracts, n° 722, 63rd Annual Meeting of Endocrine Soc.

Moeller H, Oettling G, Fiederer B, Brügmann G (1983). A quantitative assay for the cytoplasmic androgen receptor using (^{3}H)dihydrotestosterone in the presence of NAD$^+$-nucleosidase. Acta Endocrinol 102:153-160.

Morioka M, Takeda K, Mitsuhata N, Ohashi T, Ohmori H, Saito T, Kanbegawa A (1982). Endogenous androgen levels of human prostatic tissues. Folia endocrinol jap 58:876-885.

Mullins DE, Rohrlich ST (1983). The role of proteinases in cellular invasiveness. Biophys Biochim Acta 695:177-214.

Müntzing J (1980). Androgen and collagen as growth regulators of the rat ventral prostate. Prostate 1:71-78.

Neet KE, Ainslie GR Jr (1980). Hysteretic enzymes. Methods in Enzymology 64:192

Nicolson GL (1983). Cancer metastasis. Organ colonization and the cell-surface properties of malignant cells. Biophys Biochim Acta 695:113-176.

NIH Concensus Development Conference on Adjuvant Chemotherapy and Endocrine Therapy for Breast Cancer (1986). In Lippman ME (ed), NCI Monographs, NIH Publication n°1.

Norris JS, Smith RG (1983). Androgen receptors. In Agarwal MK (ed): "Principles of Receptorology". Berlin: de Gruyter, pp. 207-271.

Nozumi K, Sato R, Ito H, Maruoka M, Shimazaki J (1981). Binding of dihydrotestosterone, R 1881 and R 5020 in cytosols from normal, benign hypertrophic and cancerous human prostates. Urol Int 36:79-87.

Ojasoo T, Raynaud JP (1978). Unique steroid congeners for receptor studies. Cancer Res 38:4186-4198.

Ossowski L, Quigley JP, Reich E (1975). Proteases and Biological Control. In Reich E, Rifkins PB, Shaw E (eds), Cold Spring Harbor Laboratory pp.901

Pertschuk LP, Rosenthal HE, Macchia RJ, Eisenberg KB, Feldman JG, Wax SH, Kim DS, Whitmore WF Jr, Abrahams JI, Gaetjens E, Wise GJ, Herr HW, Karr JP, Murphy GP, Sandberg AA (1982). Correlation of histochemical and biochemical analyses of androgen binding in prostatic cancer: relation to therapeutic response. Cancer 49:984-993.

Pertschuk LP, Macchia RJ, New-York Prostate Cancer Binding Site Study Group (1984). Histochemical androgen binding assay in prostatic cancer. J Urol 131:1096-1098.

Pertuiset BF, Moguilewsky M, Magdelenat H, Martin PM, Philibert D, Poisson M (1984). Sex steroid receptors in human meningioma and glioma. In Bresciani F et al. (eds). Prog Canc Res Ther 31 pp. 561-568.

Pinsky L, Kaufman M, Chudley AE (1985). Reduced affinity of the androgen receptor for 5α-dihydrotestosterone but not methyltrienolone in a form of partial androgen resistance. J Clin Invest 75:1291-1296.

Poste G (1983). Tumor cell heterogeneity and the metastatic process. In Rich MA, Hager JC, Furmanski P (eds): "Understanding Breast Cancer". New York: Marcel Dekker pp. 119-166.

Poste G, Greig R, Tzeng J, Koestler T, Corwin S (1984). Interactions between tumor cell subpopulations in malignant tumors. In Nicolson GL, Milas L (eds): "Cancer Invasion and Metastasis: Biologic and Therapeutic Aspects". New York: Raven Press pp. 223-244.

Prins GS, Lee C (1982). Effect of protease inhibitors on androgen receptor analysis in rat prostate cytosol. Steroids 40:189

Raynaud JP, Ojasoo T, Vaché V (1979). Unusual steroids in measuring steroid receptors. In Thompson EB, Lippman ME (eds): "Steroid Receptors and the Management of Cancer". CRC Press Inc, Boca Raton pp. 215-232.

Raynaud JP, Bouton MM, Martin PM (1980). Human prostate hyperplasia and adenocarcinoma: steroid hormone receptor assays and therapy. In Schröder FH, de Voogt HJ (eds): "Steroid Receptors, Metabolism and Prostatic Cancer". Amsterdam: Excerpta Medica pp. 165-181.

Rennie PS, Bruchovsky N, McLoughlin MG, Batzold FH, Dunstan-Adams EE (1983). Kinetic analysis of 5α-reductase isoenzymes in benign prostatic hyperplasia (BPH). J steroid Biochem 19:169-173.

Robel P (1984). Hormono-dépendance de la prostate humaine. La Presse Médicale 13:2117-2119.

Robel P, Eychenne B, Blondeau JP, Jung-Testas I, Groyer MT, Mercier-Bodard C, Hechter O, Roux C, Dadoune JP (1983). Androgen receptors in rat and human prostate. Hormone Res 18:28-36.

Robel P, Eychenne B, Blondeau JP, Baulieu EE, Hechter O (1985). Sex steroid receptors in normal and hyperplastic human prostate. Prostate 6:255-267.

Robinson E (1984). The fight against the delay in the diagnosis of cancer. Biomedicine 38:321-322.

Rohr HP (1979). New methods for the quantitative histopathology analysis of the prostate at the light and electron microscopic level: stereological correlations. In Coffey DS, Isaacs JT (eds): "Prostate Cancer". Geneva: UICC Technical Report Series, Vol 48, pp. 38-55.

Roy AB (1971). The steroid 5∝-reductase activity of rat liver and prostate. Biochimie 53:1031

Sandberg AA, Karr JP (1983). Steroid hormone receptors and prostate cancer. Clinics in Oncology 2:331–343.

Schulz P, Bauer HW, Fittler F (1985). Steroid hormone regulation of prostatic acid phosphatase expression in cultured human prostatic carcinoma cells. Biol Chem, Hoppe-Seyler 366:1033–1039.

Shain SA, Boesel RW (1978). Human prostate steroid hormone receptor quantitation. Current methodology and possible utility as a clinical discriminant in carcinoma. Invest Urol 16:169

Shain SA, Boesel R, Sannayan G, Radwin H (1980). Androgen receptors in prostatic carcinoma and hyperplasia. Cancer Res Proc 21: n°662.

Shain SA, Gorelic LS, Boesel RW, Radwin HM, Lamm DL (1982). Human prostate androgen receptor quantitation: effects of temperature on assay parameters. Cancer Res 42:4849–4854.

Smith T, Chisholm GD, Habib FK (1983a). Towards a reproducible method of estimating androgen receptors in human prostate. J steroid Biochem, 18:531–534.

Smith T, Chisholm GD, Habib FK (1983b). Nuclear androgen receptor determination in human prostate. J steroid Biochem, suppl 19: n°29, 10S.

Snochowski M, Pousette Å, Ekman P, Bression D, Andersson L, Högberg B, Gustafsson JÅ (1977). Characterization and measurement of the androgen receptor in human benign prostatic hyperplasia and prostatic carcinoma. J Clin Endocrinol Metab 45:920–930.

Spandidos DA (1985). Mechanism of carcinogenesis: the role of oncogenes, transcriptional enhancers and growth factors. Anticancer Res 5:485–498.

Stebbings WSL, Vinson GP, Anderson E, Puddefoot JR, Farthing MJG (1985). Hybrid ligand method for androgen receptor measurement. J Endocr suppl 104:30.

Stoscheck CM, King LE Jr (1986). Role of epidermal growth factor in carcinogenesis. Cancer Res 46:1030–1037.

Talmadge JE (1983). The selective nature of metastasis. Cancer Metastasis Reviews 2:25–40.

Trachtenberg J (1982). Current status of androgen receptor measurements in prostatic cancer. In Paulson DF (ed): "Genitourinary Cancer 1" Vol 6. Cancer Treatment and Research pp. 239–250.

Trachtenberg J, Walsh PC (1982). Correlation of prostatic nuclear androgen receptor content with duration of response and survival following hormonal therapy in advanced prostatic cancer. J Urol 127:466–471.

Traish AM, Müller RE, Wotiz HH (1981). A new procedure for the quantitation of nuclear and cytoplasmic androgen receptors. J Biol Chem 256:12028–12033.

Traish AM, Müller RE, Wotiz HH (1986a). Binding of 7α,17α-dimethyl-19-nortestosterone (Mibolerone) to androgen and progesterone receptors in human and animal tissues. Endocrinology 118:1327–1333.

Traish AM, Müller RE, Wotiz HH (1986b). A new exchange assay for the quantitation of prostatic androgen receptor complexes (AR) formed in vivo. Fed Proc 44: n° 6224.

van Aubel O, Bolt-de Vries J, Blankenstein M, Schröder F (1986). Does the nuclear androgen receptor content from cancerous prostatic tissue predict the duration of response following orchiectomy in patients with metastatic disease of the prostate ? Urol Res 14: n°14, 158.

van Steenbrugge GJ, van Dongen JJW, de Jong FH, Gallee MPW, Schroeder FH (1986). Androgens in a transplantable human prostate cancer cell line (PC 82) : Correlation with proliferation. Urol Res 14: n° 10, 157.

Vande Woude G, Levine AJ, Topp WC, Watson JD (eds) (1984). Oncogenes and viral genes. In "Cancer cells". Cold Spring Harbor Laboratory.

Vermeulen A, van Camp A, Mattelaer J, DeSy W (1979). Hormonal factors related to abnormal growth of the prostate. In Coffey DS, Isaacs JT (eds): "Prostate Cancer". Geneva: UICC Technical Report Series, Vol 48, pp. 81–92.

de Voogt HJ, Dingjan P (1978). Steroid receptors in human prostatic cancer : A preliminary evaluation. Urol Res 6: 151–158.

de Voogt HJ, Rao BR (1983). Present concept of the relevance of steroid receptors for prostatic cancer. J steroid Biochem 19:845–849.

Walsh PC, Hutchins GM, Ewing LL (1983). Tissue content of dihydrotestosterone in human prostatic hyperplasia is not supranormal. J Clin Invest 72:1772–1777.

Weiss L (1985). Differences between primary cancers and their metastases. In "Principles of Metastasis". New York: Academic Press pp. 257–299.

Wilbert DM, Griffin JE, Wilson JD (1983). Characterization of the cytosol androgen receptor of the human prostate. J Clin Endocrinol Metab 56:113

Zava DT, Landrum B, Horwitz KB, McGuire WL (1979). Androgen receptor assay with (^{3}H)methyltrienolone (R 1881) in the presence of progesterone receptors. Endocrinology 104: 1007–1012.

Prostate Cancer, Part A: Research, Endocrine
Treatment, and Histopathology, pages 141–143
© 1987 Alan R. Liss, Inc.

BIOCHEMICAL MARKERS IN HUMAN PROSTATE

Ledenko N., Mestayer C, Bongini M., Legrand
J.C., Wright F.
Service de Biochimie, Laboratoire 413, CHU
Pitié-Salpêtrière, 91 Boulevard de l'Hôpital 75634 Paris
Cedex 13, FRANCE.*

Androgen receptors and 5 α-dihydrotestosterone (DHT) levels in prostatic carcinoma may be of value in predicting responsiveness to anti-androgenic therapy. Benign prostatic hypertrophy (BPH), another androgen dependant desease, is also characterized by a 2 to 4 fold increases in DHT and androgen receptor content. However, in both pathologies, the exact mechanism responsible for these accumulations is yet to be established and could be of value in the understanding of the initiation processes for prostatic carcinoma where DHT is also implicated.

Cytosolic and nuclear androgen receptor, microsomal 5 α-reductase (the enzyme catalyzing the transformation of testosterone to the more portent androgen DHT) 3 α and ß hydroxysteroid oxydoreductases (transformation of DHT to 3 α and 3 ß diols) were measured in prostatic tissue. Moreover blood and tissue levels of T, Δ4-androstenedione and DHT were measured for all patients studied together with tissue 3 α diol and plasma estradiol (E_2) and progestone (P).

Hormones were measured by radioimmunoassays after extraction and purification on celite microcolums. Receptors were measured with tritiated R 1881, as ligand, alone or together with a 200 fold excess of cold R 1881 (SCATCHARD).

RESULTS :

Plasma assays
BPH (n = 37)   Laboratory means for
                              young male population (n 54)

testosterone :	5.04 ±2.16	5.92 ± 1.42 ng/ml
dihydrostestosterone :	0.66 ±0.26	0.31 ± 0.17 ng/ml
Δ 4 -Androstenedione :	0.89 ± 0.4	1.10 ± 0.36 ng/ml
Estradiol :	38.60 ± 21.80	33.60 ± 9.30 ng/ml
Progesterone :	1.10 ± 0.40	1.10 ± 0.40 ng/ml

Plasma DHT alone is significantly higher in BPH
($p < 0.05$)   SD are indicated

Tissue assays	*BHP (n = 15)*	*young men(5)*
cytosolic T (ng/g tissue)	0.24 ± 0.11	0.31 ± 0.21
DH "	5.36 ± 0.46	2.2 ± 0.93
Δ 4 "	0.08 ± 0.02	0.09 ± 0.04
3 α androstanediol	1.49 ± 0.39	1.86 ± 0.98
nuclear T (ng/g tissue)	1.54 ± 0.45	1.09 ± 0.44
DHT	3.22 ± 0.56	1.45 ± 0.54
Δ4	0.22 ± 0.07	0.18 ± 0.07
3 α androstanediol	3.20 ± 0.45	3.14 ± 1.11

Tissue DHT only is significantly higher both in cytisol and nuclei from
BPH tissue versus normal prostate

Receptor assays

BPH (n = 11)   normal young
men (5)

Cytosolic receptor

		BPH (n = 11)	normal young men (5)
Kd (nM)	=	0.176 ± 0.055	0.170 ± 0.098
Bmax (fmoles/mg P)	=	26.7 ± 11.3	34.2 ± 12.7

Nuclear receptor

Kd (nM)	=	0.194 ± 0.078	0.199 ± 0.102
Bmax (fmoles/mg/P)	=	57.7 ± 21.2	19.2 ± 13.9

<u>Microsomal 5 α reductase</u>
6 pmoles of 5 α reduced metabolites of testosterone produced in
normal prostatic tissue versus 12 pmole in BHP.
<u>Microsomal 3 α and 3 β HSOR</u>
no significant difference for β HSOR between the 2 groups. Higher 3
α HSOR in BPH versus normal tissue.
These results are discussed together with the role of 3 α
androstanediol in prostate.

In conclusion, DHT production is increased in BPH by both increased
tissue 5 α reductase and androgen receptor thus retaining this more
potent androgen in the nuclear fraction of this androgen target cell and
enhancing the hyperstimulation produced by this androgenic message.

* Results supported by a grant from A.R.C., the Comité de Paris
L.N.C.C. and the Scientific Consultation CHU.-P S.

Prostate Cancer, Part A: Research, Endocrine
Treatment, and Histopathology, pages 145–172
© 1987 Alan R. Liss, Inc.

NEW CONCEPTS ON THE ANDROGEN SENSITIVITY OF PROSTATE
CANCER

Fernand Labrie, Isabel Luthy, Raymonde Veilleux,
Jacques Simard, A. Bélanger and A. Dupont

MRC Group in Molecular Endocrinology and Medicine, Laval University Medical Center,
Quebec G1V 4G2, Canada

INTRODUCTION

Since the observations of Huggins and his colleagues
in 1941 (Huggins and Hodges, 1941), orchiectomy and treatment with estrogens have been the cornerstone of the management of advanced prostate cancer. These two approaches
cause improvement for a limited time interval in 60 to 80%
of cases, thus leaving 20 to 40% of the patients without
improvement of their disease (Nesbit and Baum, 1950; Jordan
et al., 1977; Mettlin et al., 1982; Murphy et al., 1983).
Moreover, progression of the cancer almost inevitably
occurs within 6 to 24 months in those who initially responded (Resnick and Grayhack, 1975) and 50% of the patients
are then expected to die within the next 6 months after
signs of disease progression (Johnson et al., 1977; Slack
et al., 1984). In addition to the limited and questionable
improvement in survival, orchiectomy is often psychologically unacceptable while estrogens cause serious side effects such as gynecomastia, fluid retention, myocardial
ischaemia and thromboembolism with a 15% death rate due to
cardiovascular complications during the first year of estrogen administration (Glashan and Robinson, 1981).

The finding that agonists of luteinizing hormone-releasing hormone (LHRH) cause a blockade in testosterone
formation in experimental animals (Labrie et al., 1978;
Labrie et al., 1980) accompanied by a loss in prostate
weight offered the possibility of replacing orchiectomy and
estrogens. In fact, in men, following a transient period of
stimulation, serum testicular androgens are reduced to

castration levels during chronic treatment with the well-
tolerated LHRH agonists (Labrie et al., 1980; 1982; Faure
et al., 1982; Warner et al., 1983; Waxman et al., 1983).
However, although LHRH agonists make castration more
acceptable than orchiectomy and free of the serious side
effects of estrogens, one cannot expect to improve the prognosis of prostate cancer beyond the results previously
achieved with orchiectomy since their effect is also
limited to the blockade of testicular androgens (Labrie et
al., 1980; 1982; 1985a).

As already observed in the first patient with prostate
cancer treated with an LHRH agonist (Labrie et al., 1980),
one limitation to the use of LHRH agonists alone for the
treatment of androgen-sensitive diseases is the rise in
serum testicular androgens which accompanies the first 5-10
days of treatment with the unacceptable risk of disease
flare during this period (Kahan et al., 1984; Waxman et al.,
1985; The Leuprolide Study Group, 1984). In addition, in
common with orchiectomy and treatment with estrogens, treatment with LHRH agonists has no influence on the adrenal
androgens which are left unopposed and continue to stimulate
prostate cancer growth after castration.

This presentation will summarize the ten arguments and
data, which independently, illustrate and stress the need to
use, always in addition to castration, a pure antiandrogen
at all times in patients with advanced prostate cancer in
order to more completely block androgens of both testicular
and adrenal origin and maximally inhibit prostate cancer
growth. Prostate cancer is the most hormone-sensitive of all
cancers and all available means should be used to maximally
block androgens in order to obtain, not simply a response,
but the best available response.

A.   HIGH CONCENTRATIONS OF DHT REMAIN IN THE PROSTATE
     CANCER TISSUE FOLLOWING CASTRATION

As illustrated in Fig. 1, a high level of the active
androgen dihydrotestosterone (DHT) remains in the prostatic
cancer tissue following castration. Although orchiectomy,
estrogens, or LHRH agonists (through blockade of bioactive
LH) cause a 90 to 95% reduction in serum testosterone (T)
levels (Labrie et al., 1980; Warner et al., 1973; Waxman et
al., 1983; Labrie et al., 1985a), a much smaller effect is

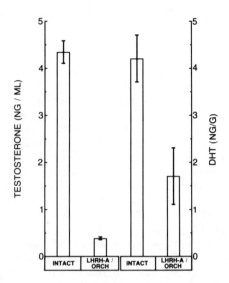

Figure 1. Effect of castration on the serum levels of T (A) and on the concentration of the active androgen DHT remaining in prostatic cancer tissue after castration (B). Note the relatively small effect (approximately 50%) of castration on intraprostatic DHT concentration as compared to the 90% fall in serum T.

observed on the really meaningful parameter of androgenic action, namely the concentration of dihydrotestosterone (DHT) in the prostatic cancer tissue.

Measurements of T and DHT levels in the serum have little or no value except as an index of testicular activity. In fact, the intraprostatic DHT concentration is the only significant parameter which indicates the level of the active androgen at its site of action in the prostatic cancer tissue itself. Unexpectedly high concentrations of DHT and 3α-diol (5α-androstane-3α,17β-diol) have been found in prostatic carcinoma after orchiectomy or DES treatment (Farnsworth and Brown, 1976; Geller et al., 1984; Bélanger et al., 1986a). This is best illustrated in Figure 1 where it can be seen that although orchiectomy causes a 90% to 95% fall in serum T level, the intraprostatic concentration of

the potent androgen DHT is reduced by only about 50%
(Farnsworth and Brown, 1976; Geller et al., 1984; Bélanger et
al., 1986a).

    Based on the intraprostatic levels of DHT measured
after castration, estrogen treatment or treatment with LHRH
agonists alone, the testes and adrenals are of approximately
equal importance in stimulating prostate cancer growth. Such
data stress the absolute need to neutralize the action of
the androgens of adrenal origin for an efficient treatment
of prostate cancer. Such high levels of DHT remaining after
surgical or medical castration are more than likely to have
an important stimulatory effect on the evolution of the
cancer. Clearly, with the knowledge of these data, a treatment limited to the blockade of androgens of testicular
origin only partially relieves the cancer from androgenic
stimulation. Moreover, measurements of serum levels of T
and DHT, although being excellent parameters of testicular
steroidogenic activity, are an inadequate index of intraprostatic androgenic activity.

B.   INTRAPROSTATIC ENZYMES CONVERT ADRENAL STEROID PRECUR-
      SORS INTO DHT

    Man is unique among species in having a high secretion
rate of adrenal steroids which are converted into active
androgens in peripheral tissues. Despite the discovery of
dehydroepiandrosterone sulfate (DHEA-S) in the serum in 1960
(Baulieu) and the fact that it is present in human serum at
far higher concentrations than any other steroid, the
biological function of this so-called adrenal androgen has
so far received little attention.

    The main androgen precursors of adrenal origin are
Δ^4-androstenedione (3 mg/day) and dehydroepiandrosterone
((DHEA, 24 mg/day) (Sanford et al., 1977)). The plasma levels
of Δ^4-androstenedione are 1.69 ± 0.88 ng/ml, whereas those of
T are 4.34 ± 0.24 ng/ml. The serum levels of DHEA and DHEA-S,
on the other hand, are 1.9 ± 0.3 ng/ml and 834 ± 147 ng/ml
(Labrie et al., 1985b). These weak adrenal androgens are
converted into strong androgens, not only in the prostatic
tissue (Acevedo and Goldziecker, 1965; Harper et al., 1974;
Voigt and Bartsch, 1986; Bélanger et al., 1986a) but also at
the peripheral level in other tissues.

Radioactive DHEA-S infused into patients is taken into prostatic tissue and transformed into DHEA, 5α-androstane-diol, T, and DHT (Harper et al., 1974)). Because DHEA-S is present in the circulation at such extremely high concentrations, only a small percentage of transformation of this steroid into DHT is sufficient to play a major role in the evolution of prostatic cancer. As expected, androstenedione, another steroid of adrenal origin, may also lead to a stimulatory response in the prostate. In fact, Acevedo and Gold-ziecker (1965) have observed that human prostatic tissue can metabolize androstenedione in vitro into T, androsterone, and 5α-androstanedione. Moreover, after in vivo infusion, Harper and associates (1974) have found an important transformation of this steroid in the prostatic tissue into T, DHT, androsterone, and 5α-androstenedione. Androst-5-ene-3β,17β-diol (Δ^5-diol), is another precursor of androgens in the prostatic tissue (Labrie et al., 1985b).

It is important to remember that direct production of T and DHT by the adrenals is minimal (Sanford et al., 1977). The importance of adrenal steroids in prostatic cancer is thus almost exclusively due to the intraprostatic metabolism of DHEA-S, DHEA, androstenedione, and Δ^5-diol into T and DHT. The low 5% level of T left in the circulation after castration is not a true image of the role of the adrenal androgens in prostate cancer tissue since T and DHT are made locally and only a small fraction is released intact in the circulation, thus corresponding to the low serum levels of both steroids measured after castration. In fact, DHT is mostly released into the blood as 3α-diol and androsterone and their glucuronide derivatives.

C. VARIABLE CONVERSION OF ADRENAL PRECURSORS INTO DHT IN DIFFERENT TUMORS

An important recent observation is that the enzymatic activity converting the adrenal steroids into DHT is highly variable between tumors. As a consequence, concentrations of on DHT similar to that found in intact men are found in the prostatic tissue of some castrated patients while, in others, DHT levels remain at more than 4 ng/g tissue after castration. In such patients, the high conversion rate of DHEA-S into DHT leads to high levels of intraprostatic DHT remaining after castration and, consequently, to the absence of clinical response of the cancer to castration.

D. HIGH SERUM LEVELS OF ANDROGEN METABOLITES OF ADRENAL
ORIGIN REMAIN AFTER CASTRATION

Table 1 shows the plasma levels of unconjugated and
glucuronated DHEA, Δ^5-diol, T, DHT, 3α-diol and androsterone
(ADT) in intact and castrated men with prostatic cancer. In
agreement with our previous results, the mean concentrations
of DHEA, which is primarily an adrenal steroid, were similar
in the two groups. As for the unconjugated steroids, the
DHEA-G concentration was similar in the two groups while the
levels of Δ^5-diol-G were diminished by 50% ($p < 0.01$) in
castrated men. Castration caused a decrease by more than 90%
($p < 0.01$) in plasma T and DHT levels as well as a diminution
of plasma 3α-diol (25%, $p < 0.05$) and ADT (42%, $p < 0.01$)
concentrations. Table 1 also indicates that except for DHT-G,
which was not detected in either intact and castrated men, T
and 5α-reduced steroid glucuronide levels, although lowered
in castrated men, remained at relatively high levels after
castration. Specifically, T-G, 3α-diol-G and ADT-G concentrations are 2.54 ± 0.31, 6.31 ± 0.72 and 11.84 ± 1.80 in intact
men and 0.72 ± 0.23, 1.79 ± 0.19 and 4.39 ± 0.69 ng/ml ($p <$
0.01), respectively, in castrated men. The most important
and original finding is however that 3α-diol-G and ADT-G,

TABLE 1. Plasma concentrations of unconjugated and glucuronated steroids in unoperated (20 pts) and castrated (18 pts)
men with prostatic cancer (Bélanger et al., 1986). Patients
were of comparable age.

Steroids	Unoperated men		Castrated patients	
	Unconjugated	Glucuronide	Unconjugated	Glucuronide
DHEA	2.40±0.34∞	4.25±0.68	1.91±0.24	4.45±0.69
Δ^5-diol	0.50±0.10	0.98±0.14	0.25±0.10*	0.40±0.06**
T	4.34±0.24	2.54±0.31	0.38±0.04**	0.72±0.23**
DHT	0.63±0.12	ND	0.05±0.01*	ND
3α-diol	0.51±0.05	6.31±0.72	0.38±0.03*	1.79±0.19**
ADT	0.38±0.02	11.84±1.80	0.22±0.04**	4.39±0.69**

∞ Mean ±SEM
*p < 0.05 unoperated vs castrated
**p < 0.01   "   "   "
ND: Not detectable

the two main metabolites of DHT, remain at 28 and 37% of control after castration, thus reflecting the high level of adrenal precursors converted into DHT in castrated men.

We can conclude from these data that adrenal androgens contribute to 30 to 40% of plasma 3α-diol-G and ADT-G in intact men. In agreement with our previous studies, the present data suggest that the measurement of these conjugated steroids provides more information on 5α-androgen formation from C-19 steroids than the unconjugated related steroids, which are at much lower plasma concentrations. Moreover, since the plasma concentrations of these steroid glucuronides are significantly correlated to those of DHEA, such data indicate that there is peripheral transformation of DHEA into androgens which are then converted into glucuronated 5α-reduced steroids.

With the measurement of additional steroids, our study is in agrement with previous reports indicating that C-19 steroids from the adrenals can be converted, in vivo, into potent androgens such as T and DHT. Furthermore, our data are in agreement with those recently published by Moghissi et al. (1984) which indicate that approximately 50% of 3α-diol-G is provided by C19-steroids from adrenal origin. Such data demonstrate the major importance of the adrenals in the pool of androgens in man.

E.   CLINICAL EVIDENCE THAT ANDROGEN-HYPERSENSITIVE TUMORS
     REMAIN AFTER CASTRATION AND DURING RELAPSE

That androgen-sensitive cancer cells remain active after surgical castration or high doses of estrogens is clearly illustrated by the finding that 33% to 39% of patients already castrated or treated with estrogens showed a positive response to the pure antiandrogen flutamide (Sogani et al., 1975; Stoliar and Albert, 1974). Moreover, after adrenal androgen suppression with aminoglutethimide in patients who had become refractory to orchiectomy and exogenous estrogens, a favorable response was observed in three of seven patients (Sanford et al., 1977). In a similar study, Robinson and coworkers found palliation in 50% of patients (Robinson et al., 1974).

The first bilateral adrenalectomy in prostatic cancer was performed by Huggins and Scott (1945) with appreciable success despite the lack of substitution therapy. Subsequently, bilateral adrenalectomy and hypophysectomy were used in advanced prostatic cancer with a significant rate of remission in previously castrated patients or those already treated with estrogens. In fact, bilateral adrenalectomy has been found to be associated with palliation in 20% to 70% of patients with advanced prostatic carcinoma who had become refractory to castration or estrogen therapy (Labrie et al., 1985b). Surgical hypophysectomy has also been found to improve transiently the disease in about 50% of patients (for review, see Labrie et al., 1985b). The benefits of additional antiandrogen therapy in relapsing patients can only be explained by the role of androgens of adrenal origin remaining at a significant level of action in the prostatic cancer after castration.

The common belief that patients in relapse after castration or treatment with estrogens have exclusively "androgen-insensitive" tumors should be abandonned. In fact, it is most likely that androgen-sensitive tumors are present at all stages of prostate cancer in all patients and that optimal androgen blockade should be performed in all cases. Instead of being "androgen-insensitive", most of (if not all) the tumors which continue to grow after castration are androgen-hypersensitive. These tumors are able to grow in the presence of the "low" level of androgens of adrenal origin left after castration. Control of the growth of these tumors requires further androgen blockade. This affirmation is supported by convincing clinical data as well as by well-established fundamental observations (Labrie et al., 1985b; Labrie and Veilleux, 1986).

Why aim for full androgen blockade? As mentioned above, this is necessary because of the presence of androgen-sensitive tumours in almost all (if not all) patients, even at the time of relapse. The observation by Fowler and Whitmore (1981) of a rapid and severe exacerbation, in 33 of 34 patients in relapse, within the first days of testosterone administration, shows extremely convincingly that prostate cancer remains almost (if not) always androgen sensitive. Moreover, as mentioned above, a second objective response is well known to be obtained in 30-45% of patients upon addition of further androgen blockade (antiandrogen, adrenalectomy, hypophysectomy, aminoglutethimide) after failure to respond to a first hormonal therapy (Labrie et al., 1985b)).

In perfect agreement with the large literature on the subject, we have recently found, in the largest series ever studied of 204 patients relapsing after orchiectomy or estrogens, a 33% objective response rate (USA National Prostatic Cancer Project criteria) to combination therapy. This indicates that in 33% of relapsing patients, growth of the prostatic cancer could have been prevented by the addition of a pure antiandrogen. In the other 66% of patients, although an objective response could not be obtained, subjective responses were seen in a significant proportion of cases. Due to the heterogeneity of the tumors, the presence of a single tumor which continues to grow classifies a patient as a non responder despite the frequent finding of a regression of the other tumors. Such a mixed response frequently improves the quality of life and is thus of significant benefit for the patients.

F.   BIOLOGICAL IMPORTANCE OF CASTRATION LEVELS OF SERUM ANDROGENS IN NORMAL AND CANCER TISSUES

A new finding of paramount importance is the biological significance of the apparently low levels of serum T and DHT which remain after surgical or medical castration in men. Castration levels of serum testosterone have so far been considered the aim as well as the biochemical evidence of the success of endocrine therapy. However, this endocrine parameter is highly misleading: as clearly demonstrated by recent data (Bartsch et al., 1983; Labrie et al., 1985b), a 90-95% inhibition of serum levels of testosterone cannot be taken as evidence for a similar inhibition of androgen action in target tissues. In fact, it has recently been demonstrated that the maintenance of serum T in castrated rats at levels similar to those found in orchiectomized men (0.2-0.4 ng/ml) causes an increase in prostate weight as high as 35-40% of the value found in intact animals (Bartsch et al., 1983; Marchetti et al., 1985). In another series of experiments, using the growth of androgen-sensitive Shionogi mammary carcinoma cells as parameter of androgen action, we have observed that castration levels of T and DHT can maintain growth of cancer cells in culture at values as high as 27 to 62% of maximal androgen-sensitive growth (Labrie and Veilleux, 1986).

As mentioned earlier, serum T levels in intact adult men usually range between 4 and 8 ng/ml while values of 0.2

to 0.4 ng/ml (5% of control) are observed after surgical or
medical castration. As an example, Fig. 2A shows respective
values of 4.49 ± 0.35 and 0.31 ± 0.02 ng/ml before and after
1 month of treatment of 12 men suffering from prostate cancer with the LHRH agonist [D-Trp[6]]LHRH ethylamide (Labrie et
al., 1985c). As illustrated in Fig. 2B, the important finding is that the apparently low castration levels of serum T
at 0.2 to 0.4 ng/ml stimulate growth of the androgen-sensitive mouse mammary carcinoma cells at 36-62% of the maximal growth rate which can be achieved at T levels corresponding to those found in intact men (4 to 8 ng/ml).

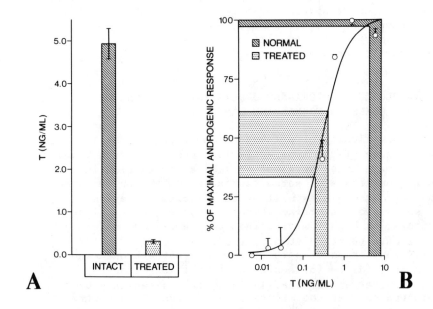

Figure 2. Effect on the growth of Shionogi mouse mammary
carcinoma cells of concentrations of testosterone (T) corresponding to the serum values found in the serum of intact
men (4-8 ng/ml) compared with growth achieved at T levels
corresponding to those obtained after surgical or medical
castration (0.2-0.4 ng/ml) (B) (Labrie and Veilleux, 1986).
Note that a 95% reduction in T concentration causes only a
38 to 64% reduction in cell growth. Panel A shows, as an
example, the serum T levels measured before and after 1
month of treatment of adult men suffering from prostate
cancer with the LHRH agonist [D-Trp[6]]LHRH ethylamide (Labrie
et al., 1985c).

The concentration of serum DHT in intact adult men usually ranges between 0.4 and 0.8 ng/ml and castration levels of DHT are at 0.04 to 0.08 ng/ml (Labrie et al., 1985c). The same group of patients shown in Fig. 2 had pre-treatment and treatment values of serum DHT of 0.55 ± 0.07 and 0.05 ± 0.03 ng/ml, respectively. Again, the impressive finding is that a reduction in serum DHT to 10% of control values decreases androgen-sensitive cell growth only from 74-84% to 27-41% of maximal androgen-sensitive cell growth (data not shown) (Labrie and Veilleux, 1986).

Contrary to the widely accepted dogma in the endocrine therapy of prostate cancer, the present data clearly demons-trate that castration levels of T and DHT retain an impor-tant stimulatory effect on androgen-sensitive growth in both normal and cancer tissue. In fact, the growth of a typical androgen-sensitive carcinoma cell line, namely the Shionogi mouse mammary carcinoma (SC-115), is stimulated at 27 to 62% of maximal growth by castration levels of T or DHT in the incubation medium. These data are in direct contradiction with the belief that the apparently low (5 to 10% of con-trol) serum concentration of serum T and DHT remaining after surgical or medical castration should have little, if any, influence on the growth of prostate cancer.

The present data obtained in an androgen-sensitive cancer cell line are in agreement with the elegant study of Barstch et al. (1983) performed in the normal rat prostate. These authors have shown, using Silastic implants of T, that the maintenance in castrated rats of serum T at the concen-tration found in the serum of castrated men leads to an approximately 10-fold higher concentration of DHT in the prostate tissue, thus causing a stimulation of prostatic weight as high as 30 to 40% of the value found in intact animals.

The physiological importance of relatively low levels of T and DHT in normal tissue had also been demonstrated in rat anterior pituitary cells in culture (Labrie et al., 1985b; Labrie et al., 1986a). Androgens are in fact well known to exert specific inhibitory effects on LHRH-induced LH release in adenohypophysial cells in culture. Using this precise and well-established in vitro system, we have obser-ved that reduction of the concentration of T in the incuba-tion medium to the values found in the serum of castrated men reduced the androgenic activity as reflected by the inhibition of LH release by only 50 to 70%.

The present data, those of Barstch et al. (1983), as
well as our previous observations (Labrie et al., 1985b;
Labrie et al., 1986; Marchetti et al., 1985), clearly demonstrate that low concentrations of androgens are highly active and that small variations of these low concentrations of
androgens can cause major changes in the responses observed
in various androgen-sensitive systems, namely cancer cell
growth (these data), growth of the normal rat prostate
(Bartsch et al., 1983; Marchetti et al., 1985) as well as
LHRH-induced LH release in normal rat gonadotrophs in culture (Labrie et al., 1985b; Labrie et al., 1986a). In these
three different systems, one common finding is that low
castration levels of T at approximately 5% of control can
maintain a high level of biological activity at 30 to 60% of
the level found under maximal stimulatory conditions. Concentrations of androgens below the adult physiological range
thus have major biological importance.

Based on the well-recognized observation that 20 to 40%
of patients with advanced prostate cancer do not respond to
surgical or chemical castration (Nesbit and Baum, 1950;
Jordan et al., 1977; Mettlin et al., 1982; Murphy et al.,
1983), it was generally believed that 20 to 40% of prostatic
carcinomas were already androgen-insensitive at the start of
treatment. As a much more likely explanation, the present
data suggest that the low but biologically important circulating levels of T and DHT remaining after castration are
responsible for most (if not all) of the uninterrupted
growth of prostatic cancer observed following standard hormonal therapy limited to the removal of testicular androgens. This is well supported by our recent observation that
less than 5% of patients with advanced prostate cancer continue to show progression of their disease when more complete androgen blockade is achieved with the pure antiandrogen
Flutamide administered in association with surgical or medical castration at start of treatment in order to more fully
block androgens (Labrie et al., 1985a; 1986a; 1986b).

The importance of adrenal androgens is particularly well
demonstrated by the finding of intraprostatic levels of DHT
as high as 1.5 ng/g tissue (3 nM) following castration or
treatment with estrogens (Geller et al., 1984; Labrie et
al., 1986b). Since the K_D value of DHT interaction with
the androgen receptor is less than 1 nM (Simard et al.,

1986; Asselin et al., 1980), it is clear that a concentration of 1.5 ng/ml or 5 nM DHT in the prostate cancer tissue is more than sufficient to exert a major stimulatory effect on cancer growth.

G. WIDE RANGE OF SENSITIVITIES OF TUMOR CELLS TO ANDROGENS

Clinical evidence in prostate cancer clearly indicates a marked heterogeneity of the sensitivity to androgens and the development of resistance to standard hormonal therapy. These data pertain to the failure of standard hormonal therapy in a proportion of previously untreated patients while a positive response can be obtained in most of these patients by further blockade of androgens (see Labrie et al., 1985b for review). In fact, while 20-40% of patients do not show a response to standard endocrine therapy (orchiectomy or estrogens), the response obtained in an important proportion of them by the addition of adrenalectomy, hypophysectomy or Flutamide clearly demonstrates that tumors were left growing under standard hormonal therapy which can be blocked by further androgen blockade. There is thus heterogeneity of androgen sensitivity among tumors present in the same patient as well as between different patients.

These clinical observations stress the importance of studying in detail the phenomenon of heterogeneity and development of true or apparent "treatment resistance" in originally androgen-sensitive cells. An excellent model for such studies is the androgen-dependent Shionogi mouse mammary carcinoma 115 (SC-115), a tumor showing rapid growth both in vivo and in tissue culture.

We have used this model to investigate the heterogeneity of androgen sensitivity in different clones obtained from a tumor as well as the changes of androgen sensitivity which occur during long-term culture of cloned cells. The present data clearly show that a wide range of hormone sensitivities are found in the clones derived from the original tumor and that, furthermore, heterogeneity develops during tissue culture of cloned cells. Such findings have major implications for the efficient treatment of prostate cancer where a population of hypersensitive cells can continue to grow in the presence of the low androgens of adrenal origin left after castration (medical or surgical).

As illustrated in Fig. 3, the 3 clones obtained from a Shionogi mouse mammary tumor show marked heterogeneity of sensitivity to DHT action. While the original tumor shows a Km value of DHT action at 0.9 nM, the Km values of DHT action in clones A, B and C were calculated at 0.024, 0.15 and 30 nM, respectively. There is thus a 1250-fold differrence in sensitivity to DHT between clones A and C obtained from a single tumor.

After 13 months in monolayer culture in the presence of 10 nM DHT, the original clone B was recloned in soft agar

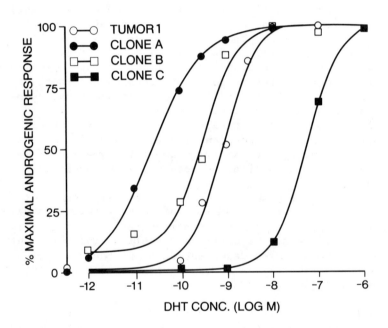

Figure 3. Effect of increasing concentrations of DHT on the maximal androgenic response (DNA content) in the 3 clones obtained from a Shionogi mouse mammary tumor. In order to facilitate visualization of differences in androgen sensitivity, all data are expressed as a percentage of the maximal response to DHT (Labrie et Veilleux, 1986). Note that there were also marked differences in basal growth in the absence of DHT as well as in the maximal response to DHT between the different clones.

and the growth sensitivity to DHT was again determined. As illustrated in Fig. 4, a marked heterogeneity of basal growth (in the absence of androgens), maximal response to DHT and sensitivity to DHT (Km values) was observed among the 10 clones obtained from one single cell. The growth rates in the absence of androgen varied by as much as 16-fold between clones 6 and 7 while the Km values ranged from 0.05 to 10 nM between clones 7 and 9 (200-fold variation).

The present data indicate that the Shionogi mouse mammary carcinoma tumors contain cell populations having a marked heterogeneity in terms of spontaneous growth in the absence of androgens as well as in terms of sensitivity of response and maximal growth responsiveness to androgens. Moreover, the present findings illustrate that such heterogeneity can develop under controlled conditions in culture in clones derived from an individual cell. Not only the

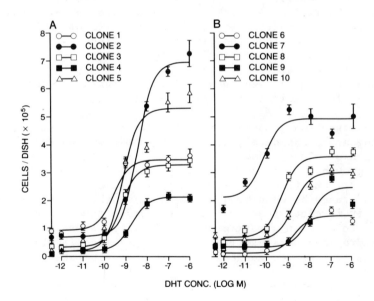

Figure 4. Effect of increasing concentrations of DHT on cell growth of 10 clones obtained after 13 months of culture of cloned cells B (Fig. 3) in medium containing 10 nM DHT (Labrie and Veilleux, 1986).

growth of the various clones shows heterogeneity in the absence of androgens but the maximal response to DHT also shows marked variations. However, the most significant observation is probably the heterogeneity of the sensitivity of cell growth to DHT. In fact, in clones obtained from the original tumor, there was a 1250-fold range of Km values of DHT action while a 200-fold range was observed in the clones obtained from a single original cell kept in culture for 13 months in the presence of DHT.

Although the origin of tumors is believed to be monoclo- nal (Dexter and Calabresi, 1982), it is clear that most, if not all, advanced tumors are composed of mixed populations of cells having a wide range of phenotypes. That heterogene- ity of androgen sensitivity analogous to the one described in this report exists in human prostate cancer is unequivoc- ally demonstrated by the clinical data showing a 30 to 50% response to adrenalectomy, hypophysectomy, Flutamide or aminoglutethimide in patients who relapse after orchiectomy or treatment with estrogens (Labrie et al., 1985b). Such a response to further androgen blockade in patients already castrated can only be explained by the presence in these patients of prostatic tumors which were still growing in the low androgenic environment provided by the adrenal androgens remaining after medical or surgical castration.

The situation in human prostate cancer thus appears to be analogous to the data presented in this study where a proportion of clones show supersensitivity to DHT with half- maximal growth at a concentration of DHT as low as 0.008 ng/ml (0.024 nM) (Fig. 2). Since the castration levels of serum DHT range between 0.04 and 0.08 ng/ml (Labrie et al., 1985b), it is clear that such hypersensitive tumors can continue to grow at a maximal rate following castration. For these androgen-hypersensitive tumors, castration levels of DHT are sufficient to maintain a maximal growth rate.

In addition to the second response observed in 30 to 50% of castrated patients following blockade of adrenal andro- gens, additional proof for the presence of androgen-super- sensitive prostatic carcinoma is provided by the recent findings that combined treatment of advanced prostate cancer with an LHRH agonist (or orchiectomy) in association with the pure antiandrogen Flutamide causes a positive response in 95% of patients (Labrie et al., 1985b; Labrie et al., 1986a; b). Since only 60 to 80% of patients were responding to castration (medical or surgical) (Nesbit and Baum, 1950; Jordan et al., 1977; Mettlin et al., 1982; Murphy et al., 1983), the increase in responders from 60-80 to 95% following the combination therapy indicates the presence of androgen-hypersensitive tumors in at least 15 to 35% of patients with advanced prostate cancer. These patients were previously thought to have "androgen-resistant" tumors at start of treatment while, on the contrary, they have androgen-hypersensitive tumors.

The approximately 5% of patients who do not respond to combination therapy might be bearing truly androgen-resistant or, alternatively, these tumors could well be even more androgen-sensitive and able to grow with the small fraction of free androgens remaining in their prostatic tumors in the presence of therapeutic doses of the antiandrogen and castration. Further blockade of adrenal androgen secretion and/or action will be needed to differentiate between these two possibilities.

The present data clearly show that tumors acquire a marked heterogeneity to androgens which has to be taken into account for the development of an effective therapeutical strategy. These pertain to the marked heterogeneity of sensitivity to androgens in the original Shionogi mouse mammary carcinoma and the clinical evidence observed in human prostate cancer. Moreover, starting with a single cloned cell, the development of similar heterogeneity can be reproduced under controlled conditions in vitro. The development of androgen-hypersensitive tumors remains the most serious problem facing the antihormonal therapy of prostate cancer and appropriate means must be found to achieve a complete antiandrogen blockade.

H.   HETEROGENEITY OF ANDROGEN RESPONSE DEVELOPS RAPIDLY AND CAN BE PREVENTED OR DELAYED BY FLUTAMIDE

While the heterogeneity of androgen responsiveness in both human prostate cancer and in an experimental model is well demonstrated (see above), one important question is how rapidly the heterogeneity of androgen responsiveness develops. As clearly observed in prostate and breast cancer, progression to treatment insensitivity is a major problem responsible for the usually partial and short-lived response to antihormonal therapy. This problem is particularly well illustrated in prostate cancer where inhibition of the secretion and/or action of adrenal androgens by adrenalectomy, hypophysectomy or the administration of Flutamide or aminoglutethimide causes a positive response of usually limited duration in only 30 to 50% of patients who have relapsed following surgical or medical castration while more than 95% of patients having received no previous treatment experience a positive response when similar complete androgen blockade is achieved at the start of treatment. Thus, while tumors resistant to the combined antihormonal therapy are present in only approximately 5% of patients having clinical stage D2 disease who received no previous treatment, the proportion of androgen-insensitive tumors increases to about 60% within the average 12 months of exposure to the adrenal androgens left after castration (Labrie et al., 1985b).

It should be mentioned that the failure to respond to antihormonal therapy seriously limits treatment alternatives since chemotherapy and radiotherapy have little success, especially at that late stage of the disease. We have thus used the androgen-sensitive Shionogi mammary cell carcinoma to study characteristics of the changes in androgen sensitivity (Luthy and Labrie, 1986).

Preincubation of Shionogi androgen-sensitive mouse mammary cells in the absence of androgen for 15 days completely eliminated the stimulatory effect of DHT on cell growth measured after 10 days of a second incubation in the presence of increasing concentrations of DHT (Luthy and Labrie, 1986). It could be seen in the same experiment that the presence of 0.03, 0.15 or 3 nM DHT during the 2-week preincubation period causes a progressive increase in both spontaneous cell growth (in the absence of androgen during the second incubation) and maximal growth response to DHT without affecting the apparent Km value of androgen action during the second incubation period.

Of potentially major therapeutic significance is the finding that preincubation with the pure antiandrogen Flutamide-OH can maintain the responsiveness of cell growth to DHT and thus prevent the rapid development of full resistance to androgens.

Although the existence of the phenomenon of treatment resistance is well demonstrated in human prostate cancer, the mechanisms involved are unknown. The only available information is that the resistance develops in approximately 60% of patients within one year after surgical or medical castration (Labrie et al., 1985b). The fact that the Shionogi mammary carcinoma can grow relatively fast both in vivo and in vitro and can be transformed from an androgen-sensitive to an "autonomous" state under both in vivo and in vitro conditions offers what appears to be the most appropriate model to study the factors involved in the development of resistance to antihormonal treatment.

Little is known about the mechanisms leading to such heterogeneity and resistance in hormone-sensitive tumors. A phenotypic mechanism could involve the selection of phenotypically altered cells (such as cell population groups affected under a low hormonal environment) or a change common to the whole cell population. The rapidity of the changes observed in the present study favors the latter possibility.

Using a well characterized model, the present data clearly demonstrae that the development of androgen resistance can be extremely rapid in the absence of androgens. Of potential major therapeutic significance is the finding that the development of androgen resistance can be prevented by simultaneous incubation with the pure antiandrogen Flutamide-OH. These preliminary data obtained with the Shionogi model offer new possibilities not only for studies of the molecular mechanisms responsible for the development of androgen resistance but also for the maintenance of androgen sensitivity in the presence of a pure antiandrogen.

I.   LOGARITHMIC NATURE OF THE BIOLOGICAL RESPONSE TO ANDROGENS FURTHER ILLUSTRATES THE IMPORTANCE OF "LOW" LEVELS OF DHT

As illustrated by the many examples presented in this section, the biological response to DHT (as well as the response to any biological stimulus) follows a logarithmic instead of a linear rule (Fig. 5). This implies that a decrease in serum DHT levels by 90% causes a much smaller inhibitory effect on the DHT-sensitive response which is decreased by less than 50% (Figs 2, 3 and 4). This observation is of major consequence since it indicates that by decreasing serum T and DHT levels by approximately 90% by medical or surgical castration, one leaves more than 50% of the androgenic stimulus on prostate cancer growth.

Another fact of major importance is that our inability to measure a steroid by presently available techniques because of lack of sensitivity should not be interpreted as meaning that the cellular mechanisms are unable to detect and respond to such apparently low levels of hormones. As illustrated in Fig. 5, the usual lower limit of sensitivity

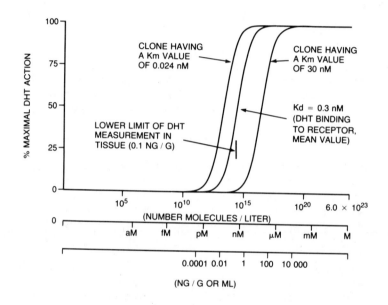

Figure 5. Dose-response curves of 2 clones of androgen-sensitive mouse mammary carcinoma SC-115 cells to increasing DHT concentrations expressed in absolute number of DHT molecules, in molarity and in ng/ml. Comparison is made with the usual mean affinity of binding of DHT to the androgen receptor. Data are from Labrie and Veilleux (1986) and Simard et al. (1986). The important observation is that levels of DHT below the lower limits of detection of current assays (0.1 ng/ml or g tissue) correspond to 1.0×10^{14} molecules of DHT per ml, thus leaving an extremely large number of DHT molecules with the potential for androgenic stimulation in normal tissues and especially in tumor cells having an hypersensitivity to androgenic stimulation (an example is the clone showing half-maximal growth at 0.008 nM DHT (left curve).

of current techniques for DHT measurement in serum or tissue is 0.1 ng/ml or g tissue. It should be realized that approximately 1×10^{14} molecules of DHT per ml or g tissue are left at this concentration of the androgen, thus leaving an extremely large number of DHT molecules free to stimulate cancer growth. As illustrated in this Figure, maximal growth of a clone of hypersensitive mouse mammary cells (SC-115) was obtained at DHT concentrations below the detection limits of presently available assays, the half-maximal stimulation being measured at 0.024 nM or 0.008 ng/ml DHT (Labrie and Veilleux, 1986).

J.   CONCLUSIONS

The antihormonal therapy of prostate cancer is based on the principle that prostate cancer development and growth is sensitive to androgens as originally suggested by Huggins and Hodges (1941). The second and recently established principle (Labrie et al., 1982; Labrie et al., 1985b) which is the basis for combined antihormonal therapy is that two sources, namely the testes and the adrenals, contribute about equally to the total amount of androgens active in the prostate (both normal and tumoral). A third fundamental principle recently elaborated (Labrie and Veilleux, 1986) is that androgen-sensitive tumors develop hypersensitivity to androgens, thus requiring a more efficient blockade of androgens for inhibition of their growth.

If one accepts that androgens stimulate prostate cancer growth, the next logical step in the treatment of this disease is to eliminate, as much as possible, all androgenic influences on prostate cancer with the best available drugs. Since the testes represent approximately 50% of androgens and appropriate means to eliminate this source of androgens are readily available, this should be an essential component of any antihormonal therapy of prostate cancer. With to-day's knowledge, the choice is between orchiectomy and the use of LHRH agonists. For the patients who accept surgical castration, this is certainly most valid. However, LHRH agonists are now widely available and there is no doubt that these peptides are a well-tolerated, safe and an efficient way to achieve a complete blockade of testicular androgen secretion (Labrie et al., 1980; Labrie et al., 1985a; Labrie et al., 1985b; Labrie et al., 1985c; Labrie et al., 1986a; 1986b).

Due to their high rate of serious cardiovascular side effects (Glashan and Robinson, 1981), estrogens, in our opinion, are no longer justified. In addition to a death rate as high as 15% due to estrogens during the first year of treatment (Glashan and Robinson, 1981), a finding which is sufficient by itself to prohibit their use, there is also evidence that estrogens can increase the level of prostatic androgen receptors, thus increasing the local activity of androgens (Moore et al., 1979; Mobbs et al., 1983). The elimination of approximately 50% of the androgens active in prostate cancer can thus be easily achieved by orchiectomy or treatment with LHRH agonists without any side-effect other than those related to the blockade of testicular androgens, namely hot flashes and a decrease or loss of libido.

The next easy and also highly efficient step is the oral administration of a pure antiandrogen such as Flutamide. For reasons discussed above, the administration of the antiandrogen should, without exception, be started at the same time as orchiectomy or first injection of the LHRH agonist. From our current knowledge on the pharmacokinetics of action of the antiandrogen, the first pill or tablet of Flutamide should be administered 2 hours before injection of the LHRH agonist or orchiectomy. The antiandrogen has a double beneficial action: firstly, it inhibits by approximately 50% the serum levels of the four adrenal steroids DHEA-S, DHEA, Δ^4-dione and Δ^5-diol, thus decreasing to the same extent the level of androgens from adrenal origin in the prostate cancer (Labrie et al., 1985b; Bélanger et al., 1984); secondly, it competes with the remaining adrenal androgens for the androgen receptor (Simard et al., 1986).

While medical or surgical castration causes a decrease in free intraprostatic DHT from approximately 3.0 to 1.5 ng/g tissue (Fig. 1), the addition of Flutamide causes a major additional decrease estimated to leave approximately 0.2 ng free DHT/g tissue. The combination of castration and Flutamide at the dose of 250 mg every 8 hours thus causes an estimated 95% decrease in intraprostatic free DHT. It should be mentioned that this approximately 95% blockade of androgens in prostate cancer tissue is achieved very easily with minimal or no side effect. It should be added that these values of free active DHT are approximate and based on the calculated affinities of DHT and Flutamide for the androgen receptor and the concentration of the respective substances in the prostate (Bélanger, Dupont and Labrie, unpublished data). Important variations also occur between patients as well as between individual tumors in each patient in terms of DHT and androgen receptor levels.

For the future, the next question is the usefulness of further androgen blockade after combination therapy. The response is most likely yes if the benefits of the added drug are not compensated by side-effects which affect the quality of life. The approximately 5% active DHT or 0.20 ng DHT/g tissue left in the cancer tissue after combination therapy can well play an important role in prostate cancer growth. The importance of these low levels of DHT is likely to vary with each tumor and different areas of the same tumor. In fact, although 0.20 ng DHT/g tissue is at the lower limit of current assays, it might well be in the range of sensitivities of some tumors or clones. As illustrated in Figs. 2, 4 and 5, the response of prostate cancer to androgens is logarithmic, thus further stressing the importance of low levels of DHT.

In summary, based on our current endocrinological, urological and biochemical knowledge, the drug that should be used in all cases of advanced prostate cancer is a pure antiandrogen such as Flutamide. It is the single most efficient inhibitor of androgen action in prostate cancer. However, this drug should never be used alone but always in combination with an LHRH agonist or surgical castration. With this combination therapy, excellent results are obtained with minimal side effects limited to hot flashes and a decrease or loss of libido. Although further androgen blockade might well be desirable and research efforts should be devoted to this subject, the other presently available drugs can only achieve a partial blockade of adrenal androgen secretion. All other drugs have an efficiency inferior to that of Flutamide, a drug that blocks most efficiently both adrenal androgen secretion and action (Labrie et al., 1985b; Bélanger et al., 1984). If one elects to use further blockade of adrenal secretion, these other drugs or measures should always be in addition to the combination therapy with Flutamide, a minimal standard therapy which should be continued for life.

Clinical trials on the benefits of combination therapy versus combination therapy plus aminoglutethimide and low dose hydrocortisone should be undertaken. It is also possi-

ble that the addition of an inhibitor of testicular androgen
secretion during the first two weeks of treatment with LHRH
agonists in order to block the transient rise in serum
androgens could be advantageous. This drug, like aminoglutethimide, however, should never be used alone but always in
combination with Flutamide and an LHRH agonist (or orchiectomy) since its inhibitory effect on adrenal steroid secretion is weaker than what can be more easily achieved with
Flutamide without side effect.

None of the above-mentioned drugs should be used alone,
combination therapy with an LHRH agonist (or orchiectomy) in
association with Flutamide being the minimal and standard
antihormonal regimen that should be used in all patients
suffering from advanced prostate cancer. Why leave tumors
grow under the influence of androgens when a well-tolerated
drug able to block these androgens is available? The time
for partial blockade of androgens in prostate cancer is
something of the past and unacceptable according to the most
up-to-date endocrine and biochemical scientific data available and are summarized above. The goal of all of us treating
advanced prostatic cancer should be the best possible response and not simply a response. We should not be satisfied
with a simple response as observed after castration but we
should only accept the best response available with combination therapy.

Since the combined antiandrogen blockade provides a
much higher rate of positive response at the start of treatment (95 vs 60-80%), and provides additional years of excellent quality of life with no side effects other than those
related to the blockade of androgens (hot flashes and a
decrease or loss of libido), it seems most logical to propose that the combination therapy with Flutamide should be
given as first treatment with no exception to all patients
having advanced prostate cancer and should be continued
without interruption for life. For all those who have received previous hormonal therapy, the combination treatment
remains the best approach since it permits a positive response in a large proportion of patients (33%, Labrie et al.,
1986c) with a good quality of life and a prolongation of
survival for those who respond. In order to decrease the
development of resistance to treatment, compliance is an
essential requirement: the combination therapy with Flutamide + LHRH agonist (in non castrated patients) should thus be
taken for life without any interruption.

REFERENCES

Acevedo HF, Goldziecker JW (1965). Further studies on the
metabolism of 4-[4-^{14}C]androstane-3,17-dione by normal and
pathological human prostatic tissues. Biochim Biophys Acta
97: 564.
Asselin J, Mélançon R, Moachon G, Bélanger A (1980). Characteristics of binding to estrogen, androgen, progestin and
glucocorticoid receptors in 7,12-dimethylbenz(a)anthrace-
ne-induced mammary tumors and their hormonal control.
Cancer Res 40: 1612.
Bartsch W, Knabbe M, Voigt KD (1983). Regulation and com-
partmentalization of androgens in rat prostate and muscle.
J Steroid Biochem 19: 929.
Baulieu EE (1960). Esters sulfates de stéroïdes hormonaux.
Isolement de l'ester sulfate de 5-androstene-3β,1-17-one
dehydroepiandrosterone (dans une tumeur cortico-surréna-
lienne). CR Acad Sci (Paris) 251: 1421.
Bélanger A, Dupont A, Labrie F (1984). Inhibition of basal
and adrenocorticotropin-stimulated plasma levels of adrenal androgens after treatment with an antiandrogen in
castrated patients with prostatic cancer. J Clin
Endocrinol Metab 59: 422.
Bélanger A, Labrie F, Dupont A (1986a). Androgen levels in
prostatic tissue of patients with carcinoma of the
prostate treated with the combined therapy using an LHRH
agonist and a pure antiandrogen. Eur J Cancer & Clin Oncol
22: 742.
Bélanger A, Brochu M, Cliche J (1986b). Levels of plasma
steroid glucuronides in unoperated and castrated men with
prostatic cancer. J Clin Endocrinol Metab 62: 812.
Dexter DL, Calabresi P (1982). Intraneoplastic diversity.
Biochim Biophys Acta 694: 97.
Farnsworth WE, Brown JR (1976). Androgen of the human prostate. Endocr Res Commun 3: 105.
Faure N, Labrie F, Lemay A, Bélanger A, Gourdeau Y, Laroche
B, Robert G (1982). Inhibition of serum androgen levels by
chronic intranasal administration of a potent LHRH agonist
in adult men. Fertil Steril 37: 416.
Fowler JE, Whitmore WF Jr (1981). The response of metastatic
adenocarcinoma of the prostate of exogenous testosterone.
J Urol 126: 372.
Geller J, Albert JD, Nachtsheim DA, Loza DC (1984). Comparison of prostatic cancer tissue dehydrotestosterone
levels at the time of relapse following orchiectomy or
estrogen therapy. J Urol 132: 693.

Glashan RW, Robinson MRG (1981). Cardiovascular complications in the treatment of prostatic carcinoma. Brit J Urol 53: 624.

Harper ME, Pike A, Peeling WB, Griffiths K (1974). Steroids of adrenal origin metabolized by human prostatic tissue both in vivo and in vitro. J Endocrinol 60: 117.

Huggins C, Scott WW (1945). Bilateral adrenalectomy in prostatic cancer. Ann Surg 122: 1031.

Huggins C, Hodges CV (1941). Studies of prostatic cancer. I. Effect of castration, estrogen and androgen injections on serum phosphatases in metastatic carcinoma of the prostate. Cancer Res 1: 293.

Johnson DE, Scott WW, Gibbons RP, Prout GR, Schmidt JD, Chu TM, Gaeta J, Sarott J, Murphy GP (1977). National randomized study of chemotherapeutic agents in advanced prostatic carcinoma: progress report. Cancer Treat Rep 61: 317.

Jordan WP, Blackard CE, Byar DP (1977). Reconsideration or orchiectomy in the treatment of advanced prostatic carcinoma. South Med J 70: 1411.

Kahan A, Delrieu F, Amor B, Chiche R, Steg A (1984). Disease flare induced by D-Trp^6-GnRH analogue in patients with metastatic prostatic cancer. Lancet 1: 971.

Labrie F, Auclair C, Cusan L, Kelly PA, Pelletier G, Ferland L (1978). Inhibitory effects of LHRH and its agonists on testicular gonadotropin receptors and spermatogenesis in the rat. In Hansson V (ed): Endocrine Approach to Male Contraception, Int J Androl (suppl 2): 303-308.

Labrie F, Bélanger A, Cusan L, Séguin C, Pelletier G, Kelly PA, Lefebvre FA, Lemay A, Raynaud JP (1980). Antifertility effects of LHRH agonists in the male. J Androl 1: 209.

Labrie F, Dupont A, Bélanger A, Cusan L, Lacourcière Y, Monfette G, Laberge JG, Emond JP, Fazekas ATA, Raynaud JP, Husson JM (1982). New hormonal therapy in prostatic carcinoma: combined treatment with an LHRH agonist and an antiandrogen. Clin Invest Med 5: 267.

Labrie F, Dupont A, Bélanger A, Lachance R, Giguère M (1985a). Long-term treatment with luteinizing hormone-releasing hormone agonists and maintenance of serum testosterone to castration concentrations. Brit Med J 291: 369.

Labrie F, Dupont A, Bélanger A (1985b). Complete androgen blockade for the treatment of prostate cancer. In De Vita Jr VT, Hellman S, Rosenberg SA (eds): Important Advances in Oncology, Philadelphia: JB Lippincott Company, p 193.

Labrie F, Dupont A, Bélanger A, Giguère M, Lacourcière Y, Emond J, Monfette G, Bergeron V (1985c). Combination therapy with Flutamide and castration (LHRH agonist or orchiectomy) in advanced prostate cancer: a marked improvement in response and survival. J Steroid Biochem 23: 833.

Labrie F, Veilleux R (1986). A wide range of sensitivities to androgens develops in cloned Shionogi mouse mammary tumor cells. The Prostate 8: 293.

Labrie F, Dupont A, Bélanger A, St-Arnaud R, Giguère M, Lacourcière Y, Emond J, Monfette G (1986a). Treatment of prostate cancer with gonadotropin-releasing hormone agonists. Endocr Rev 7: 67.

Labrie F, Dupont A, Bélanger A, Giguère M, Borsanyi JP, Lacourcière Y, Emond J, Monfette G, Lachance R (1986b). The importance of combination therapy with Flutamide and castration (LHRH agonist or orchiectomy) in previously untreated as well as previously treated patients with advanced prostate cancer. In: Hormonal Manipulation of Cancer: Peptides, growth factors and (anti)-steroidal agents. Raven Press, New York, in press.

Luthy I, Labrie F (1986c). The development of androgen resistance in mouse mammary tumor cells can be prevented by the antiandrogen Flutamide. The Prostate (in press).

Marchetti B, Plante M, Poulin, R. & Labrie F (1985). Dramatic response of prostate weight and ornithine decarboxylase to low levels of testosterone in castrated rats. J. Steroid Biochem. 36: 32S.

Mettlin C, Natarajan N, Murphy GP (1982). Recent patterns of care of prostatic cancer patients in the United States: results from the surveys of the American College of Surgeons Commission on Cancer. Int Adv Surg Oncol 5: 277.

Mobbs BG, Johnson IE, Connolly JG, Thompson J (1983). Concentration and cellular distribution of androgen receptor in human prostatic neoplasia: can estrogen treatment increase androgen receptor content? J Steroid Biochem 19: 1279.

Moghissi E, Ablan F, Horton R (1984). Origin of plasma androstanediol glucuronide in men. J Clin Endocrinol Metab 59: 417.

Moore RJ, Gazak JM, Wilson JD (1979). Regulation of cytoplasmic dihydrotestosterone binding in dog prostate by 17β-estradiol. J Clin Invest 63: 351.

Murphy GP, Beckley S, Brady MF, Chu M, DeKernion JB, Dhabuwala C, Gaeta JF, Gibbons RP, Loening SA, McKiel CF, McLeod DG, Pontes JE, Prout GR, Scardino PT, Schlegel JU, Schmidt JD, Scott WW, Slack NH, Soloway M (1983). Treatment of newly diagnosed metastatic prostate cancer

patients with chemotherapy agents in combination with
hormones versus hormones alone. Cancer 51: 1264.

Nesbit RM, Baum WC (1950). Endocrine control of prostatic
carcinoma: clinical and statistical survey of 1818 cases.
JAMA 143: 1317.

Resnick MI, Grayhack JT (1975). Treatment of stage IV carcinoma of the prostate. Urol Clin North Amer 2: 141.

Robinson RMG, Shearer RJ, Fergusson JD (1974). Adrenal suppression in the treatment of carcinoma of the prostate.
Br J Urol 46: 555.

Sanford EJ, Paulson DF, Rohner TJ, Drago JR, Santen RJ,
Bardin CW (1977). The effects of castration on adrenal
testosterone secretion in men with prostatic carcinoma. J
Urol 118: 1019.

Sciarra F, Sorcini G, Di Silverio F, Gagliardi V (1971).
Testosterone and 4-androstenedione concentration in peripheral and spermatic venous blood of patients with prostatic adenocarcinoma. J Ster Biochem 2: 313.

Simard J, Luthy I, Guay J, Bélanger A, Labrie F (1986).
Characteristics of interaction of the antiandrogen Fluta-
mide with the androgen receptor in various target tissues.
Mol Cell Endocrinol, in press.

Slack NH, Murphy GD, NPCP Participants (1984). Criteria for
evaluating patient responses to treatment modalities for
prostatic cancer. Urol Clin North Amer 11: 337.

Sogani PC, Ray B, Whitmore WF Jr (1975). Advanced prostatic
carcinoma: flutamide therapy after conventional endocrine
treatment. Urology 6: 164.

Stoliar B, Albert DJ (1974). SCH 13521 in the treatment of
advanced carcinoma of the prostate. J Urol 111: 803.

The Leuprolide Study Group (1984). Leuprolide versus
diethylstilbestrol for metastatic prostate cancer. New
Engl J Med 311: 1281.

Voigt KD, Bartsch W (1986). Intratissular androgens in
benign prostatic hyperplasia and prostatic cancer. J
Steroid Biochem, in press.

Warner B, Worgul TJ, Drago J, Demers L, Dufau M, Max D,
Santen RJ, Abbott Study Group (1973). Effect of very high
doses of D-Leucine[6]-gonadotropin-releasing hormone proethylamide on the hypothalamic-pituitary testicular axis
in patients with prostatic cancer. J Clin Invest 71:
1842.

Waxman JH, Was JAH, Hendry WF, Whitfield HN, Besser GM,
Malpas JS, Oliver RTD (1983). Treatment with gonadotropin-releasing hormone analogue in advanced prostatic
cancer. Brit Med J 286: 1309.

Waxman JH, Man A, Hendry WF, Whitfield HN, Tiptaft RC, Paris
AMI, Oliver RT (1985). Importance of early tumour exacerbation in patients treated with long acting analogues of
gonadotrophin releasing hormone for advanced prostatic
cancer. Brit Med J 291: 1387.

Prostate Cancer, Part A: Research, Endocrine
Treatment, and Histopathology, pages 173–197
© 1987 Alan R. Liss, Inc.

CURRENT CONCEPT FOR IMPROVING TREATMENT OF PROSTATE CANCER
BASED ON COMBINATION OF LH-RH AGONISTS WITH OTHER AGENTS

Andrew V. Schally, Tommie W. Redding, Jose I.
Paz-Bouza, Ana Maria Comaru-Schally, and
Georges Mathe
Endocrine, Polypeptide and Cancer Institute
VA Medical Center and Tulane University School of
Medicine, New Orleans, LA 70146 U.S.A.;
Institut de Cancerologie et d'Immunogenetique
(ICIG), 94800 – Villejuiff, FRANCE

Various experimental approaches for the treatment of
prostate cancer based on the use of analogs of luteinizing
hormone-releasing hormone LH-RH alone or in combination
with analogs of somatostatin and other peptides or with
chemotherapeutic agents are being investigated in animal
models of prostate tumors and human prostate cancer lines
transplanted to nude mice. The results obtained may
provide a rationale for testing these combinations of
compounds in patients with prostate cancer.

EFFECTS OF CHRONIC ADMINISTRATION OF LH-RH AGONISTS

Some LH-RH analogs substituted in position 6, 10 or
both, are much more active than LH-RH and also possess
prolonged activity (Schally and Kastin, 1971; Fujino et
al., 1974; Konig et al., 1975; Corbin et al., 1978; Schally
et al., 1980ab; Rivier et al., 1981a; Schally and Coy,
1983;). The most important LH-RH agonists and their
potencies are listed in Table 1. Although an acute
injection of superactive agonists of LH-RH induces a marked
and prolonged release of LH and FSH, paradoxically, chronic
administration produces dramatic inhibitory effects through
a process of "down regulation" of pituitary membrane
receptors for LH-RH, desensitization of the pituitary
gonadotrophs and reduction in gonadal receptors for LH and
FSH (Johnson et al., 1976; Auclair et al., 1977; Corbin et
al., 1978; Sandow et al., 1978; Hsueh and Erickson, 1979;

TABLE 1

LH-RH AGONISTS UNDERGOING CLINICAL TRIALS IN PATIENTS WITH TUMORS

LH-RH	STRUCTURE										RELATIVE POTENCY	ROUTE OF ADMINISTRATION
	1	2	3	4	5	6	7	8	9	10		
	p-Glu	His	Trp	Ser	Tyr	Gly	Leu	Arg	Pro	Gly-NH$_2$	1	—
Buserelin (Hoechst)		—————————————				D-Ser(TBU)—————————————				Ethylamide	100	SC,IN
Nafarelin (Syntex)		—————————————				D-(2-Nal) —————————————					100	SC,IN
Leuprolide (Abbott-Takeda)		—————————————				D-Leu —————————————				Ethylamide	50	SC
Lutrelin (Wyeth)		—————————————				D-Trp-7-N-Me-Leu —————				Ethylamide	100	
ICI-118630		—————————————				D-Ser(TBU)—————————————				Az-Gly-NH$_2$	50	SC,IM (DEPO)
Histrelin (Ortho)		—————————————				D-His(Bzl)—————————————				Ethylamide	100(?)	
Decapeptyl† (Triptorelin) (Debiopharm) (Lederle-American Cyanamid) (Ferring) (Ipsen-Beaufour Int.)		—————————————				D-Trp —————————————					100	MICROCAPSULES*

* Once a month, i.m. (SC, subcutaneous; IN, Intranasal; IM, Intramuscular)
† D-Trp-6-LH-RH Ethylamide (Generic) is also used by some groups

Revised and modified from Eisenberg et al, Journal of Clinical Oncology Vol 4, No 3:414-424, 1986.

Schally et al., 1980b; Sundaram et al., 1981; Corbin, 1982). In male animals this inhibition of pituitary–gonadal axis is manifested by a marked decrease in the secretion of LH, FSH, suppression of testicular steroidogenesis, a reduction in plasma testosterone levels, and fall in the weights of testes, seminal vesicles, and prostate (Corbin et al., 1978; Sandow et al., 1978; Hsueh and Erickson, 1979; Schally et al., 1980b). In men, a persistent suppression of Leydig cell function, manifested by a fall in serum testosterone and 5α–dihydrotestosterone (DHT), has been observed after chronic administration of D–Trp–6–LH–RH and other LH–RH agonists (Wiegelman et al., 1977; Happ et al., 1978; Bergquist et al., 1979; Linde et al., 1981; Tolis et al., 1981).

A highly simplified schematic representation of how LH–RH agonists affect pituitary-gonadal axis and the prostate is shown in Fig. 1. LH–RH agonists also exert some direct effects on the prostate (Hierowski et al., 1983). These phenomena form the basis for oncological applications of LH–RH agonists.

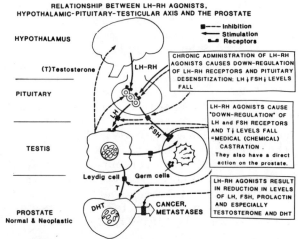

NOTE: Estrogen (DES) also inhibits the pituitary LH and FSH release and suppresses the prostate directly but stimulates prolactin and has major side effects.

Figure 1. Taken in part but adapted and modified from "Clinical Studies Using Luteinizing Hormone Releasing Hormone (LHRH)" by CA Paulsen et al., Population Center for Research in Reproduction, Dept of Medicine, U of Washington, Seattle. Used by permission from Dr. A Paulsen.

EXPERIMENTAL AND CLINICAL USE OF LH-RH AGONISTS IN PROSTATE CANCER

It is well established that about 70% of human prostate cancers are testosterone-dependent (Huggins et al., 1941; Whitmore, 1956; Walsh, 1975; Murphy, 1981). The treatment of advanced (stage C or D) prostate cancer is usually based upon androgen dependence of the tumor (Huggins et al., 1941; Whitmore, 1956; Walsh, 1975; Murphy, 1981). Endocrine therapy for carcinoma of the prostate includes orchiectomy, hypophysectomy, and administration of estrogens or antiandrogens (Geller and Albert, 1983). However, surgical castration is associated with a psychological impact while estrogens have cardiovascular, hepatic, and mammotropic side effects. The mortality from cardiovascular disease may be significantly increased in patients receiving Diethylstilbestrol (D.E.S.) therapy (Hedlund et al., 1980; Jacobi and Wenderoth, 1982), especially in doses higher than 3mg/day. A new, radically different endocrine therapy without apparent toxicity, is based on the use of agonistic analogs of LH-RH (Schally et al., 1983; 1984ab). The potential utility of D-Trp-6-LH-RH and other LH-RH agonists in the treatment of prostate carcinoma and other hormone-sensitive tumors in man was first demonstrated in studies in rat models of prostate cancer (Redding and Schally, 1981).

The finding that prolonged treatment with agonistic analogs of LH-RH can result in testicular inhibition and chemical castration prompted us to use this method in an attempt to induce the regression of prostate tumors in rat models (Redding and Schally, 1981). Treatment of male rats bearing the Dunning R3327H prostate adenocarcinoma with D-Trp-6-LH-RH reduced the percentage increase in tumor volume to one-third, and decreased actual tumor weight by 58% as compared to untreated controls. Serum LH, FSH, prolactin, and testosterone levels were significantly reduced after treatment with D-Trp-6-LH-RH.

The demonstration that D-Trp-6-LH-RH inhibits the growth of prostate tumors in rats led to clinical trials. The first successful palliative treatment of advanced prostatic carcinoma by agonistic analogs of LH-RH was shown in a collaborative trial carried out in 1979-81 at the Royal Victoria Hospital in Montreal (Tolis et al., 1982). The only side effects consisted of a decrease in libido and climacteric-like vasomotor phenomena. This trial demonstrated for the first time that superactive agonistic LH-RH analogs are efficacious therapeutic agents in patients with androgen-sensitive prostatic adenocarcinoma. These findings have been confirmed and extended by other clinical trials on the use of LH-RH agonists in patients with prostate cancer in Europe and North America (Warner et al., 1983; Labrie et al., 1983ab; Comaru-Schally et al., 1984; Borgmann et al., 1983; Mathe et al., 1984; Waxman et al., 1983; Walker et al., 1983; Ahmed et al., 1983; Allen et al., 1983; Gonzalez-Barcena et al., 1985; Koutsilieris and Tolis, 1983). In these trials, in addition to D-Trp-6-LH-RH (Decapeptyl), the agonists D-Ser(Bu^t)^6-des-Gly-NH$_2$^{10}-LH-RH ethylamide (HOE 766, Buserelin), D-Leu-6-des-Gly-NH$_2$^{10}-LH-RH ethylamide (Leuprolide) and Ser(bu^t)^{6}AZ-Gly^{10}-LH-RH(I.C.I. 118630 Zoladex) were used. These clinical results have been presented by others. And only some recent collaborative studies with D-Trp-6-LH-RH will be summarized here.

Gonzalez-Barcena, et al. (1985) treated twenty patients with stage D$_2$ prostatic carcinoma for up to 18 months with D-Trp-6-LH-RH. The analog was give s.c. once daily at a dose of 1,000 μg/day for the first 7 days. Subsequently, the dose was reduced to 100 μg/day. All patients had bone pain and high levels of acid and alkaline phosphatase. After the first week of D-Trp-6-LH-RH administration, major decreases in bone pain and reversal of the signs of prostatism were observed. Acid phosphatase gradually fell, achieving normal values after 12 weeks. Initial plasma testosterone was within normal limits, but during treatment with D-Trp-6-LH-RH it fell to castration levels. Resting values of PRL, GH, TSH, and cortisol did not show significant changes (Gonzalez-Barcena, et al., 1985). After TRH, TSH increased in five patients, but five did not respond. However, at 2 and 4 months, all patients released TSH in response to TRH. Two patients died during the treatment with D-Trp-6-LH-RH despite initial subjective responses and decreases in testosterone levels. The rise in acid phosphatase levels in these two patients was accompanied by a general deterioration, suggesting the emergence of an androgen-independent cancer (Gonzalez-Barcena et al., 1985). One patient who developed progressive hepatic, bone, and pulmonary metastases in spite of previous orchiectomy was also treated with the analog. Three months later his acid phosphatase levels were within normal values, and partial regression of metastases was observed.

In follow-up studies, Gonzalez-Barcena, et al. (1986), treated forty patients with Stage D$_2$ prostatic carcinoma for up to 30 months with D-Trp-6-LH-RH. As in the first study, the analog was given s.c. once daily at a dose of 1 mg/day for the first 7 days and subsequently, the dose was reduced to 100 µg/day.

Blood samples were taken before the injection of the analog and 1,2,4, and 6 hours later. Serum LH, FSH, and testosterone levels were measured by RIA. The initial administration of 1 mg D-Trp-6-LH-RH caused a marked elevation of LH and FSH that lasted more than 24 hours. One month later, and throughout the therapy, however, the basal values of LH and FSH were in the subnormal range and no increase in serum gonadotropins levels was obtained after administration of the analog. Initial plasma testosterone was within normal limits, but during treatment with D-Trp-6-LH-RH it fell to castration levels, and no increases were seen during the six hours following the injection of the analog. These results show that chronic administration of D-Trp-6-LH-RH at the doses used, blocks the pituitary-gonadal axis and that the escape phenomenon from the effects of the LH-RH agonists-induced blockade does not occur under our conditions, in contrast to the observations of Kerle et al. (1984) with the I.C.I. Analog Zoladex.

Mathe et al. (1986) treated eighty-one patients with prostatic carcinoma, mostly at stage D, with LH-RH agonist D-Trp-6-LH-RH (Decapeptyl) daily s.c. for 3 months in order to evaluate the incidence of remissions according to WHO recommendations for oncologic trials. The findings were compared to those obtained with other hormonal therapies of prostatic carcinoma according to the statistical method of "expected response rate" as adapted by Lee and Wesley for phase II trials. Treatment with D-Trp-6-LH-RH greatly reduced serum LH and testosterone levels without raising serum prolactin. After 1-2 weeks of therapy, there was relief of subjective symptoms and a reversal of the signs of prostatism, as well as marked decrease in bone pain. At 90 days, 52 patients had complete relief of prostatism and 21 had only mild signs and symptoms. Seventy patients were experiencing no bone pain and an additional 6 had only mild pain. Prostatic size evaluated by rectal examination and transabdominal ultrasonography reverted to normal in 26.4% of patients (complete remission) and was reduced by more than 50% in an additional 17.6% (partial remission); the overall rate of complete plus partial regression of prostatic enlargement being 44%. Scans showed a major improvement of bone lesions in 14.8% of cases. Prostatic acid phosphatase levels were decreased by more than half in 61% of the patients. No flare-up of the disease was encountered and there were no side effects, except for impotence. Statistical analyses of results indicated that the incidence of complete and partial regression (CR and PR) observed with D-Trp-6-LH-RH was not significantly different from that recorded in previous studies for another LH-RH analog, Buserelin. However, CR and PR obtained with D-Trp-6-LH-RH (44%) was significantly higher than that for orchiectomy (22%). The treatment of prostatic carcinoma with D-Trp-6-LH-RH avoids the cardiovascular and mammotropic side effects of estrogens, hepatic effects of some antiandrogens and the psychological impact of orchiectomy. These and other results demonstrated that D-Trp-6-LH-RH and other LH-RH agonists can be used as an effective endocrine therapy for advanced prostate carcinoma (Mathe et al., 1986).

EXPERIMENTAL STUDIES WITH LH-RH ANTAGONISTS

While repeated chronic administration of LH-RH agonists is required to induce a paradoxical inhibition of LH and FSH release and reduction in the levels of sex steroids, similar effects can be obtained with a single administration of LH-RH antagonists (Schally et al., 1980b; Rivier et al., 1981b; Schally and Coy, 1983). Antagonistic analogs of LH-RH were developed for contraception. Modern antagonists possess modifications in positions 1, 2, 3, 6, and 10 (Rivier et al., 1981a; Schally, 1983). These antagonists act on the same receptor sites as LH-RH and cause an immediate inhibition of the release of gonadotropins and sex steroids. A series of potent LH-RH antagonists has been synthesized and tested chronically in animals and acutely in human beings (Schally, 1983). In women and primates, these antagonists disrupt the menstrual cycle and block ovulation. In male rats, administration of LH-RH antagonists has been shown to decrease gonadotropin and testosterone levels and reduce the weights of testes and accessory sex organs (Rivier et al., 1981b).

Successful suppression of prostate tumors by chronic administration of the agonist D-Trp-6-LH-RH prompted us to investigate whether inhibitory analogs would also have an effect (Redding et al., 1982; Schally et al., 1983). Several antagonistic analogs including: N-Ac-D-p-F-Phe^1,p-Cl-D-Phe^2,D-Trp-^{3,6},D-Ala-^{10}-LH-RH, N-Ac-D-p-Cl-Phe^{1,2},D-Trp-3,D-Phe^6,D-Ala^{10}-LH-RH, and N-Ac-D-p-Cl-Phe^{1,2},D-Trp^3,D-Arg^6,D-Ala^{10}-LH-RH have been used in our studies on rat models of prostate tumors. In rats bearing the Dunning R3327H prostate adenocarcinoma, treatment with these antagonists decreased the percentage increase in tumor volume and diminished actual tumor volume compared to controls. Tumor weights were also markedly decreased. Tumor doubling time was three-to four-fold longer in rats receiving inhibitory analogs than in controls. Serum LH, FSH, and testosterone levels were significantly decreased after treatment with inhibitory analogs (Redding et al., 1982; Schally et al., 1983).

The inhibition of prostate carcinomas by antagonistic LH-RH analogs is probably due to the suppression of plasma levels of testosterone, although LH-RH analogs might also act directly on prostatic tumors (Hierowski et al., 1983). The use of antagonistic analogs of LH-RH for the treatment of prostate cancer would avoid the transient stimulation of the release of gonadotropins and testosterone that occurs initially in response to LH-RH agonists, thus preventing the temporary clinical flare-up of the disease (Schally et al., 1984ab). However, because of some side effects such as edema and erythema, no chronic clinical studies have been performed so far with LH-RH antagonists in the fields of contraception or cancer. A clinical evaluation of more recent LH-RH antagonists, which might be free of side effects in the treatment of prostate cancer, and a comparison of their therapeutic efficacy with D-Trp-6-LH-RH and other agonists would be most interesting.

DEVELOPMENT OF LONG-ACTING DELIVERY SYSTEMS FOR D-TRP-6-LH-RH

The therapy for prostate cancer was made more practical and efficacious by the development of a long-acting formulation of microcapsules of D-Trp-6-LH-RH for controlled release over a period of 30 days (Redding et al., 1984; Asch et al., 1985; Mason-Garcia et al., 1985). The delayed-release formulation was in the form of microcapsules prepared by a phase separation process. The resulting product was a free-flowing powder of spherical particles consisting of Decapeptyl (2% w/w) distributed in a polymeric matrix of 53:47 (mol %) of a biodegradable, biocompatible polymer (DL-lactide-co-glycolide) (98% w/w). The microcapsules were loaded in disposable syringes and sterilized with a 2 Megarad dose of gamma radiation. This procedure did not affect the biological activity of the peptide. Just before intramuscular administration, the microcapsules were suspended in an injection vehicle containing 2% carboxymethylcellulose and 1% Tween 20 in water. Once-a-month intramuscular injection of D-Trp-6-LH-RH decreased the growth of the androgen-dependent Dunning R3327H prostate tumors in rats and suppressed serum testosterone levels more effectively than daily subcutaneous administration of unencapsulated D-Trp-6-LH-RH. The once-a-month use of microcapsules makes the therapy with D-Trp-6-LH-RH more convenient and it should also better ensure patient compliance.

Roger et al. (1985), provided evidence for the efficacy of periodic administration of Decapeptyl microcapsules for suppressing testicular secretion in patients with prostate cancer. Each patient received, intramuscularly, an injection equivalent to 3mg Decapeptyl in microcapsules designed to deliver, in a controlled fashion, a daily dose of 100 µg D-Trp-6-LH-RH for 30 days. Seven men with a prostatic carcinoma received subcutaneously 500 µg Decapeptyl/day for seven days and in addition received on days 8, 28, and 56 an IM injection of Decapeptyl microcapsules. Plasma LH and FSH peaked on day 2. In 5 men high testosterone levels were maintained from day 2 to day 4, and then fell abruptly on day 6. In the other two subjects, testosterone secretion was completely suppressed after the second IM injection.

Parmar et al. (1985), compared the safety and efficacy of a delayed release formulation of D-Trp-6-LH-RH microcapsules with orchiectomy in the treatment of advanced prostatic carcinoma. Forty-one patients were randomly assigned to D-Trp-6-LH-RH and 38 patients to orchiectomy. Suppression of testosterone and reduction in prostatic acid phosphatase were similar in both groups. Overall, 87% of the patients in the D-Trp-6-LH-RH group and 81% of the orchiectomy group had an objective response to treatment. Side effects related to the decrease in testosterone were similar in both groups. Three patients in the D-Trp-6-LH-RH group experienced a disease "flare" in the first 10 days of treatment, which resolved completely with the fall in testosterone to castrate levels. There was a trend on follow-up towards decreased psychological morbidity in the D-Trp-6-LH-RH group. It was concluded that the slow-release preparation of D-Trp-6-LH-RH microcapsule is equally efficacious as orchiectomy and offers an important new method free of side effects in the management of advanced prostatic carcinoma (Parmar et al., 1985).

EFFECTS OF COMBINATIONS OF LH–RH AGONISTS WITH ANTIANDROGENS

The existing results warrant continuation of large scale clinical trials with LH-RH agonists to establish their long-term efficacy. For the treatment of advanced prostate carcinoma, however, it is possible that the therapeutic response could be improved by combining LH-RH agonists with other compounds including antiandrogens, peptides such as somatostatin analogs or PIF and various chemotherapeutic agents.

Antiandrogens, which neutralize the effect of endogenous androgens, have been used in the management of prostate cancer in man (Walsh and Korenman, 1971; Smith et al., 1973; Stoliar and Albert, 1974; Sogani et al., 1975; Neumann and Schenck, 1976; Menon and Walsh, 1980; Rost et al., 1981; Geller and Albert, 1983; Raynaud et al., 1984). In some clinical trials, a combination of HOE 766 with antiandrogens RU-23908 or Flutamide was used for treatment of patients with stage C and D_2 prostate carcinoma (Labrie et al., 1983ab; 1984ab). It was stated that the combined treatment with the LH-RH analog and antiandrogen is more effective than the analog alone (Labrie et al., 1984a). On the basis of these results we decided to study the effects of a simultaneous administration of the antiandrogen flutamide and microcapsules of the agonist D-Trp-6-LH-RH in the Dunning R3327H rat prostate adenocarcinoma model to determine whether the combination of these two drugs might inhibit tumor growth more effectively than single agents

(Redding and Schally, 1985). Microcapsules of D-Trp-6-LH-RH, calculated to release a controlled dose of 25µg/day for a period of 30-days, were injected intramuscularly once a month. Flutamide was administered s.c. at a daily dose of 25 mg/kg. The therapy was started 100 days after the tumor transplantation and continued for 60 days. Tumor weights and volumes were significantly reduced in rats treated with Decapeptyl microcapsules or flutamide alone, but microcapsules inhibited tumor growth more than the antiandrogen. The combined treatment of flutamide and Decapeptyl microcapsules significantly decreased tumor weight and volume, but did not exert a synergistic effect on tumor growth, the reduction being smaller for the combination than for the Decapeptyl alone. There was a significant elevation of serum testosterone, LH, and prolactin in rats treated with flutamide. On the other hand, in rats given microcapsules of D-Trp-6-LH-RH, testosterone fell to castration levels within 7 days and remained at nondetectable values, serum LH and prolactin levels also being suppressed in this group. The combined administration of microcapsules and flutamide also significantly decreased serum testosterone to nondetectable levels by day 7 and suppressed serum LH and prolactin (Redding and Schally, 1985). Our findings raise doubts whether the combination of microcapsules of an agonist like D-Trp-6-LH-RH with small doses of antiandrogens offers an advantage over the use of LH-RH agonists alone in the treatment of prostatic carcinoma. Until additional results become available, the benefits gained from adding antiandrogen to therapy with LH-RH agonists remain controversial.

COMBINATION OF LH-RH AGONISTS WITH SOMATOSTATIN ANALOGS OR PIF (PROLACTIN INHIBITING FACTOR)

Prolactin has been shown to stimulate prostate growth to enhance metabolic processes in the prostate and to potentiate the response of the prostate to 5-dihydrotestosterone (DHT) (Grayhack et al., 1955; Grayhack, 1963; Thomas and Keenan, 1976; Negro-Vilar, et al., 1977; Muntzing et al., 1977; Holland and Lee, 1980; Assimos et al., 1984; Blankenstein et al., 1985; Coert et al., 1985; Johnson et al., 1985). Consequently, prolactin could be involved in prostate cancer as a cofactor. Inhibition of both testosterone and prolactin would thus be expected to suppress prostate cancers more effectively than a deficiency of androgen alone.

Somatostatin analogs and peptides with PIF (prolactin inhibiting factor) activity inhibit prolactin release (Schally et al., 1986). Somatostatin analogs also suppress growth hormone secretion and have direct antiproliferative effect on cells resulting in growth inhibition (Mascardo and Sherline, 1982; Schally et al., 1984a, 1986ab; Cai et al., 1985; Hierowski et al., 1985) (Fig. 2). The reduction in prolactin levels produced by the administration of a suitable somatostatin analog or a peptide with PIF activity combined with the decrease in serum testosterone which results from chronic treatment with LH–RH agonists may inhibit growth of prostate tumors better than LH–RH agonists alone (Cai et al., 1986; Schally et al., 1986b). Decrease in GH levels induced by somatostatin analogs might also contribute to an additional inhibition of tumor growth. A simplified schematic representation of how somatostatin analogs or PIF could be used alone or together with LH–RH agonists for the treatment of prostate cancer is shown in Fig 2.

PROPOSED USE OF SOMATOSTATIN ANALOGS AND PIF FOR THE TREATMENT
OF PROSTATE CANCER IN COMBINATION WITH LH–RH AGONISTS

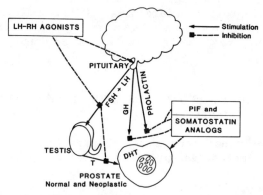

Prolactin enhances metabolic and proliferative processes in the prostate and may potentiate the action of DHT. Somatostatin analogs and/or PIF inhibit prolactin release. Somatostatin analogs also suppress growth hormone and have direct antiproliferative effect on cells (growth inhibition)

Figure 2.

Evidence obtained in animal models of prostate tumors is in agreement with this hypothesis. In Dunning R3327H model of prostate adenocarcinoma in Copenhagen-Fisher rats, twice daily s.c. administration of 25 µg D-Trp-6-LH-RH or the analog L-5F-Trp-8,D-Cys-14-somatostatin significantly reduced the tumor volume (Schally et al., 1986a). The combination of somatostatin analog with D-Trp-6-LH-RH resulted in even greater reduction in tumor volume than that which was obtained with the LH-RH agonist alone (Schally et al., 1986a).

Modern superactive octapeptide analogs of somatostatin including D-Phe-Cys-Tyr-D-Trp-Lys-Val-Cys-Thr-NH$_2$ (RC-121), in doses of 2.5 µg b.i.d. significantly decreased the weight and volume of Dunning R3327H prostate cancers and when given in combination with once-a-month D-Trp-6-LH-RH microcapsules potentiated the effects of the latter. The investigation of microcapsules of somatostatin analog D-Phe-Cys-Tyr-D-Trp-Lys-Val-Cys-Trp-NH$_2$ (RC-160) designed for a controlled release of this analog over a 30-day period, revealed that they inhibited the growth of Dunning prostate tumors when given alone. Combination of injectable microcapsules of D-Trp-6-LH-RH with microcapsules of RC-160 resulted in a synergistic potentiation of the inhibition of tumors. The combination of LH-RH agonists with somatostatin analogs could result in an increase in the therapeutic response in prostate cancer. It is possible that somatostatin analogs could be developed for use as adjuncts to Decapeptyl in the treatment of prostate cancer in man.

COMBINATION OF LH-RH AGONISTS WITH CHEMOTHERAPY

Long-acting delivery systems based on microcapsule formulation of D-Trp-6-LH-RH in biodegradable polymer poly (DL-Lactide-co-glycolide) for once-a-month administration, suppress testosterone levels over a 30-day period, make the treatment more convenient and efficacious as compared with daily administration and ensure patient compliance (Redding et al., 1984; Schally et al., 1984a; Parmar et al., 1985). This approach could become the method of choice for the endocrine treatment of prostate carcinoma. Still, the duration of remissions may be limited, as hormonal manipulations do not prevent the ultimate growth of hormone-independent cells (Geller and Albert, 1983; Mukamel et al., 1980; Schmidt et al., 1980; Isaacs et al., 1981; Murphy et al., 1983; Isaacs, 1984). Fig. 3 shows a highly simplified schematic representation of these phenomena. It is well established for other hormonal approaches that, in the majority of patients, the duration of remission is limited and a relapse to androgen-ablation therapy eventually occurs (Murphy et al., 1983). The mechanism responsible for the relapse of prostate cancer after surgical or medical castration is attributed to a selective proliferation of clones of androgen-independent cancer cells, which pre-existed within a predominantly androgen-sensitive but heterogeneous tumor (Isaacs et al., 1981; Isaacs, 1984). While hormone-dependent tumor cells stop growing after androgen ablation, the testosterone-insensitive cells are able to proliferate and eventually become predominant (Isaacs, 1984). Thus, the aim of combining hormonal therapy with chemotherapy would be to delay or prevent this situation and to prolong the survival. The use of both approaches, endocrine and chemotherapeutic, given together, may increase the rate of response and its duration.

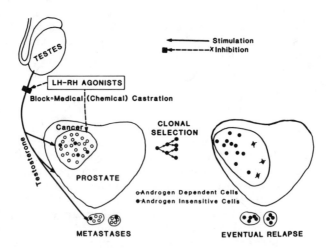

THERAPY OF PROSTATE CANCER WITH LH-RH AGONISTS ONLY

Figure 3.

The effect of combining hormonal treatment consisting of long-acting microcapsules of the agonist D-Trp-6-LH-RH with the chemotherapeutic agent cyclophosphamide was investigated in the Dunning R3327H rat prostate cancer model (Schally and Redding, 1985). Microcapsules of D-Trp-6-LH-RH calculated to release 25µg/day were injected intramuscularly once a month. Cyclophosphamide (Cytoxan) (5 mg/kg of body weight) was injected intraperitoneally twice a week. The treatment was started 2 months after transplantation, when the developing tumors measured 60-70mm^3 and continued for 100 days. The microcapsules of D-Trp-6-LH-RH reduced tumor volume more than Cytoxan did, and the combination of the two drugs appeared to completely arrest tumor growth. Tumor weights also were diminished significantly, but the decrease in weight was smaller in the Cytoxan-treated group than in rats that received the microcapsules. The combination of Cytoxan plus the microcapsules was much more effective than the single agents in reducing tumor weights (Schally and Redding, 1985). Testes and ventral prostate weights were significantly diminished and serum testosterone and prolactin values were reduced by administration of microcapsules of D-Trp-6-LH-RH alone or in combination with Cytoxan (Schally and Redding, 1985). Novantrone (Mitoxantrone), an agent belonging to the same class of anthracenedione antibiotics as Adriamycin, but less toxic, was also used in combination with microcapsules of D-Trp-6-LH-RH. Again, the combination with Novantrone (0.25 mg/kg i.v. every 21 days) led to a better inhibition of prostate cancer than D-Trp-6-LH-RH microcapsules alone and in fact, arrested tumor growth. Pathological examination of the tumors showed a very important decrease in the number of cells and also an increment in the connective tissue in the group treated with the combination of microcapsules with Novantrone. These histological results suggest that the combination therapy inhibits the growth of the tumoral cells and that these cells are replaced by connective tissue. The fibroblastic proliferation may indicate a favorable response to therapy.

These results in rats suggest that combined administration of long-acting microcapsules of D-Trp-6-LH-RH with a chemotherapeutic agent, started soon after the diagnosis of prostate cancer is made, might inhibit the proliferation of androgen-dependent and independent cells (Fig. 4), improve further the therapeutic response, and increase the survival rate. A simultaneous or sequential administration of hormonal treatment based on microcapsules of the LH–RH agonist and chemotherapy should be superior to either modality alone, since a single approach affects only a portion of the tumor population. The timing of such combined therapy may be of great importance as suggested by studies in experimental rat models (Isaacs, 1984) and in patients (Mukamel et al., 1980; Schmidt et al., 1980). Since the response to chemotherapy might be potentiated by an early and transitory increase in testosterone levels after initial administration of LH–RH agonists, our present view is that the combined therapy should be initiated together, with chemotherapy being given several hours after the first administration of LH–RH agonists (Mathe et al., 1986).

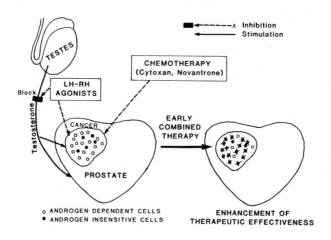

COMBINED THERAPY OF PROSTATE CANCER WITH LH–RH AGONISTS AND CHEMOTHERAPY

Figure 4.

Direct Effects of LH–RH Analogs on Prostate Tumors

Our findings indicate that D–Trp–6–LH–RH could have some direct inhibitory effect on prostate tumors. We have been unable to find LH–RH receptors in normal rat prostate tissue, but we observed binding of D–Trp–6–LH–RH to plasma membranes from Dunning R3327H prostate tumors (Hierowski et al., 1983). The binding of a powerful antagonist, Ac-D-p-Cl-Phe-1,2,D-Trp-3,D-Lys-6,D-Ala-10-LH-RH to plasma membranes from the same rat prostate tumors was also observed (Hierowski et al., 1983). Recently, we also showed that D-Trp-6-LH-RH inhibits directly the growth of several human prostate cancer cell lines in vitro. Addition of 10^{-5} to 10^{-6} M concentration of D-Trp-6-LH-RH significantly inhibited the uptake of tritiated thymidine in LNCAP, DU-145 and PC-3 cell lines. These findings support the view that LH-RH analogs, in addition to their main effect which is exerted on the pituitary, and a possible action on the gonads also act directly on prostatic tumors.

CONCLUSIONS

Clinical results accumulated so far indicate that long-term therapy with agonists of LH-RH is the preferred alternative to surgical castration or therapy with estrogens in men with advanced prostate cancer. Our experimental findings suggest that combination of once-a-month controlled delivery system of D-Trp-6-LH-RH with chemotherapy or with somatostatin analogs could further improve therapeutic response in men with prostatic cancer. These approaches will be tried clinically in the near future. Methods based on the use of LH-RH agonists in combination with somatostatin analogs or with modern chemotherapeutic agents might supplement or replace present procedures for the treatment of hormone-sensitive prostate cancers. An increase in the survival rate of patients with prostate cancer appears as an attractive target for future clinical trials.

ACKNOWLEDGEMENTS

We thank the National Hormone and Pituitary Program (NHPP) for the gifts of materials used in radioimmunoassays. The experimental work described in this paper was supported by the National Institutes of Health Grants AM07467 and CA 40003 (to A.V.S.) and by the Medical Research Service of the Veterans Administration. We thank Ms. Nancy Meadows for the preparation of figures.

REFERENCES

Ahmed SR, Brooman PJC, Shalmet SM, Howell A, Blacklock NJ, Rickards D (1983). Treatment of advanced prostatic cancer with LHRH analog ICI 118630: clinical response and hormonal mechanisms. Lancet ii:415–518.

Allen JM, O'Shea JP, Mashiter K, Williams G, and Bloom SR (1983). Advanced carcinoma of the prostate: treatment with a gonadotrophin releasing hormone agonist. Br Med J 286:1607–1609.

Asch RH, Rojas FJ, Bartke A, Schally AV, Tice T, Siler-Khodr TM, Klemcke HG, Bray RE, Hogan MP (1985). Prolonged suppression of plasma LH levels in male rats after a single injection of an LH–RH agonist in poly(DL-lactide-co-glycolide) in microcapsules. J Androl 6:83–88.

Assimos D, Smith C, Lee C, Grayhack JT (1984). Action of prolactin in regressing prostate: independent of action mediated by androgen receptors. Prostate, 5:589–595.

Auclair C, Kelly PA, Coy DH, Schally AV, Labrie F (1977). Potent inhibitory activity of (D–Leu–6–Des–Gly–NH$_2$) LH–RH ethylamide on LH/hCG and PRL testicular receptor levels in the rat. Endocrinology 101:1890–1893.

Bergquist C, Nillius SJ, Bergh T, Skarin G, Wide W (1979). Inhibitory effects on gonadotropin secretion and gonadal function in men during chronic treatment with a potent stimulatory luteinizing hormone-releasing hormone analogue. Acta Endocrinol 91:601–608.

Blankenstein MA, Bolt-de Vries J, Coert A, Nievelstein H, Schroder FH (1985). Effect of long-term hyperprolactinemia on the prolactin receptor content of the rat ventral prostate. Prostate, 6:277–283.

Borgmann V, Nagel R, Al-Abadi H, Schmidt-Gollwitzer M (1983). Treatment of prostatic cancer with LH–RH analogs. Prostate, 4:553–568.

Cai RZ, Szoke B, Fu D, Redding TW, Colaluca J, Torres-Aleman I, Schally AV (1985): In: Synthesis and Evaluation of Activities of Octapeptide Analogs of Somatostatin: Ninth American Peptide Symposium, Toronto. In Deber CM, Hruby VJ, Koppel KD (eds), "Peptides, Structure and Function," Rockford, IL: Pierce Chemical Co, pp 627–630.

Cai RZ, Szoke B, Lu R, Fu D, Redding TW, Schally AV (1986). Synthesis and biological activity of highly potent octapeptide analogs of somatostatin. Proc Natl Acad Sci USA 83:1896–1900.

Corbin A (1982). From contraception to cancer: A review of the therapeutic applications of LH–RH analogs as antitumor agents. Yale J Biol Med 55:27–47.

Corbin A, Beattie CW, Tracy J, Jones R, Foell TJ, Yardley J, Rees RWA (1978). The anti-reproductive pharmacology of LH–RH and antagonistic analogs. Int J Fertil 23:81–92.

Coert A, Nievelstein H, Kloosterboer HJ, Loonen P, Van der Vries J (1985). Effect of hyperprolactinemia on the accessory sexual organs of the male rat. Prostate 6:269–276.

Comaru-Schally AM, Ramalho A, Leitao PR, Schally AV (1984). Clearance of lung metastases of prostate carcinoma after treatment with LH–RH agonist. Lancet ii:281–282.

Fujino M, Fukuda T, Shanagawa S, Kobayashi S, Yamazaki I, Nakayama R, Seely JH, White WF, Rippel RH (1974). Synthetic analogs of luteinizing hormone releasing hormone (LH–RH) substituted in positions 6 and 10. Biochem Biophs Res Commun 60:406–413.

Geller J, Albert JD, (1983). Comparison of various hormonal therapies for prostatic carcinoma. Sem Oncol 10 (Suppl. 4):34–41.

Gonzalez-Barcena D, Perez-Sanchez P, Ureta-Sanchez S, Dominguez HB, Graef-Sanchez A, Morales MB, Comaru-Schally AM, Schally AV (1985). Treatment of advanced prostatic carcinoma with D-Trp-6-LH–RH. Prostate 7:21–30.

Gonzalez-Barcena D, Perez-Sanchez P, Berea-Dominguez H, Graef-Sanchez A, Becerril-Morales M, Comaru-Schally AM, and Schally AV (1986). Persistent blockade of the pituitary-gonadal axis in patients with prostatic carcinoma during chronic administration of D-Trp-6-LH–RH. Prostate, in press.

Grayhack JT (1963). Pituitary factors influencing growth of the prostate. Natl Cancer Inst Monogr, 12:189–199.

Grayhack JT, Bunce PL, Kearns JW, Scott WW (1955). Influence of the rat pituitary on prostatic response to androgen in the rat. Bull Johns Hopkins Hosp 96:154–163.

Happ J, Scholz P, Weber T, Cordes U, Schramm P, Neubauer M, Beyer J (1978). Gonadotropin secretion in eugonadotropic human males and postmenopausal females under long-term application of a potent analog of gonadotropin-releasing hormone. Fertil Steril 30:674–678.

Hedlund PO, Gustafson H, Sjogren S (1980). Cardiovascular complications to treatment of prostate cancer with estramustine phosphate (Estracyl) or conventional estrogen. A follow-up of 212 randomized patients. Scand J Urol Nephrol Suppl 55:103-105.

Hierowski MT, Liebow C, duSapin K, and Schally AV (1985). Stimulation by somatostatin of dephosphorylation of membrane proteins in pancreatic cancer MIA PaCa-2 cell line. FEBS Lett 179:252-256.

Hierowski MT, Altamirano P, Redding TW, Schally AV (1983). The presence of LH-RH-like receptors in Dunning R-3327H prostate tumors. FEBS Lett. 154:92-96.

Holland JM, Lee, C (1980). Effects of pituitary grafts on testosterone stimulated growth of rat prostate. Biol Reprod 22:351-355.

Hsueh AJW, Erickson GF (1979). Extra-pituitary inhibition of testicular function by luteininzing hormone-releasing hormone. Nature 281:66-67.

Huggins C, Stevens RE, Hodges CW (1941). Studies on prostatic carcinoma. II. The effect of castration on advanced carcinoma of the prostate gland. Arch Surg 43:209-211.

Isaacs JT (1984). The timing of androgen ablation therapy and/or chemotherapy in the treatment of prostatic cancer. Prostate 5:1-17.

Isaacs JT, Coffey DS (1981). Adaptation versus selection as the mechanism responsible for the relapse of prostatic cancer to androgen ablation therapy studied in the Dunning R-3327-H adenocarcinoma. Cancer Res 41:5070-5075.

Jacobi GH, Wenderoth UK (1982). Gonadotropin-releasing hormone analogues for prostate cancer: untoward side effects of high-dose regimens acquire a therapeutical dimension. Eur Urol 8:129-134.

Johnson B, Gendrich RL, White WF (1976). Delay of puberty and inhibition of reproductive processes in the rat by a gonadotropin-releasing hormone agonist analog. Fertil Steril 27:853-860.

Johnson MP, Thompson SA, Lubaroff DM (1985). Differential effects of prolactin on rat dorsolateral prostate and R3327 prostatic tumor sublines. J Urol 133:1112-1120.

Kerle D, Williams G, Ware H, Bloom SR (1984). Failure of long-term luteinizing hormone releasing hormone treatment for prostatic cancer to suppress serum luteinizing hormone and testosterone. Br Med J 289:468-469.

Konig W, Sandow J, Geiger R (1975). Structure-function relationships of LH-RH/FSH-RH. In Walter R, Meienhofer J (eds): "Peptides: Chemistry Structure and Biology," Ann Arbor: Ann Arbor Science Pub, Inc, pp 883-888.

Koutsilieris M, Tolis G. (1983). Gonadotropin releasing hormone agonistic analogs in the treatment of advanced prostatic carcinoma. Prostate 4:569–577.

Labrie F, Belanger A, Dupont A, Emond J, Lacoursiere Y, Monfette G (1984a). Combined treatment with LHRH agonist and pure antiandrogen in advanced carcinoma of prostate. Lancet ii:1090.

Labrie F, Dupont A, Belanger A, Lacoursiere Y, Raynaud JP, Gareau J, Fazekas ATA, Monfette G, Girard JG, Emond J, Houle JG (1983a). New approach in the treatment of prostate cancer: Complete instead of only partial removal of androgens. Prostate 4:579–594.

Labrie F, Dupont A, Belanger A, Emond J, Monfette G (1984b). Simultaneous administration of pure antiandrogens, a combination necessary for the use of luteinizing hormone-releasing hormone agonists in the treatment of prostate cancer. Proc Natl Acad Sci USA, 81:3861–3863.

Labrie F, Dupont A, Belanger A, Lefebvre FA, Cusan L, Monfette G, Laberge JG, Emond JP, Raynaud JP, Husson JM, Fazekas ATA (1983b). New hormonal treatment in cancer of the prostate: Combined administration of an LHRH agonist and an antiandrogen. J Steroid Biochem 19:999–1007.

Linde R, Doelle GC, Alexander N, Kirchner F, Vale W, Rivier J, Rabin D (1981). Reversible inhibition of testicular steroidogenesis and spermatogenesis by a potent gonadotropin-releasing hormone agonist in normal men. N Engl J Med 305:663–667.

Mascardo RN, Sherline P (1982). Somatostatin inhibits rapid centrosomal separation and cell proliferation induced by epidermal growth factors. Endocrinology 111:1394–1396.

Mason-Garcia M, Vigh S, Comaru-Schally AM, Redding TW, Somogyvari-Vigh A, Horvath J, Schally AV (1985). Radioimmunoassay for D-Typ[6] analog of luteinizing hormone-releasing hormone: measurement of serum levels after administration of long-acting microcapsule formulation. Proc Natl Acad Sci USA 82:1547–1551.

Mathe G, Schally AV, Comaru-Schally AM, Mauvernay RY, VoVan ML, Machover D, Misset JL, Court B, Bouchard P, Duchier J, Morin P, Keiling R, Schwarzenberg L, Kerbart P, Achille E, Tronc JC, Fendler JP, Pappo E, Metz R, Prevot G (1986). A phase II trial with D-Trp-6-LH-RH in prostatic carcinoma: a comparison with other homonal agents. Prostate, in press.

Mathe G, VoVan ML, Duchier J, Misset JL, Morin P, Keiling R, Schwarzenberg L, Kerbrat P, Achille E, Tronc JC, Machover D, Fendler, JP, Pappo E, Metz R, Prevot G, Comaru-Schally AM, Schally AV (1984). On oriented phase-II trial of D-Trp-6-LH-RH in patients with prostatic carcinoma. Med Oncol Tumor Pharmacother 1:119-122.

Menon M, Walsh PC (1980). Hormonal therapy for prostatic cancer. In Murphy, GP (ed): "Prostatic Cancer," Littleton, MA: PSG Publishing Co., Inc., pp 175-199.

Mukamel E, Nissenkorn I, Servadio C (1980). Early combined hormonal and chemotherapy for metastatic carcinoma of prostate. Urology 16:257-260.

Muntzing J, Kirdani R, Murphy GP, Sandberg AA (1977). Hormonal control of zinc uptake and binding in the rat dorsolateral prostate. Invest Urol 14:492-495.

Murphy GP (1981). Prostate cancer: continuing progress. Cancer J Clin 31:96-110.

Murphy GP, Beckley S, Brady MF, Chu TM, deKernion JB, Dhabuwala C, Gaeta JF, Gibbons RP, Loening SA, McKiel CF, McLeod DG, Pontes JE, Prout GR, Scardino PT, Schlegel JU, Schmidt JD, Scott WW, Slack NH, Soloway MS (1983). Treatment of newly diagnosed metastatic prostatic cancer patients with chemotherapy agents in combination with hormones versus hormones alone. Cancer 51:1264-1272.

Negro-Vilar A, Saad WA, McCann, SM (1977). Evidence for a role of prolactin in prostate and seminal vesicle growth in immature male rats. Endocrinology 100:729-737.

Neumann F, Schenck B. (1976). New antiandrogens and their mode of actions. J Reprod Fertil (Suppl.) 24: 129-145.

Parmar H, Lightman SL, Allen L, Phillips RH, Edwards L, Schally AV (1985). Randomised controlled study of orchidectomy vs. long-acting D-Trp-6-LH-RH microcapsules in advanced prostatic carcinoma. Lancet ii:1201-1205.

Raynaud JP, Bonne C, Moguilewsky M, Lefebvre FA, Belanger A, Labrie F (1984). The pure antiandrogen RU 23908 (Anandron), a candidate of choice for the combined antihormonal treatment of prostatic cancer: A Review. Prostate 5:299-311.

Redding TW, Coy DH, Schally AV (1982). Prostate carcinoma tumor size in rats decreases after administration of antagonists of luteinizing hormone-releasing hormone. Proc Natl Acad Sci USA 79:1273-1276.

Redding TW, Schally AV (1981). Inhibition of prostate tumor growth in two rat models by chronic administration of D-Trp-6-LH-RH. Proc Natl Acad Sci USA 78:6509-6512.

Redding TW, Schally AV (1985). Investigation of the combination of the agonist D-Trp-6-LH-RH and the antiandrogen flutamide in the treatment of Dunning R-3327H prostate cancer model. Prostate 6:219-232.

Redding TW, Schally AV, Tice TR, Meyers WE (1984). Long-acting delivery systems for peptides: inhibition of rat prostate tumors by controlled release of (D-Trp^6) luteinizing hormone-releasing hormone from injectable microcapsules. Proc Natl Acad Sci USA 81:5845-5848.

Rivier J, Rivier C, Perrin M, Porter J, Vale WW (1981a). GnRH analogs: Structure-activity relationships. In: Zatuchni GI, Shelton JD, Sciarra JJ (eds): LHRH peptides as female and male contraceptives. Philadelphia, Harper and Row, pp 13-23.

Rivier C, Rivier J, Vale W (1981b). Effect of a potent GnRH antagonist and testosterone propionate on mating behavior and fertility in the male rat. Endocrinology 108:1998-2001.

Roger M, Duchier J, Lahlou N, Nahoul K, Schally AV (1985). Treatment of prostatic carcinoma with D-Trp-6-LH-RH: plasma hormone levels after daily subcutaneous injections and periodic administration of delayed release preparations. Prostate 7:271-282.

Rost A, Schmidt-Gollwitzer M, Hantlemann W, Brosig W (1981). Cyproterone acetate, testosterone, LH, FSH, and prolactin levels in plasma after intramuscular application of cyproterone acetate in patients with prostatic cancer. Prostate 2:315-322.

Sandow J, VonRechenberg W, Jerzabek G, Stoll W (1978). Pituitary gonadotropin inhibition by a highly active analog of luteinizing hormone-releasing hormone. Fertil Steril 30:205-209.

Schally AV (1983). Current status of antagonistic analogs of LH-RH as a contraceptive method in the female. PARFR Vol 2. No. 5.

Schally AV, Arimura A, Coy DH (1980a). Recent approaches to fertility control based on derivatives of LH-RH. In Munson PL, Diczfalusy J, Glover J, Olson RE (eds): "Vitamins and Hormones," New York: Academic Press, pp 257-323.

Schally AV, Cai RZ, Torres-Aleman I, Redding TW, Szoke B, Fu D, Hierowski MT, Colaluca J, Konturek S (1986a). Endocrine, gastrointestinal and antitumor activity of somatostatin analogs: Washington Spring Peptide Symposium. In Moody TW (ed): "Neural and Endocrine Peptides and Receptors," New York: Plenum, (in press).

Schally AV, Coy DH (1983). Stimulatory and inhibitory analogs of LH-releasing hormone: basic and clinical studies. In: McCann SM, Dhindsa DS (eds): "Role of Peptides and Proteins in Control of Reproduction," New York: Elsevier Biomedical, pp 89-110.

Schally AV, Coy DH, Arimura A (1980b). LH-RH agonists and antagonists. Int J Gynaecol Obstet 18:318-324.

Schally AV, Comaru-Schally AM, Redding TW (1984a). Antitumor effects of analogs of hypothalamic hormones in endocrine-dependent cancers. Proc Soc Exp Biol Med 175:259-281.

Schally AV, Kastin AJ (1971). Stimulation and inhibition of fertility through hypothalamic agents. Drug Ther 1:29-32.

Schally AV, Redding, TW (1985). Combination of long-acting microcapsules of the D-tryptophan-6-analog of luteinizing hormone-releasing hormone with chemotherapy: investigation in the rat prostate cancer model. Proc Natl Acad Sci USA 82:2498-2502.

Schally AV, Redding TW, Cai RZ, Paz JI, Ben-David M, Schally AM (1986b). Somatostatin analogs in the treatment of various experimental tumors. In Klein, J (ed): "International Symposium on Hormonal Manipulation of Cancer: Peptides, Growth Factors and New (Anti) Steroidal Agents," New York: Raven Press, in press.

Schally AV, Redding TW, Comaru-Schally AM (1984b). Potential use of analogs of luteinizing hormone-releasing hormones in the treatment of hormone-sensitive neoplasms. Cancer Treatment Reports 68:281-289.

Schally AV, Redding TW, Comaru-Schally AM (1983). Inhibition of prostate tumors by agonistic and antagonistic analogs of LH-RH. Prostate 4:545-552.

Schmidt JD, Scott WW, Gibbons R, Johnson DE, Prout GR, Jr, Loening S, Soloway M, deKernion J, Pontes JE, Slack NH, Murphy GP (1980). Chemotherapy programs of the National Prostatic Cancer Project (NPCP). Cancer 45:1937-1946.

Smith RB, Walsh PC, Goodwin WE (1973). Cyproterone acetate in the treatment of advanced carcinoma of the prostate. J Urol 110:106-108.

Sogani PC, Ray B, Whitmore WF, Jr. (1975). Advanced prostatic carcinoma: Flutamide therapy after conventional endocrine treatment. Urology 6:164-166.

Stoliar B, Albert DJ (1974). Sch 13521 in the treatment of advanced carcinoma of the prostate. J Urol 111:803-807.

Sundaram K, Cao YQ, Wang NG, Bardin CW, Rivier J, Vale W (1981). Inhibition of the action of sex steroids by gonadotropin-releasing hormone (GnRH) agonists: A new biological effect. Life Sci 28:83–88.

Thomas JA, Keenan EJ (1976). Prolactin influences upon androgen action in male accessory sex organs. In Singhal RL, Thomas JA (eds): "Cellular Mechanisms Modulating Gonadal Hormone Action, Advances in Sex Hormone Research," Baltimore: University Park Press, Vol 2, pp 425–470.

Tolis G, Ackman A, Stellos A, Mehta A, Labrie F, Fazekas A, Comaru-Schally AM, Schally AV (1982). Tumor growth inhibition in patients with prostatic carcinoma treated with luteinizing hormone-releasing hormone agonists. Proc. Natl. Acad. Sci USA 79:1658–1662.

Tolis G, Mehta A, Comaru-Schally AM, Schally AV (1981). Suppression of androgen production by D-tryptophan-6-LH-RH in man. J Clin Invest 68:819–822.

Walker, K.J., Nicholson, R.I., Turkes, AO, Turkes, A., Robinson, M., Crispin, Z., and Dris, S. (1983): Therapeutic potential of the LHRH agonist, ICI 118630, in the treatment of advanced prostatic carcinoma. Lancet, ii:413–415.

Walsh PC (1975). Physiological basis for hormonal therapy in carcinoma of the prostate. Urol Clin N Amer 2:125–140.

Walsh PC, Korenman, SG (1971). Mechanism of androgenic action effect of specific intracellular inhibitors. J Urol 105:850–851.

Warner B, Worgul TJ, Drago J, Demers L, Dufau M, Max D_6, Santen RJ (1983). Effect of high dose D-Leucine^6- Gonadotropin-releasing hormone proethylamide on the hypothalamic-pituitary testicular axis in patients with prostatic cancer. J Clin Invest 17:1842–1853.

Waxman JH, Wass JAH, Hendry WF, Whitfield HN, Besser GM, Malpas JS, and Oliver RTD (1983). Treatment with gonadotrophin releasing hormone analog in advanced prostatic cancer. Br Med J 286:1309–1312.

Whitmore WJ Jr. (1956). Hormone therapy in prostatic cancer. Amer J Med 21:697–713.

Wiegelman W, Solbach HG, Kley HK, Kruskemper HL (1977). LH and FSH response to long-term application of an LH-RH analog in normal males. Horm Metab Res 9:521–522.

Prostate Cancer, Part A: Research, Endocrine
Treatment, and Histopathology, pages 199–206
© 1987 Alan R. Liss, Inc.

DECAPTETYL IN THE TREATMENT OF METASTATIC PROSTATIC CANCER. COMPARATIVE STUDY WITH PULPECTOMY

H. Botto, F. Richard, F. Mathieu,
M. Camey
Centre Médico-chirurgical Foch
40, rue Worth, 92151 Suresnes, FRANCE

INTRODUCTION

For more than 40 years, the treatment of advanced prostatic cancer has been based on endocrine therapy and/or suppression of the patient's androgen secretion. Surgical testicular pulpectomy, disguised castration, is the simplest method of endocrine therapy and has been proven to be effective. Other medical modalities can be used with an apparently equivalent level of efficacy : oestrogens and, more recently, antiandrogens and LHRH analogues.

The aim of this study was to evaluate the efficacy of an LHRH analogue, Decapeptyl [D-Trp6-LHRH (Ipsen-Biotech)] compared with that of pulpectomy in this indication.

MATERIAL AND METHODS

1. Patients

80 patients of various ages with stage C or D prostatic cancer were included in this study. Patients who had previously received another form of endocrine or radiotherapy treatment or those with another active neoplastic lesion or with a life expectancy of less than 4 months or with confirmed hepatic or renal failure were excluded from this study. However, endoscopic resection of the prostate did not constitute a criterion of exclusion.

The criteria of evaluation were as follows :

- clinical symptoms : urinary symptoms (prostatism, dysuria, frequency), pain, general status (appetite, sleep, functional activity) ; classical elements (rectal examination, IVP, histology obtained by aspiration biopsy or transurethral resection) ;
- transrectal prostatic ultrasonography in preference to suprapubic ultrasonography, every 3 months;
- radioimmunoassay of plasma testosterone and acid phosphatase (PAP);
- bone scintigraphy, chest x-ray and hepatic ultrasonography every six months.

2. Treatment
The patients were randomised to receive either Decapeptyl or surgical testicular pulpectomy. Each treatment group initially consisted of 40 patients.

All patients were followed for at least 18 months or until death. Decapeptyl was administered subcutaneously at a dose of 100 mcg per day for 7 days. The long-acting form was introduced on the 8th day by means of an intramuscular injection of 3 mg of available peptide in the form of sustained-release microcapsules providing a daily dosage of about 100 mcg. The second long-acting injection was administered on the 28th day and the subsequent injections were administered every 4 weeks.

3. Withdrawals from the study
Patients in the two groups were withdrawn from the study when the therapeutic efficacy was found to be inadequate after one month of treatment (especially when pain was not modified) or much later in the study following:

- recurrence of pain,
- development of aggravation of metastases,
- development of hypercalcaemia,
- gradual increase in the PAP level during the first trimester.

4. Statistical analysis
Statistical analysis was performed using the t test for unmatched series for the quantitative data and the Chi squared test for the qualitative data. The actuarial survival curves of the two groups were compared by the log rank method.

RESULTS

The 80 patients had a follow-up period of at least 12 months : the mean age of the patients was 69.85 ± 9.59 years (Decapeptyl) and 72.55 ± 6.91 years (pulpectomy). The 2 groups presented all of the histological types.

1. Clinical results

Urinary symptoms
An overall improvement was observed. The improvement in the severity of dysuria with Decapeptyl was faster, more marked and more prolonged. Intensity was scored from 0 to 4 with the following results :

TABLE I

	D0	D15	M1	M3	M6	M12
Decapeptyl	2.487	1.641	1.051	0.650	0.595	0.375
n =	39	39	39	39	37	24
Pulpectomy	2.775	2.050	1.600	1.189	1.108	0.619
n =	40	40	40	37	37	21
Significance	NS	NS	$p < 0.05$	$p < 0.01$	$p < 0.02$	NS

NS = not significant
n = number of patients
D = Day
M = Month

Volume of the prostate
The volume of the prostate, evaluated by ultrasonography regressed in both groups (see Table). This regression was more marked in the Decapeptyl group, although this group had a larger initial volume of D0.

	D0	M1	M3	M6	M12
Decapeptyl	56.333	30.484	22.273	17.633	11.875
n =	30	31	33	30	16
Pulpectomy	37.194	26.407	20.645	20.690	19.846
n =	36	27	31	29	13
Significance	p < 0.05	NS	NS	NS	p< 0.05

NS = not significant
n = number of patients

Pain
Like dysuria, pain regressed in both groups and analysis of its severity
according to the same scoring system (0 to 4) revealed the following
results :

	D0	D15	M1	M3	M6	M12
Decapeptyl	1.6	0.950	0.450	0.425	0.459	0.167
n =	40	40	40	40	37	24
Pulpectomy	1.150	0.725	0.550	0.324	0.432	0.619
n =	40	40	40	37	37	21
Significance	NS	NS	NS	NS	NS	p < 0.05

NS = not significant
n = number of patients

These results were corroborated by the analgesic consumption and the
bone scan changes.

* The analgesic consumption was scored from 0 to 4 :

	D0	D15	M1	M3	M6	M12
Decapeptyl	0.925	0.622	0.371	0.343	0.353	0.174
n =	40	37	35	35	34	23
Pulpectomy	0.750	0.526	0.389	0.242	0.364	0.474
n =	40	38	36	33	33	19
Significance	NS	NS	NS	NS	NS	NS

NS = not significant
n = number of patients

* Bone scan : the following results were obtained at 6 months - 1 year in the patients with increased bone uptake on D0 :

	Decapeptyl n = 24	Pulpectomy n = 22
Resolution	4	2
Improvement	6	6
No change	13	7
Deterioration	1	7

Other clinical signs

The general performance status, based on evaluation of sleep, functional activity, appetite and weight changes, was improved in both groups with no significant difference between the 2 groups.

2. Laboratory parameters

Testosterone
The results demonstrate that castration levels (testosterone < 0.5 mcg/ml) were obtained rapidly in both groups.
At 1 month, 38 of the 39 patients assessed were castrated in the pulpectomy group and 35 out of 40 in the Decapeptyl group. At 2 months, all of the patients in the Decapeptyl group were castrated, while 3 patients in the pulpectomy group showed a transient rise in testosterone levels. In the Decapeptyl group, castration was maintained throughout the study in all but one of the subjects. In the pulpectomy group, the serum testosterone levels increased in 3 patients.

A purely laboratory "flare up" was detected in the Decapeptyl group : a transient increase in testosterone of no clinical significance was seen in one patient on D15. This patient has been followed for 15 months with no signs of recurrence.

Prostatic acid phosphatases (PAP)

Although the mean PAP level was very different in the 2 groups at the start of the study (56.3 ng/ml versus 21.360 ng/ml), virtually normal values were obtained in the majority of patients after 2 months of treatment (histogram). At 12 months, the PAP level was normal (< 7 ng/ml) in 24 out of 27 patients in the Decapeptyl group and in 15 out of 19 patients in the pulpectomy group.

The case of hormonal "flare up" described above was not accompanied by a concomitant increase in PAP.

3. Overall course

Withdrawals from the study or patients lost to follow-up

A number of patients from the 2 groups were withdrawn from the study either because of deterioration in the symptoms or because of personal problems :
- in the Decapeptyl group : 12 cases, including 6 because of deterioration,
- in the pulpectomy group : 22 cases, including 10 because of deterioration.

Recent data concerning outcome was available for some of these patients : these patients were included in the analysis of survival when they had not received any other form of treatment.

Disease progression or recurrence

Laboratory or symptomatic recurrences occurred in :
. 9 cases in the Decapeptyl group after a mean of 7 ± 6.3 months
.11 cases in the pulpectomy group after a mean of 6.82 ± 5 months

Survival

13 patients in each group died during the study. However, 3 patients in the Decapeptyl group and 1 patient in the pulpectomy group died from a cardiovascular cause.
- the mean survival after inclusion in the study for the 10 patients in the first group was 14.6 ± 7.9 months
- the mean survival for the 12 patients in the second group was 10.6 ± 5.5 months.

The actuarial survival curve demonstrated a slight difference which was not significant. By the direct method, the survival rate for Decapeptyl was 80% at 12 months and 69% at 18 months compared with 70% at 12 months and 65% at 18 months for pulpectomy.

4. Tolerance

Local tolerance : the subcutaneous and intramuscular injections of Decapeptyl were well tolerated locally.
Systemic tolerance : the only side effects - which actually reflect castration - were hot flushes and/or impotence in more than one half of cases. These effects never required suspension of treatment. No cardiovascular complications were observed, even in patients with a history of cardiovascular disease :
. two cases of moderate and transient increase in the systolic and diastolic blood pressure were observed at the very beginning of treatment, in 2 previously normotensive patients,
. the heart rate remained stable during treatment.
No allergic reactions were reported.

No haematological effects were detected (antithrombin III - plasminogen - factor VII).
No adverse drug interactions were observed.

CONCLUSION

On the basis of this study, we can conclude on the efficacy of treatment with the sustained-release form of Decapeptyl in prostatic cancer in comparison with pulpectomy. Decapeptyl induces biochemical castration at least as rapidly and as completely as surgical pulpectomy. Moreover, analysis of the survival curves shows that Decapeptyl ensures a survival time at least equal to that offered by pulpectomy.

The local and systemic tolerance of sustained-release Decapeptyl was excellent throughout the study, without any active hormono-clinical flare-up.

Finally, the sustained-release form of Decapeptyl simplifies treatment and eliminates the septic risk, while ensuring constant therapeutic impregnation.

These results are in accordance with those of other studies conducted on Decapeptyl in the same indication (Parmar - de Sy - Boccardo - Tolis). They also confirm the studies performed with other LHRH analogues regardless of their respective durations of action.

Prostate Cancer, Part A: Research, Endocrine
Treatment, and Histopathology, pages 207–220
© 1987 Alan R. Liss, Inc.

METASTATIC PROSTATE CANCER UNDER LONG TERM PERNASAL BUSERELIN OR INTRAMUSCULAR DECAPEPTYL DEPOT TREATMENT

U. K. Wenderoth, H.-W. Spindler, W. Ehrenthal,
H. v.Wallenberg, J. Happ, G.H. Jacobi,
Department of Urology, Johannes Gutenberg-University Medical School, Langenbeckstraße 1,
D-6500 Mainz, Federal Republic of Germany

During the last five years a large number of publications emerged in the literature on the palliative effect of LHRH analogues given to patients with prostate cancer who would have otherwise been treated by either orchiectomy or oestrogens (Borgman et al., 1982; Happ et al., 1986; Labrie et al., 1983; Papadopoulos et al., 1986; Parmar et al., 1985; Roger et al., 1985).

In recent years we have used the subcutaneously and pernasally applicable LHRH analogue Buserelin in 122 patients with advanced prostatic carcinoma (Jacobi and Wenderoth, 1982; Wenderoth et al., 1982; Wenderoth and Jacobi, 1983; Wenderoth and Jacobi, 1985). In the last two years we have also gained experience with patients treated by intramuscular injections of a depot formulation of another analogue, i.e. Decapeptyl, the D-Trp 6-LHRH.

We herein report our endocrine and clinical follow-up results accumulated over five years.

Patients and Tumor Characteristics

From October 1981 to May 1986 a total of 151 patients with advanced prostatic adenocarcinoma were treated, 122 in the Buserelin-group and 29 in the Decapeptyl-group. The following analysis is based only on patients fully evaluable endocrinologically as well as clinically.

Buserelin - October 1981 - May 1986: 85 patients
Decapeptyl - April 1984 - May 1986: 22 patients
These 107 patients had all newly diagnosed untreated

tumors proven by biopsy.

Grade of tumor differentiation was assessed by using the W.H.O. grading system: 6.5 % grade I, 21.5 % grade II, and 72 % grade III.

Before treatment tumors were classified in stages after investigating their extention by sonography, computer tomography, chest x-ray, bone scan, bone survey if necessary, prostate specific acid phosphatase (PAP-EIA, ABBOTT), as well as prostate specific antigen (PSA-RIA, Diagnostic Products Corp.) in the majority of cases.

Using the TNM-system 76 patients (71 %) had bone metastases with or without lymph node involvement (M1), 31 patients (29 %) had locally advanced lesions of categories T3-4 N0 M0.

Treatment Evaluation

All patients had measurable lesions in order to objectively assess treatment response. This was achieved by using the criteria of the E.O.R.T.C. as well as those of the American National Prostatic Cancer Treatment Group (NPCTG).

A total of 40 patients (31 in the Buserelin-group and 9 in the Decapeptyl-group) suffered from metastatic bone pain suitable for the assessment of subjective treatment response. Hormone monitoring was different in the two treatment groups.

Buserelin-group: Serum testosterone was measured before treatment, weekly during the first month, and 3-monthly thereafter for up to 42 months. Serum-LH was determined under basal conditions and one hour after stimulation with 25 µg of native LHRH. These LHRH-stimulation tests were performed in 14 patients before treatment, and every 6 months for the following 3 years.

Other hormone investigations consisted of sereal measurements of the adrenal steroids Delta-4-androstenedione and DHEA-S, Cortisol, Thyroxine, and Prolactin in serum.

Decapeptyl-group: Serum testosterone and LH were measured in all patients initially and at the following treatment intervals: 6,12,24,48 hours; 1,2,3,4,5 weeks, and in 5-weekly intervals thereafter over 65 weeks, corresponding to 13 injections. In 8 patients serum levels of Decapeptyl during 6 i.m. injections were measured by

RIA using two different antibodies (Happ et al., 1986).

Treatment

Buserelin (Suprefact^R, Behringwerke) was either used subcutaneously for the initial 6–14 days and continued pernasally, or given per nasal spray from the beginning. The majority of patients received 3x500 µg per day s.c., the detailed dose regimen is summarized in Table 1. All different doses have proved equi-effective in achieving castrate levels of serum testosterone 4 weeks after treatment.

Dose Regimen

Buserelin
- 2 x 200 µg/d s.c. 14 days ⎫ and 3 x 400 µg/d
- 3 x 1000 µg/d s.c. 6 days ⎬ p.n.
- 3 x 500 µg/d s.c. 6 days ⎭ thereafter
- 3 x 300 µg/d p.n. contineously

Decapeptyl
- D-Trp 6-LHRH 3.2 mg microencapsulated in 119 mg Lyophilisate injected i.m. every 5 weeks

TABLE 1: Dose regimen used in 85 patients under Buserelin and 22 patients under Decapeptyl depot treatment.

D-Trp-6-LHRH (Decapeptyl^R Depot, Ferring) was used as slow - release formulation of 3 mg in about 170 mg microcapsules. This dose was injected intramuscularly every 5 weeks.

Endocrine Data

Buserelin-group (fig. 1): Serum testosterone increased from initially 4.8 + 2.2 ng/ml to 5.6 + 2.4 ng/ml after 2 weeks of treatment. This was followed by an abrupt fall into the castrate range (0.5 ng/ml) after 4 weeks of treatment. Serum testosterone measured in 3-monthly intervals showed average values ranging between 0.4 + 0.1 and 0.2 + 0.1 ng/ml.

Buserelin

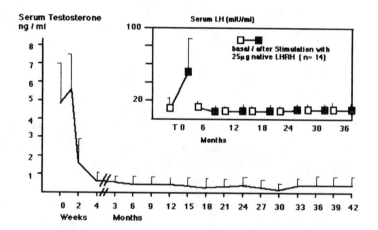

Figure 1: Serum testosterone (mean value + standard deviation) of serum testosterone in 85 patients treated with Buserelin; the inset depicts the LHRH stimulation results (for details see text!).

Serum-LH was initially 13 + 9 mIU/ml and reached by the stimulation with native LHRH 53 + 34 mIU/ml.

After initiation of treatment the stimulation tests were repeated every 6 months and showed basal levels ranging from 2 + 0.5 to 5 + 2 mIU/ml, the stimulatory LH levels ranged from 2 + 0.5 to 6 + 8 mIU/ml.

FSH was also determined during these stimulation tests with virtually the same pattern.

Pretreatment values of Delta-4-androstenedione and DHEA-S were 4.8 + 1 nMol/l and 1.2 + 0.5 mg/l, respectively, and did not change significantly throughout the study.

Initial values for serum thyroxine was 8 ± 1 µg/dl, for serum cortisol 15 ± 3 µg/dl, and for serum prolactin 7 ± 3 µg/l. All three hormones remained virtually identical over 36 months of treatment.

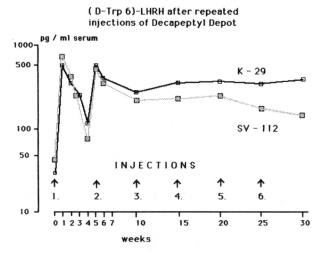

(D-Trp 6)-LHRH after repeated injections of Decapeptyl Depot

Figure 2: Serum levels of Decapeptyl during 6 i.m. injection intervals in 8 patients; K-29 and SV-112 are different antibodies used in the RIA for internal control.

Decapeptyl-group: Serum levels of Decapeptyl reached peak levels of an average of 1700 pg/ml 3 hours after i.m. injection. Thereafter serum Decapeptyl decreased with a calculated half-life of 4.8 hours to 500 pg/ml in the first week, and declined to 80 - 100 pg/ml up to the second injection (fig. 2). During repeated applications in 5-weekly intervals a moderate accumulation with minimum concentrations of about 400 pg/ml serum were found. Compared to the Buserelin-group testosterone reached the peak stimulation level already at day 3, from initially 4.5 ± 1.2 ng/ml to 6.3 ± 1.8 ng/ml. Down-regulation was fully in progress after one week of treatment and castrate levels were universally reached at 3 weeks. During following 5-weekly injections testosterone levels changed between 0.2 and 0.3 ng/ml and this castrate range was maintained in all patients (fig. 3). In all patients, serum LH preceded testosterone in the stimulation peak about 40 hours, the state of down-regulation was achieved 3 weeks after treatment (fig. 3).

Decapeptyl

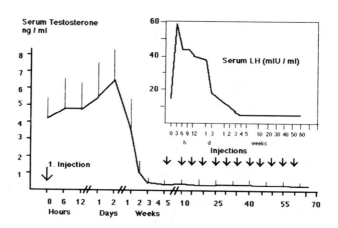

Figure 3: Serum testosterone (mean value ± standard deviation) of 22 patients treated with Decapeptyl; the inset shows the mean values of serum LH for the same patients.

Change from Buserelin to Decapeptyl: A group of 4 patients treated pernasally with Buserelin for 11 to 26 months and responding objectively asked for a change to the depot form of Decapeptyl because of the inconvenience of the nasal spray. These cases are not included in the 2 aforementioned groups. After their last pernasal Buserelin application serum testosterone was determined in hourly intervals for 6 hours, and the first Decapeptyl injection was given intramuscularly. Testosterone was determined in 3-hourly intervals for up to 12 hours, and weekly thereafter (fig. 4). During this therapy change testosterone remained within the castrate range of 0.5 ng/ml.

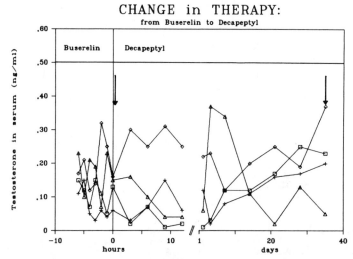

CHANGE in THERAPY:
from Buserelin to Decapeptyl

Figure 4: Testosterone levels of 4 patients who changed
from long term pernasal Buserelin treatment to
intramuscular Decapeptyl treatment (for details
see text!).

Clinical Data

In all patients objective clinical response was first
assess 6 months after initiation of treatment. Patients
under Buserelin therapy have a follow-up ranging from 2
to 4.5 years, patients under Decapeptyl ranging from 15
to 24 months. For both treament groups rates for objective and subjective response are given in table 2. The
average duration of response is 23 months in the Buserelin-group, and 14 months in the Decapeptyl-group.
Subjective response was assessed after 2 months of
therapy and in 32 of 40 patients a significant relief of
metastatic bone pain was encountered.
Table 3 summarizes objective responses comparing data
according to the E.O.R.T.C. and NPCTG criteria. Over
all response is 52 % using E.O.R.T.C. criteria, and 81 %
according to the less rigid NPCTG criteria, in which the
"stable disease"- category is keyed as objective response.

Clinical Response
(E.O.R.T.C. Criteria)

Objective	Buserelin (n= 85)	Decapeptyl (n=22)
Partial and complete response	54 %	51 %
No Change	25 %	33 %
Progression	21 %	16 %
Subjective	25/31 (81%)	7/9 (78%)

TABLE 2: Response rates of the two treatment groups assessed 6 months after initiation of treatment.

Different Response Criteria
Mainz June 1986 (n = 107)

NPCTG		E.O.R.T.C.
Partial and complete Response 53%	81 % 52 %	Partial and complete Response 52 %
Stable Disease 28%		No Change 30 %
Progression 19%	19 % 48 %	Progression 18%

TABLE 3: Comparison of clinical response based on different response criteria of the National Prostatic Cancer Treatment Group (NPCTG) and the E.O.R.T.C.; note, that the "no-change"-category of the E.O.R.T.C. is named "stable disease" by the NPCTG.

Follow-Up by the Use of Serum Tumor Markers

In the Decapeptyl treated group all patients had measurements of serum PAP and PSA at each interval of hormone determination. If the initial values are taken as 100 %, all patients responded to the treatment with an initial increase and subsequent abrupt fall of PAP and PSA paralleling the corresponding testosterone level (fig. 5).

DECAPEPTYL–Depot: Long Term Evaluation
of Testosterone, PSA and PAP

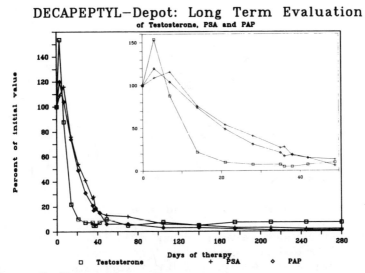

Figure 5: Mean values of serum testosterone, PSA and PAP in 22 patients treated with intramuscular injections of Decapeptyl depot; the inset shows the course of PSA and PAP in good correlation to testosterone; all values are expressed as percentage of initial pretreatment values.

During the time of clinical response PAP and PSA values remaind below the 20 % margin of initial pretreatment values. Patients who experienced clinical relapse showed, however, a steadily increase of both tumor markers, while testosterone remaind within the castrate range (fig. 6). This early sign of progression was observed 3 months before the first clinical evidence of relapse was demonstrable.

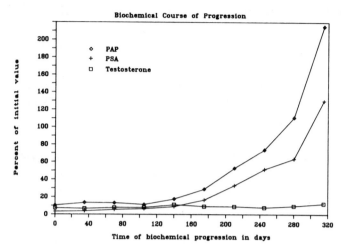

Figure 6: Mean values of serum testosterone, PSA and PAP in 5 patients under Decapeptyl depot treatment, who experienced clinical relapse. Time To is the standardized starting point of increasing PAP and PSA values, while serum testosterone remains within the castrate range.

If PAP or PSA were plotted against serum testosterone for the time up to clinical relapse, clear-cut logarithmic correlations between either tumor marker and the individual testosterone level could be computed (figs. 7 and 8). There is an excellent linear correlation between PAP and PSA with a correlation coefficient of r=0.99.

Side Effects

There were two sudden deaths of unknown cause 2 weeks after initiation of Buserelin therapy. Despite close clinical follow-up there was no case of satisfactorally documented so-called "flair-up" based on objective clinical parameters. Five primarily symptomatic patients reported continuity of symptoms during the first 3 weeks of treatment with pain relief thereafter. Vice versa, however, 4 patients reported a significant relief of bone pain while still in the phase of testosterone as well as tumor marker stimulation during the first 2 weeks. Bone pain alone as well as PAP or PSA increase are certainly insufficient parameters to characterize the dubious term of "flair-up".

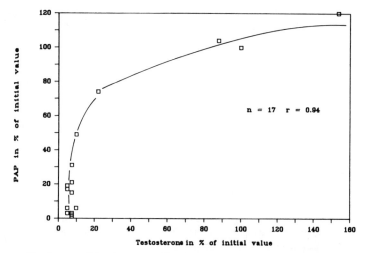

Figure 7: Logarithmic correlation of PAP versus testosterone in 22 patients under Decapeptyl depot
treatment up to the time to progression; n=17
represents pairs of mean %-values of PAP and
testosterone.

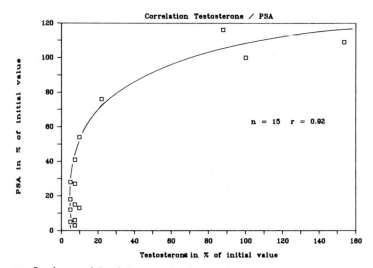

Figure 8: Logarithmic correlation of PSA versus testosterone in 22 patients under Decapeptyl depot
treatment up to the time to progression; n=15
represents pairs of mean %-valus of PSA and
testosterone.

Both LHRH-analogues were equally well tolerated, with hot flashes as the only unexpected untoward reactions in about 3/4 of all patients.

Critical Comment and Summary

Three major assumptions emerged from these clinical and endocrine long term studies.

First, Buserelin given pernasally in the conventional doses and Decapeptyl microcapsules administered intramuscularly in 5-week intervals are equally effective in terms of their long term castration effect in previously untreated patients with prostatic carcinoma. However, Decapeptyl causes complete LH and subsequent testosterone down-regulation one week earlier as compared to Buserelin. Furthermore this treatment is more convenient, and the compliance is better.

The somewhat superior rates of objective response of Buserelin over Decapeptyl - although without statistical significant difference - are most likely due to the longer follow-up of Buserelin treated patients. This is also underlined by the different duration of response in the two treatment groups. Both LHRH-analogues are equally well tolerated.

Second, in groups of prostate cancer patients with far advanced disease treated with palliative intention only true subjective or objective remission should by considered as a positive treatment response. No change in tumor burden or in the severe symptomatology of such patients must be rated as therapy failure and evaluated equal to progression. This modus of evaluation of treatment response is used by the E.O.R.T.C. In all well documented studies of patients treated with LHRH-analogues as monotherapy rates of partial plus complete remission between 50 % and almost 60 % are found, leaving the remainder 25 - 30 % for the "no-change"-category and about 20 % for progression. The National Prostatic Cancer Treatment Group (NPCTG), however, adds patients without change in tumor burden or symptomatology (so-called stable disease) to the group of objective remission and calls this entire group "objective response". Under such circumstances LABRIE and coworkers (Labrie et al., 1983) have repeatedly reported response rates well above 90 % by using an LHRH-analogue in combination with an antiandrogen. The comparison of our monotreatment data using both E.O.R.T.C. as well as NPCTG criteria shows an improvement of the objective response category from 52 % (E.O.R.T.C.) to 81 % (NPCTG). Thus such a modus of reporting treatment data minimizes markedly the high response rate calculated after the combination therapy.

Third, our results comparing PAP und PSA as the two most useful tumor markers with the corresponding testosterone levels suggest a close correlation. It is tempting to conclude that during the initial phase of testosterone stimulation, the phase of down-regulation and the subsequent period of treatment response, peripheral testosterone has some unknown regulatory effect on the formation of these prostate specific products PAP and PSA and on their release from the cancer cells. It is conceivable that not all prostate cancer cells behave uniformly in this regard. Relapsing cell clons, however, which escape from testosterone deprivation and cause clinical tumor progression also escape from this tumor marker/androgen interrelationship.
Our data on five relapsing patients show that PAP and PSA concentrations increased while serum testosterone remained in the castrate range. Thus, PAP and PSA acquire under such circumstances true tumor marker function. Initial increase and subsequent decrease of PAP and PSA during the early phase of LHRH-treatment are of no prognostic value, since such changes are uniformly seen in all patients and only reflect their interrelation to the change in serum testosterone.

References

Borgmann V, Hardt W, Schmidt-Gollwitzer M, Adenauer H, Nagel, R (1982). Lancet i:1097-1099.
Happ J, Schultheiss H, Jacobi GH, Wenderoth UK, Buttenschön K, Miesel R, Spahn H, Hör G (1986). Rotterdamm: Int Symp Hormonal Manipulation of Cancer, Abstr. 108.
Jacobi GH, Wenderoth UK (1982). Eur Urol 8:129-134.
Labrie F, Dupont A, Bélanger A, Lacoursiere Y, Raynaud JP, Husson JM, Gareau J, Fazekas ATA, Sandow J, Monfette G, Girard JG, Emond J, Houle JG (1983). Prostate 4:579-594

Papadopoulos I, Kleinschmidt K, Weißbach L (1986). Akt Urol 17:(in press)

Parmar H, Lightman SL, Allen L, Phillips RH, Edwards L, Schally AV (1985). Lancet ii:1201-1205.

Roger M, Duchier J, Lahlou N, Nahoul K, Schally AV (1985). Prostate 7:271-282.

Wenderoth UK, Happ J, Krause U, Adenauer H, Jacobi GH (1982). Eur Urol 8:343-347.

Wenderoth UK, Jacobi GH (1983). World J Urol 1:40-48.

Wenderoth UK, Jacobi GH (1985). Akt Urol 16:58-63.

Prostate Cancer, Part A: Research, Endocrine
Treatment, and Histopathology, pages 221–227
© 1987 Alan R. Liss, Inc.

LONG TERM THERAPY WITH A DEPOT LHRH ANALOGUE (ZOLADEX[R]) IN
PATIENTS WITH ADVANCED PROSTATIC CANCER.

L. Denis, F. Keuppens, C. Mahler (Belgium),
F.M.J. Debruyne, E.H.J. Weil (Netherlands),
G. Lunglmayr (Austria), D. Newling, M.R.G.
Robinson, B. Richards, P.H. Smith, P. Whelan
(United Kingdom).

Analogues of luteinizing hormone releasing hormone
(LHRH) have become well established as an alternative means
of treatment of advanced prostatic cancer (1). Chronic
release of these compounds leads to a reduction of serum
testosterone into castrate range in patients with prostatic
cancer. This study deals with the endocrine and clinical
effects of a depot formulation of LHRH (Zoladex[R] depot) in
a multinational, multicenter phase II open study.

OBJECTIVES OF THE STUDY

The aims of the study are :
- to document patient acceptability of this depot formulation and any adverse drug reactions.
- to confirm the initial and long term suppression of serum
testosterone to castrate levels.
- to determine the subjective and objective response rates
and duration of responses.

PATIENTS AND METHODS

All patients had histological confirmed proof of prostatic cancer. Radiological and / or bone scan evidence of
bone metastases, evidence of soft tissue metastasis or
tumor extension through the prostatic capsule together with
a minimul life expectancy of six months was one of the inclusion criteria. Informed consent was obtained from all
patients.
All previously treated patients were excluded from the
study. Patients were evaluated for subjective and objective

assessment. The subjective assessment included urological
symptoms, activity score, pain and analgesia use. The urological symptoms recorded included daytime frequency, nyct-
uria, hesitancy, dysuria, urgency and flow scored from 0
to 3. The other subjective scores are listed in table 1.
The total subjective score consists of the sum of the mean
total score of urological symptoms and the other scores.
A subjective response was based on no increase in any of
the four scores and a decrease of the total score by 4 or
pain and analgesic score by 2. The subjective assessment
was evaluated every month for three months and 12 weekly
after three months. The presence or absence of libido, erections, hot flushes and breast swelling and tenderness as
well as any concomitant symptoms were investigated at the
same time intervals.

TABLE 1. Non urological subjective scoring system

Activity Score :

Full activity	0
Restricted activity	1
Restricted to home	2
Confined to bed	3
Total nursing required	4

Bone Pain Score :

None	0
Mild	1
Moderately severe	2
Severe	3
Intolerable	4

Analgesic Score :

No analgesics	0
Occasional non-narcotic analgesia	1
Regular non-narcotic analgesia	2
Occasional narcotic analgesia	3
Regular narcotic analgesia	4

The objective assessment included prostatic dimensions and
T category · Patients without metastases were assessed by
computed tomography or ultrasound. Other parameters included
serum total and prostatic acid phosphatase, bone scan and /
or radiographic assessment of bone metastases, measurable
soft tissue disease and weight of the patient. The objective
response criteria are listed in table 2. Objective assessment was performed every 12 weeks with repeat assessment
of the imaging techniques after 24 weeks treatment and
every 24 weeks thereafter.

TABLE 2. Objective response criteria

Complete Objective Regression :
No evidence of residual tumour.

Partial Objective Regression :
No evidence of disease progression and any of the following:
Primary tumour : A decrease in a) T category or
                                b) product of length and
                                   width by 50% or
                                c) volume by 35%
Bone metastases : A decrease in radiological or bone scan
                  evidence of metastases.
Extra-skeletal metastases : Reduction in size by 35%.
Acid phosphatase : Return to normal or reduction by 80%.

Stable Disease :
Lack of objective progression and insufficient evidence for
partial objective regression.

Objective Progression :
Any of the following:
Primary tumour : A increase in a) T category or
                                b) product of length and
                                   width by 50% or
                                c) volume by 35%
Bone   : Appearance of new metastases on X-ray or
                 bone scan.
Extra-skeletal   Appearance of new metastases or increase
metastases   : by 35% of any existing measurable meta-
                 stases.

Blood samples were taken for hematological, biochemical and endocrinological (LH, FSH and testosterone) examinations, performed every 4 weeks for 12 weeks and 12 weekly thereafter. Extra serum was deepfrozen after 24 weeks sampling to determine the possible formation of antibodies to the drug.

Zoladex[R] depot is presented as a white cylindrical rod in which the drug is dispersed in a matrix of d, l-lactide-glycolide-copalymer. This rod was administered every 28 days by subcutaneous injection into the anterior wall using a pre-loaded syringe with a 16 gange needle. Initially the first fifty patients were entered at three doses (0.9 mg, 1.8 mg or 3.6 mg) which were randomly allocated. All subsequent patients were entered at the optimal 3.6 mg dose (2). Treatment and points included adverse drug reactions, patients unwilling to continue treatment, withdrawal from study by the investigator, death of patient and objective progression of prostatic cancer as defined by the response criteria.

RESULTS

One hundred and fifty eight patients were entered into the study with a mean age of 71.7 years (50-87). Distant metastases were present in 112 (71%). The mean duration of treatment was 22.5 weeks and at the time of analysis 117 patients were still on study. Fourteen patients were withdrawn because of objective progression, thirteen died of other causes, five were lost to follow-up and nine were withdrawn for other reasons.

ADVERSE EFFECTS

A transient increase in bone pain developed in four patients while one patient developed ureteric obstruction and one paraplegia during the first months of treatment. Both patients recovered and continued the study in partial remission at the three months evaluation. One patient developed an itchy, maculo-papular rash which subsided after arrest of the next injection. This is the only patient withdrawn from the study for adverse effects. The depot formulation was well tolerated locally. Except for five minor complaints of redness no local side effect developed and specifically no one single abscess formation was noted after any of the estimated 900 depots administered.

Endocrine side effects related to the serum testosterone

reduction brought decrease in libido and erection in 70% of the patients where these were present. Breast swelling and tenderness occurred in 5 (3%) of the patients. Hot flushes were reported by 47% of the patients. All endocrine effects were specifically requested by the physician.

ENDOCRINE RESULTS

Twenty four hours after the first injection LH levels reached a peak value (37.3 $\pm$ 5E 0.5 UI/l). Within a week they lowered to their initial level and maximal suppression was achieved in all patients after three weeks (4.1 $\pm$ 5E 0.7 IU/l). Subsequent injections of the drug elicited no further increase of LH and maintained the suppression. FSH levels rose rapidly in a similar way as LH to reach a peak 24 hours after the first injection (16.2 $\pm$ 5E 2.5 IU/l). After 3 weeks suppression was maximal (2.9 $\pm$ 5E 0.3 IU/l) and was maintained by additional injections. Serum testosterone (T) rose to a maximum (16.9 $\pm$ 5E 1.4 nmol/l) three days after the first injection of Zoladex depot. In the majority of patients castrate levels ($\leqslant$ 2 nmol/l) were achieved by day 21. After 28 days all patients except two in the 1.8 mg dose group and one in the 0.9 mg dose group were in castrate range and remained without significant fluctuations at this levels.
Serum prolactin and serum hormone binding globuline were followed for 6 months in a group of 50 patients. No significant changes were noted. No antibody formation to the preparation was detected.

CLINICAL RESULTS

At time of the present evaluation the mean duration of treatment was 22.5 weeks (between 4 - 54 weeks) and there are 117 patients continuing therapy. Of the 41 patients that went of treatment, 14 were withdrawn because of objective signs of progression, 13 died, 9 were withdrawn for other reasons and 5 were lost to follow-up.
Of the 199 evaluable patients 63 (53%) achieved a partial remission, 23 (19%) had stable disease and in 33 (28%) there was disease progression. Subjective response as assessed by the clinicians in 71 patients with symptomatic disease at the start of treatment was found in 48 (68%) of the patients.

DISCUSSION

Not one instance of failure to place the drug in the subcutaneous fat was reported in these series. A few red spots were recorded but no abscess formation or serious local side effect were recorded. The expected endocrine reactions as loss of libido and erections, occasional hot flushes and breast tenderness were recorded after specific questioning of the patients on these side effects. This confirms our previous report that patient acceptability was high (2) and may confirm the observation that the majority of patients comply better with injections than with intranasal sniff (3).

The transient rise in T coincided with flare-up symptoms in two patients. A possible relation to pain exacerbation could be suspected on retrospective analysis. Although rare the adverse effects of rise in T has been reported (4) and we decided to continue this study with a concomitant therapy of diethylstilbestrol (3x1 mg daily) or cyproterone acetate (3x50 mg daily) during the first week of treatment. A precaution that we advice in all patients with far advanced disease.

The subjective and objective response rates obtained in this study compare favorably to similar treatment regimens with other potent LHRH analogues (3,5,6) or with classic orchidectomy / estrogen treatment (7).

Summarizing we conclude that this form of medical castration carries less side effects than the tested drugs available and compete with the psychic stress of surgical castration. Randomized prospective trials are organized to answer this question (EORTC 30843 LHRH vs LHRH and anti-androgen vs orchidectomy ; EORTC 30853 LHRH and anti-androgen vs orchidectomy). Another important aspect is the reversibility of treatment which could suggest this form as treatment as firstline treatment to be followed by the cheaper orchidectomy after definite proof of positive response. Again prospective studies should be organized to answer this question.

REFERENCES

Schröder FH, Richards B (eds) (1985) Therapeutic principles in metastatic prostatic cancer. Alan R Liss, New York.
Robinson MRG, Denis L, Mahler C, Walker K, Stitch R, Lunglmayr G (1985) An LH-RH analogue (Zoladex) in the management of carcinoma of the prostate: a preliminary report

comparing daily subcutaneous injections with monthly depot injections. Eur J of Surg Onc 11: 159-165.

Present CA, Soloway MS, Klioze SS, Kosola JW, Yakabow AL, Mendez RG, Kennedy PS, Wyres MR, Neassig VL, Ford KS (1985) Buserelin as primary therapy in advanced prostatic carcinoma. Cancer 56: 2416-2419.

Kahan A, Delrieu F, Amor B, Chiche R, Steg A (1984) Disease flare induced by D-Trp6-LHRH analogue in patients with metastatic prostatic cancer. Lancet 1: 971.

Debruyne FMJ, Karthaus HFM, Schröder FH, De Voogt HJ, De Jong FH, Klijn JGM (1985) Results of a Dutch phase II trial with the LHRH agonist Buserelin in patients with metastatic prostatic cancer. Schröder FH, Richards B (eds) Therapeutic principles in metastatic prostatic cancer. Alan R Liss, New York, 251.

Warner B, Worgul TJ, Drago J, Demers L, Dufau M, Max D, Santen RJ, members of the Abbott Study Group (1983) Effect of very high dose d-leucine^6-gonadotropin-releasing hormone proethylamide on the hypothalamic-pituitary testicular ascis in patients with prostatic cancer. J Clin Invest 71: 1842.

Denis L, Murphy GP, Prout GR, Schröder F (eds) (1984) Controlled trials in urologic oncology. Raven Press, New York.

Prostate Cancer, Part A: Research, Endocrine
Treatment, and Histopathology, pages 229–237
© 1987 Alan R. Liss, Inc.

TREATMENT OF ADVANCED CARCINOMA OF THE PROSTATE BY LHRH-AGONISTS

Hubert I. Claes, Ludo Vandenbussche, Raoul L. Vereecken

Department of Urology, University Clinics St.-Pieter, Louvain, Belgium.

Thirty-four patients with advanced prostate carcinoma were treated by LHRH agonists: seventeen by LHRH agonist I.C.I. 118630 Zoladex (group 1), seven by LHRH agonist I.C.I. 118630 in combination with cyproterone acetate (group 2), five by Hoe 766 Buserelin (group 3) and five by Hoe 766 in combination with cyproterone acetate (group 4).

The Zoladex injections as well as the Buserelin injections and sprays were well tolerated without local irritation or discomfort. Side effects like breast swelling or tenderness, or signs of toxicity were neglectable. All patients became impotent but did not complain about that. An aggravation of bone pain complaints, especially around the second week was noted in group 1 and 3 but never in group 2 and 4. The subjective and objective evaluation of the four groups after one, three and six months are compared and discussed.

INTRODUCTION

Endocrine treatment of prostatic carcinoma has been used for over 40 years. Orchidectomy or oestrogens were until some years ago the most common methods of achieving androgen deprivation but oestrogens are associated with a high incidence of cardiovascular problems, while orchidectomy has psychological problems. A more recent method of achieving androgen deprivation is the use of LHRH analogues. Such analogues, which are more potent than natural LHRH, cause an initial stimulation of FSH and LH release but when given repeatedly cause a down-regulation of pituitary LHRH receptors (Auclair et al., 1977a; 1977b) with consequent reductions in serum LH and testosterone in male patients (Linde et al., 1981). Thus, LHRH analogues produce a "medical" castration which is reversible on cessation of therapy. This study used the LHRH analogue I.C.I. 118630 (Zoladex) and Hoe 766 (Buserelin). They differ from natural LHRH at position six in the decapeptide chain where glycine is replaced by D-serine (t-Bu) and at position ten where glycine amide is replaced by azaglycine amide (= Zoladex) or by ethylamide (= Buserelin).

PATIENTS AND METHODS

Thirty-four patients entered this open trial to evaluate the endocrinological effects and efficacy of I.C.I. 118630 or Hoe 766. Seventeen patients were treated by LHRH agonist I.C.I. 118630 (group 1), seven by LHRH agonist I.C.I. 118630 in combination with cyproterone acetate (group 2), five by Hoe 766 (group 3) and five by Hoe 766 in combination with cyproterone acetate (group 4).

TABLE 1. Mean age of every patient group.

ZOLADEX	72.4 YEARS (RANGE 56-81)
ZOLADEX + CYPROTERONE ACETATE	71.0 YEARS (RANGE 61-90)
BUSERELIN	73.8 YEARS (RANGE 70-80)
BUSERELIN + CYPROTERONE ACETATE	69.6 YEARS (RANGE 53-77)

All patients had histologically proven advanced (stages C and D) prostatic cancer and, with the exception of transurethral resection in some patients, had received no prior therapy. The average ages as well as the tumour differentiation of the four groups were similar (Table 1 and 2).

In group 1, five patients began therapy with daily sub-cutaneous injections of 250 mcg and two started with 1.8 mg depot monthly; the other ten patients received the I.C.I. 118630 depot of 3.6 mg four-weekly from the start of treatment. Three months after the start of the trial, all patients received the 3.6 mg depot monthly. All the patients of group 2 received the I.C.I. 118630 depot four-weekly in combination with cyproterone acetate 2 x 100 mg daily during two weeks. The group 3 patients were treated by Hoe 766 3 x 500 mcg/day subcutaneously during one week and afterwards 12 x 100 mcg/day intranasally. In group 4, the patients received the same treatment of group 3 but in combination with cyproterone acetate 3 x 50 mg daily during four weeks.

TABLE 2. Histological grading of each patient group.

	N PATIENTS	HIGH DEGREE (G1)	MEDIUM DEGREE (G2)	LOW DEGREE (G3)
ZOLADEX	17	7	4	6
ZOLADEX + CYPROTERONE ACETATE	7	2	4	1
BUSERELIN	5	1	2	2
BUSERELIN + CYPROTERONE ACETATE	5	2	2	1

Objective responses to therapy were assessed every three months, and were based on the National Prostatic Cancer Project criteria (Schmidt et al., 1980). Bone metastases were evaluated by radioisotopic scan and X-ray. Lymph node and local extension were evaluated by CT scan. Subjective response to therapy was assessed by the clinician and by assessing scores for urological symptoms, pain, analgesic requirement and activity. These were performed before, during and after cessation of therapy. Testosterone and prostatic acid phosphatase were measured before treatment at 4, 8 and 12 weeks and every three months thereafter.

RESULTS

Endocrine results. In general, the time to achieve castrate levels of testosterone was 4 to 8 weeks. Only three patients never reached this castrate level because of an insufficient cooperation of the patient (Table 3). Comparing the four groups, we observe that an association of the LHRH-analogue with cyproterone acetate leads to faster achievement of castrate levels of testosterone (Table 4).

When reached, castrate levels persisted throughout the trial except for one patient in group 1, whose testosterone returned to the normal range after receiving his fourth depot (Zoladex). This persisted, despite two further administrations of depot. The patient was then withdrawn from the study.

TABLE 3. Time to achieve the castrate levels of testosterone in the four groups.

	N PTS	WEEK 4	WEEK 8	NEVER
ZOLADEX	17	10	7	0
ZOLADEX + CYPROTERONE ACETATE	7	7	0	0
BUSERELIN	5	2	1	2
BUSERELIN + CYPROTERONE ACETATE	5	3	1	1

TABLE 4. Evolution of mean serum testosterone during first four weeks.

	PRE TREAT (N PTS)	DAY 8 (N PTS)	DAY 15 (N PTS)	DAY 22 (N PTS)	DAY 29 (N PTS)
ZOLADEX	457.3 (17)	382.8 (4)	248.8 (6)	120.8 (5)	113.2 (17)
ZOLADEX + CYPROTERONE ACETATE	616.0 (7)	401.3 (6)	100.5 (6)	38.5 (6)	18.0 (7)
BUSERELIN	574.4 (5)	404.4 (5)	147.0 (5)	176.2 (5)	145.8 (5)
BUSERELIN + CYPROTERONE ACETATE	566.0 (5)	286.5 (5)	61.8 (5)	30.4 (5)	72.8 (5)

Objective response. As shown in figure 1, there are more partial regressions and less progressions in the groups associated with cyproterone acetate.

Subjective response. A favourable subjective response occurred faster and more frequently in the groups where cyproterone acetate was given (Fig. 2). Moreover, the transient increase in bone pain which occurred in ten of the seventeen patients of group 1 and in three of five patients in group 3 didn't happen in these two groups.

Tolerability. Fourteen patients reported hot flushes, but they were never described as severe. In the majority of patients the hot flushes decreased in intensity as therapy was continued. Other side effects noted, included a developing of breast swelling in three patients (only in one case associated with tenderness) and a decrease in libido in 7 patients (Table 5). The subcutaneous injections of the depot I.C.I. 118630 and Hoe 766, as well as the intranasal spray (Hoe 766) were well tolerated locally. No patients were withdrawn from therapy due to side effects.

FIG. 1. Objective response to therapy of the four groups after three, six and twelve months.

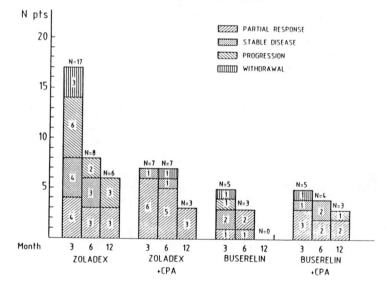

FIG. 2. Subjective response to therapy of the four groups after one and three months.

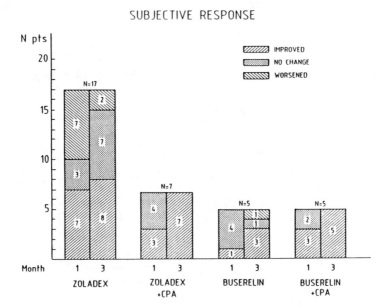

TABLE 5. Side effects noted in the four patient groups.

	N PTS	HOT FLUSHES	BREAST SWELLING	BREAST TENDERNESS	LIBIDO PRE	LIBIDO DECREASE	ERECTIONS PRE	ERECTIONS DECREASE
ZOLADEX	17	12	1	0	5	4	5	4
ZOLADEX + CPA	7	1	2	1	2	2	1	1
BUSERELIN	5	0	0	0	0	0	0	0
BUSERELIN + CPA	5	1	0	0	1	1	1	1

DISCUSSION

Our investigation of 34 patients, treated for more than 6 months, has proved the LHRH analogues Zoladex and Buserelin to be potent to reduce serum testosterone to levels similar to those seen in castrated men within 4-8 weeks, and maintain this level for 6 months and longer under continuous therapy with subcutaneous Zoladex injections or intranasal Buserelin application (Vance, 1984 and Borgmann, 1983).

One patient of group 1 showed a rise in testosterone to within the normal range following administration of the fourth depot. The reasons for this are unclear. It is possible that either the depot was not successfully administered or that the LHRH receptor had become refractory (Kerle et al., 1984).

The hot flushes, which are similar to those found at the female menopause and which are also observed after orchidectomy, are probably due to acute hormonal withdrawal.

A transient increase in bone pain was seen in ten of the seventeen patients of group 1 and in three of the five patients in group 3. These transient increases in bone pain may be related to the initial stimulation of testosterone release following the first administration of the analogue (Ahmed et al., 1985; Allen et al., 1983; Labrie et al., 1980). These phenomena are not generally regarded as a contraindication of LHRH therapy unless the patients have acute ureteric obstruction or if boney metastases are likely to cause spinal compression. The most recent results from Labrie (1985) showing that combination therapy with an anti-androgen can suppress the initial stimulation in bone pain, had led us to adopt this method of treatment (group 2 and 4) and we didn't notice any increase in pain in these patient groups during the first three months.

Although there seems to be a slight advantage as well in objective as in subjective response for the patients treated in combination with cyproterone acetate, our series are too small and the follow-up too short to draw any conclusion about this.

Both Zoladex and Buserelin were well tolerated. No patient did complain about the four-weekly Zoladex injections and intranasal application of Buserelin was not too complicated for most of the patients (only 3 nearly senile elderly patients were not able to use the intranasal spray properly).

It is a decisive advantage of both LHRH analogues in the treatment of advanced prostatic cancer that it offers an alternative to both orchidectomy with its psychical stress and oestrogen therapy with its negative side effects.

REFERENCES

Ahmed SR, Grant J, Shalet SM, Horwell A, Chowdhury SD, Wheaterson T, Blacklock NJ (1985). Preliminary report on use of depot formation of LHRH analogue ICI 118.30 ('Zoladex') in patients with prostatic cancer. Br Med J 290: 185-187.

Allen JM, O'Shea JP, Masheter K, Williams G, Blook SR (1983). Advanced carcinoma of the prostate: treatment with a gonado-trophin releasing hormone agonist. Br Med J 286: 1607-1609.

Auclair C, Kelly PA, Labrie F, Coy DH, Schally AV (1977a). Inhibition of testicular leutenizing hormone receptor level by treatment with a potent leutenizing hormone-releasing hormone agonist or human chorionic gonadotrophin. Biochem Biophys Res Commun 76: 855-862.

Auclair C, Kelly PA, Coy DH, Schally AV, Labrie F (1977b). Potent inhibitory activity of |D-Leu^6,Des-Gly-NH$_2^{10}$| LHRH ethylamide on LH-hCG and PRL testicular receptor in the rat. Endocrinology 101: 1890-1893.

Borgmann V, Nagel H, Al-Abadi M, Schmidt-Gollwitzer M (1983). Treatment of prostatic cancer with LH-RH analogues. The Prostate 4: 553-568.

Kerle D, Williams G, Ware H, Bloom SR (1984). Failure of long term luteinizing hormone releasing hormone treatment for prostatic cancer to suppress serum luteinizing hormone and testo-sterone. Br Med J 289: 468-469.

Labrie F, Cusan L, Seguirs C, Bélanger A, Pelletier G, Reares J, Kelly PA, Lemay A, Raynaud JP (1980). Antifertility effects of LHRH agonist in the male rat and inhibition of testicular steroido-genesis in man. Brit J Fertil 25(3): 157-170.

Labrie F, Dupont A, Bélanger A (1985). Complete androgen blockade for the treatment of prostate cancer. In: Important Advances in Oncology. Ed. J.B. Lippincott Company, Philadelphia.

Linde R, Doelle GC, Alexander M, Kirchner F, Vale W, Rivier J, Rabin D (1981). Reversible inhibition of testicular steroidogenesis and spermatogenesis by a potent gonadotrophin-releasing hormone agonist in normal men: An approach toward the development of a male contraceptive. New Engl J Med 305: 663-667.

Schmidt JD et al. (1980). Chemotherapy programs of the National Prostatic Cancer Project (NPCP). Cancer 45: 1937-1946.

Vance MA, Smith JA (1984). Endocrine and clinical effects of LHRH-A in prostatic cancer. Clin Pharmacol Ther 36(3): 350-354.

Prostate Cancer, Part A: Research, Endocrine
Treatment, and Histopathology, pages 239–241
© 1987 Alan R. Liss, Inc.

RESULTS OF LONG TERM TREATMENT OF ADVANCED PROSTATIC CANCER
WITH THE LHRH ANALOGUE BUSERELIN

D. Fontana, D.F. Randone, G.C. Isaia*, M. Colombo
M. Giusti*, M. Bellina, L. Rolle, G. Fasolis

Urologic Clinic – *IInd Medical Clinic
University of Turin, Italy

It is well known that about 75% of advanced prostatic
cancers respond, at least initially, to androgen suppression
therapy (Schirmer, 1965). The availability of LHRH analogues
and the demonstration of their efficacy in suppressing
gonadal function without resulting in estrogenic side effects
nor in psychological problems of orchiectomy has prompted to
assess this therapy as primary treatment of advanced (Faure,
1982; Waxman, 1983; Wenderoth, 1983) prostatic cancer.

Between July 1983 and October 1985, 36 patients with
advanced prostatic cancer entered an open, noncomparative
study on the use of LHRH analogue Buserelin (500 mcg. x 3
daily subcutaneously and then 400 mcg x 3 daily intranasally).
Of these patients, 29 (11 C, 18 D; 6 G1, 17 G2, 6 G3) are
fully evaluable with a follow up of 6–36 months ($\bar{x}$ = 17,
2 months). The mean pre-treatment blood testosterone levels
were 3,5 $\pm$ 2,1 ng/ml (assay at 8 a.m. Biomedica Sorin Kit
direct method). The values were unsignificantly higher at
the end of the first week and then decreased to 0,49 $\pm$ 0,49
ng/ml (p 0,001) at the forth week of treatment without
significant variation for the rest of treatment. Serum LH
(basal and after stimulus: 0,1 mg I.V. of Relefact Hoechts)
decreased while PRL, 17β OH Estr., Cortisol and the weak
adrenal androgens: DHEAs and Androstenedione (basal and
after stimulus: 0,25 mg I.V. Synacthen) did not significantly change.

The response to treatment (N.P.C.P. criteria) was the
following:

PROGRESSION: 10/29 (34,5%)
STABLE DISEASE: 3/29 (10,5%)
PARTIAL RESPONSE: 16/29 (55 %)

The death rate within two years of treatment was 17% (5/29).

The mean values of Testosterone and Prostatic Acid Phosphatase were not significantly different in the progression and responders groups. Therefore, progression of the disease seems not to be related to lack of androgenic suppression.

In 78% of patients with bone pain (60% of cases) symptoms either improved or totally disappeared. Micturition and general health condition also markedly improved. No case of clinical evidence of flare up of the disease was observed; in the first month of treatment, hot flushes were present in 60% of patients. Loss of libido and erection were observed in all patients.

The patients compliance was fairly good as 4/36 (11%) were lost to follow up between the first and ninth month of treatment.

The other patients are not evaluable because of Hypersensitivity (Schirmer, 1965), development of a new tumor (Schirmer, 1965), withdrawal of the drug after one week of treatment (Schirmer, 1965).

In conclusion, in agreement with other authors (Koutsillieris, 1985), our study shows that the LHRH analogue Buserelin can be safely employed as primary treatment in advanced prostatic cancer.

REFERENCES

Faure N, Labrie F, Lemary A (1982). Inhibition of serum androgen levels by chronic intranasal and subcutaneous administration of a potent LHRH agonist in adult men. Fertil Steril 37:416-424.

Koutsillieris M, Tolis G (1985). Long term follow up of patients with advanced prostatic carcinoma treated with either Buserelin (HOE 766) or orchiectomy: classification of variables associated with disease outcome. The Prostate 7:31-39.

Schirmer HKA, Murphy GP, Scott W (1965). Hormone therapy for prostatic cancer and the clinical course of the disease.

Urol Digest 4:15-21.
Waxman JH, Wass JA, Hendry WF (1983). Treatment with gonadotrophin releasing hormone analogue in advanced prostatic cancer. Br Med J 286:1309-1312.
Wenderoth UK, Jacobi GH (1983). Gonadotrophin releasing hormone analogues for palliation of carcinoma of the prostate. World J Urology 1:40-48.

Prostate Cancer, Part A: Research, Endocrine
Treatment, and Histopathology, pages 243–244
© 1987 Alan R. Liss, Inc.

LH-RH ANALOGUE TREATMENT OF ADVANCED PROSTATIC CANCER

Alcini E., D'Addessi A., Vacilotto D.
Surgical Dept. Urological Division, Catholic University
of Sacred Heart- Policlinico "A. Gemilli", Largo A.
Gemelli 1, 00168 Rome - ITALY

The authors present 12 patients with advanced prostatic carcinoma treated with LH-RH analogue (ICI 118,630 - Zoladex Depot) from November 84 to October 85. Evaluable patients were 9, followed up > 12 weeks. Tumor stage was T2M+ (3 cases), T3M0 (1), T3M+ (6), T4M0 (1), T4M+ (1); mean age 71 years (57-84) grade G1(2), G2(8), G3(2).

Subjective parameters for evaluation were urological symptoms, performance status, bone pain, use of analgesics. Objective ones were T-stage, prostate dimension, TAP and PAP, bone scan evaluation of metastases.

The drug was administered by subcutaneous injection : 3,6 mg every 28 days. Response to therapy was recorded at 4, 8, 12, 24, 48 weeks and every 6 months thereafter.

Four possible objective responses were defined complete (CR), partial (PR), stable disease (SD), progression (PROG).

RESULTS
Nine of 12 patients are evaluable (follow up > 12 weeks at 31 Jan.86). One patient died after 6 weeks from renal failure probably due to rapid local progression of cancer. Two other patients had PR for 20-24 weeks (decreased tumor volume), bu subsequently developed bone metastases.

Serum LH decreased from a mean value of 19.70 to 11.06 UI/1 after 12 weeks. Serum testosterone strikingly decreased from 6.7 to 0.8

mg/ml after 4 weeks, remaining depressed below castration levels defined as 1 mg/ml.

Seven of 8 patients (88%) showed a good subjective response starting from 9th week.

PRs at 12 weeks were 6 (66%) : 4 are stable up to now, while 2, as we said, had progression after 20-24 weeks. PRs was obtained after 7-6 weeks of treatment.

Three of 3 and 4 of 5 (80%) patients presenting with respectively high TAP and PAP showed reduction >80%. No patients developed any modification in laboratory parameters.

Ten of 12 patients presenting libido before therapy reported a reduction. However, 4 of 10 patients able to have erection before treatment reported no modification of this function.

There was no local or general reaction to the drug and no patient showed cardiovascular or clotting disorders, often affecting traditional hormonotherapy.

Time and numbers must confirm efficacy of LH-RH analogue therapy. Our series shows good short-term disease control without serious side effects.

Prostate Cancer, Part A: Research, Endocrine
Treatment, and Histopathology, pages 245–247
© 1987 Alan R. Liss, Inc.

INDUCTION AND MAINTENANCE OF CASTRATION BY AN LHRH ANALOGUE: D-Trp6 LHRH OR DECAPEPTYL

J. Fretin, F. Demerle, A. Jardin
Urologie, Hôpital du Kremlin-Bicêtre
Paris

A trial was conducted in 16 patients aged between 58 and 84 years with previously untreated stage D2 prostatic adeno- carcinoma in order to determine the conditions of installation and stability of the castration induced by D-Trp6 LHRH or DECAPEPTYL prescribed as single agent therapy.

Three modalities of administration were studied and identical results were obtained whether treatment was commenced and continued with the subcutaneous form at a dose of 0.1 mg/day or with the sustained release form (S.R.) consisting of a monthly injection of 3.75 mg or monthly injections were administered after 7 days of daily injections :
- after an early (from Day 2), moderate and brief (not exceeding Day 8) initial phase of stimulation, castration was gradually induced and was complete (T < 0.50 ng/ml) by Day 28 (Figures 1 and 2). None of the patients presented a clinical deterioration or recrudescence of pain.
- the stability of the castration was confirmed on the basis of the 14 hour serum testosterone levels for 11 patients treated with the S.R. form and 3 patients treated with the subcutaneous form (Figures 3 and 4) : no escape phenomena were noted.
- the blood level of D-Trp6 LHRH, determined in several patients, was between 0.15 and 0.45 ng/ml. It must be maintained at a constant level in order to ensure continual desensitisation of the specific receptors.

Conclusion : D-Trp6 LHRH or DECAPEPTYL induces castration within 3 to 4 weeks, which is subsequently maintained without escape. The dosage of 0.1 mg/day or 3.75 mg/month (S.R. form) is sufficient to obtain this result.

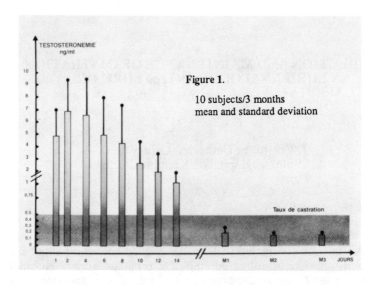

Figure 1.

10 subjects/3 months
mean and standard deviation

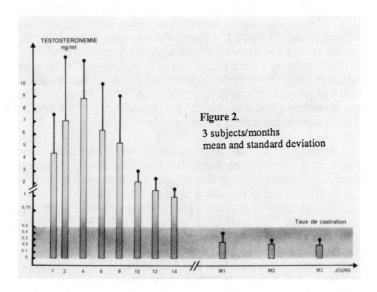

Figure 2.

3 subjects/months
mean and standard deviation

MAINTIEN DE LA CASTRATION					
	TO	T3	T6	T12	T24
DUC... (1)	0,20	0,20	0,20	0,20	0,25
COL... (2)	0,30	0,20	0,20	0,15	0,15
DUP... (3)	0,15	0,10	0,05	0,05	0,05
FAY... (4)	0,05	0,10	0,05	0,05	0,05
GAY... (5)	0,30	0,20	0,20	0,15	0,10
DOU... (6)	0,30	0,40	0,30	0,30	0,15
BAR... (7)	0,15	0,20	0,20	0,20	0,15
GIR... (8)	0,35	0,35	0,30	0,25	0,35
PER... (9)	0,20	0,20	0,15	0,10	0,20
BEA... (10)	0,20	0,35	0,15	0,15	0,35
LHE... (11)	0,15	0,25	0,25	0,25	0,25
m	0,21	0,23	0,19	0,17	0,19
s	0,09	0,10	0,08	0,08	0,03
FRO... (12)	0,15	0,10	0,20	0,15	0,15
POO... (13)	0,15	0,20	0,20	0,20	0,15

Figure 3. 24 hour cycle established in
-11 patients treated with the S.R. form
- 2 patients treated with the subcutaneous form

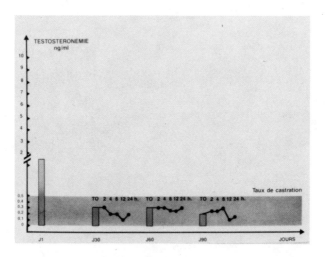

Figure 4. 24 hour cycle at D.30, D.60, and D.90 in one
subject treated with 100 mcg/day s.c.

Prostate Cancer, Part A: Research, Endocrine
Treatment, and Histopathology, page 249
© 1987 Alan R. Liss, Inc.

TREATMENT OF ADVANCED PROSTATIC CANCER WITH A LONG-ACT-
ING FORMULATION OF D-TRP-6 LH-RH. AN ITALIAN PROSTATIC
CANCER PROJECT (P.O.N.CA.P.) STUDY.
Presented by F.Boccardo(project secretary and study co-
ordinator)-Istituto Nazionale per la Ricerca sul Cancro
Genova-Italy.

 95 previously untreated patients(pts)with stage C and
D prostatic ca.were treated for up to 24 mos (median 16
mos)with the long acting formulation of D-TRP-6 LH-RH,
that was injected i.m. every 4 wks until disease pro-
gression.Treatment produced a significant decrease in
LH levels and suppression of testosterone(T)within the
3rd wk.T remained within castrate levels in the long
run.Repeated serial measurements in 7 pts after 6 or mo
re mos of treatment showed that the initial spike of LH
and T levels was no longer evident.86 pts are currenlty
(march 1986)evaluable for overall response according to
the NPCP-USA criteria.In C and D1 groups(n=33)69.7% show
ed partial response(PR),27.3% were stable(S),and 3% pro-
gressed(P).In D2 group(n=53)figures were 37.7%,49.1%
and 13.2% respectively. Response in different involved
sites is shown below:

	PROSTATE	(%)	NODES	(%)	BONE	(%)
CR	1/86	(1.2)	5/17	(29.4)	–	–
PR	42/86	(48.8)	6/17	(35.3)	7/53	(13.2)
S	42/86	(48.8)	6/17	(35.3)	38/53	(71.7)
P	1/86	(1.2)	–	–	8/53	(15.1)

Median progression free survival was 12 mos in D2 pts,
while it has not yet been reached in C and D1 pts (p=
0.0008-log rank test).So far no difference in survival
was evident between the 2 groups.Loss of libido(75%)and
hot flushes(50%)were the commonest side-effects.The increase of PAP after the 1st wk was accompained by mild
bone pain in 8 pts and by dysury in 3 of them. The slow
release preparation of D-TRP-6 LH-RH offers an important
alternative in the management of advanced prostatic can
cer.

Prostate Cancer, Part A: Research, Endocrine
Treatment, and Histopathology, pages 251–253
© 1987 Alan R. Liss, Inc.

PRELIMINARY REPORT ON A PHASE II MULTICENTRIC STUDY ON DEPOT LH-RH ANALOGUE IN ADVANCED PROSTATIC CANCER.

BONO A.V[1]., POZZI E[1]., BIANCO A[2].,
MORELLLI A[3].BOLGAN A.[4], ALBANO D[5]
FRUGONI A[6], USAI E[7].
1 - Urol.Dept.Regional Hosp., Varese;
2 - Inst.of Oncology. Univ of Naples,
3 - M.Vittoria Hosp.,Turin;
4 - S.Giovanni e Paolo Hosp., Venice;
5 - S.Spirito Hosp., Casale;
6- Urol.Dept.S.Paolo Hosp., Savona;
7- Inst. of Urol.,Univ.of Cagliari. Italy

The preliminary data coming from a multicentric Phase II study with a Depot preparation of LH-RH Analogue (ICI 118.63O) are presented. Criteria for inclusion into the study were : histologically proven Prostatic Cancer, no previous or concomitant treatments, life expectancy over 3 months clinical stages C, D1 and D2.

The drug was administered subcutaneously every 4 weeks in Depot preparation containing 3.6 mg of active Analogue.Pre-treatment studies consisted in : prostatic biopsy, transrectal ultrasound or prostatic and pelvic CT scan, I.V.P., abdominal CT scan or ultrasound, chest X-ray, wholebody bone scan, renal and liver function determinations, blood counts, hormonal evaluations (Testosterone, LH), Pap-RIA

As indicator lesion the prostate was allowed as well as any other visceral metastasis. The prostate was measured by CT scan or transrectal ultrasound at 6 cm from anal ring (bidimensional). Osseous pain was assessed by the patient himself through linear analogue scale. Urological disturbances were assessed by uroflow or examiner evaluation.
During the follow-up, indicator lesion diameters, clinical T category, LH, Testosterone, liver and renal functions, Pap-RIA, bone or other pain were registered at 4th, 8th, and 12th weeks and every 12 weeks thereafter.Whole body bone scan, chest X-ray and any other necessary examination were performed at the 12th and 24th weeks and every 24th week thereafter. Side-effects such as impotence,hot flashes, etc.. were carefully registered at each course.

At a cut-off analysis performed on 30 April 1986, 80 patients were introduced into study. 51 of them were considered evaluable having been treated for a minimum of 3 courses.

Out of the 80 pts. recruited, 5 were considered to be ineligible for the following reasons: Stage B = 3 cases Radiotherapy on the indicator = 1, concomitant rectal carcinoma = 1.

The 38% of patients experienced a certain amount of hot flashes, usually in the evening and at night - which however did not affect their social life - and a sharp reduction or abolition of erection (50% of cases) and libido (48%) to which "castrate" hormonal levels were related. In 5% of cases some breast swelling was noticed, in 12%, tenderness of mammary areas in only one (1.9%) a transient rise of serum testosterone.

Other reversible side-effects not clearly related to the treatment were observed in 3 patients : diffuse muscular pain = 1 pt; leg edema = 1 pt; hyperthricosis = 1 pt.

In two additional patients, jaundice developed. In one a choledochal stone was removed by endoscopy and treatment continued.In the other, a hepatic dysfunction was detected and it was interpreted as secondary to anti-inflammatory therapy given for rheumatoid arthritis and not related to the treatment. This case was eliminated from the study.

Neither temporary progressions in volume of indicator lesions nor in urologic disturbances nor in pain were registered.

In the present series evaluable patient distribution in stages was = Stage C = 5 pts; Stage D1 = 1 pt; Stage D2 with visceral metastases = 2 pts; Stage D2 -bone metastases = 43 pts. In 48 patients therefore the primary tumor was the indicator lesion whereas in 3 measurable visceral or lymph-node deposits were measured.

The mean follow-up was on 22 weeks and the following responses were registered :

Stage C : PR 1/5 NC 3/5 PD 1/5
Stage D1 : NC 1/1
Stage D2, visceral metastases : PR 2/2 (both on the liver
after the 3d and 5th course)
Stage D2, bone metastases : PR 13/43 (30.2%), NC 23/43
(53.5%) PD 7/43 (16.2%).

Increase in the Performance Status (WHO) was seen in 43% of cases, with relief of pain usually in bony segments and with urologic symptoms improvement in 15%.

The median duration of response in responders was of 16 weeks.

In conclusion, the therapeutic regimen tested in advanced prostatic cancer, even if it did not give any CR during the short period of observation so far available,has proved very efficient in reducing the symptoms and in improving the quality of life. The only and foreseen side-effect was the impairment of sexual activity.

The rate of responses (30.2% of PR in stage D2 patients) together with the extremely low rate of PD during the follow-up seems highly favourable.

Prostate Cancer, Part A: Research, Endocrine
Treatment, and Histopathology, pages 255–260
© 1987 Alan R. Liss, Inc.

TREATMENT OF ADVANCED PROSTATIC CANCER WITH LHRH-ANALOGUES.
PREVENTION OF "FLARE-UP" PHENOMENON.

Ch. BOUFFIOUX[*], L. DENIS[**], C. MAHLER[***], J. de LEVAL[*].

(*) Urological Department, CHU Sart-Tilman, Liège (Belgium)
(**) Urological Department, Az Middelheim, Antwerp (Belgium)
(***) Endocrinological Department, Az Middelheim,
      Antwerp (Belgium)

A. Introduction.

Several studies have demonstrated the efficacy of LHRH-
analogues in advanced carcinoma of the prostate.
However, during the initial phase of the treatment, LHRH-
analogues produce a stimulation of the pituitary gonadal
axis provoking a transient increase of plasma testosterone
levels during the first week of treatment (1,2,3).
Thereafter, the suppression of the LH secretion leads to a
fall of plasma testosterone that reaches the levels found
in surgically castrated men within 3 weeks (see figure).

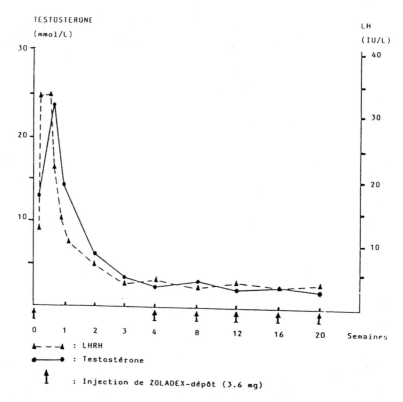

TESTOSTERONE (mmol/L) — LH (IU/L)

♦ – – ♦ : LHRH
●――● : Testostérone
↑ : Injection de ZOLADEX-dépôt (3.6 mg)

Effect of ICI 118,630 (Depot-Zoladex, 3.6 mg) on LH (――)
and testosterone (----) plasma levels. Arrows indicate the
injections of the LHRH-analogue every 4 weeks.

There is much concern about this initial rise of testosterone
levels. It could cause an acceleration of the growth of the
tumor and impair the favourable effects of subsequent
androgen depression.

B. Review of the literature.

Most of the studies with LHRH-analogues (BUSERELIN[R],
ZOLADEX[R], leuprolide, decapeptyl) do not mention any initial
worsening of the patient's condition indicating a possible
deletary effect of the initial rise of testosterone levels.
But there are some reports that clearly indicate a disease

flare by LHRH-analogues in patients with metastatic
prostatic cancer.

KAHAN et al (4) report 2 cases where the administration
of D-Trp^6-LHRH-analogue resulted in excruciating pain,
progressive delirious state and in patient 2 a sudden paraplegia due to spinal cord compression by epidural
metastases. Both patients died in the following 2 weeks.

FAURE et al (5) report 2 cases among 14 patients where a
transient increase of the metastatic algic syndrome was
observed.

DEBRUYNE et al (6) report 27 % of flare-up in patients
treated by ZOLADEX^R alone when clinical (pain) and
biological (phosphatases) parameters are considered, but
no serious deterioration was observed.

ROBINSON et al (7) in a multicentric study with ZOLADEX^R
including 250 patients observed 4 cases of transient
increase of metastatic pain requiring major analgesics,
1 case of ureteric obstruction and 2 paraplegia requiring
a laminectomy.

C. Personal experience.

In Antwerp, L.D. and C.M. observed in a first series of
patients treated with LHRH-analogues alone (ICI 118,630 –
DEPOT-ZOLADEX^R) one case of paraplegia due to a burden of
vertebral metastases occurring one week after the start of
the treatment and that required a laminectomy. They also
noticed a transient increase of osseous metastatic pain in
about 4 % of the patients.

In a second series of patients, DES 3.0 mg/day was
systematically associated to the LHRH-analogues; the
treatment was initiated the day before the first injection

of DEPOT-ZOLADEX^R and discontinued after 2 weeks. With this association, no complication nor temporary initial worsening of the patient's condition was noticed, so far, in more than 30 patients.

In Liège, we have treated 34 patients with advanced prostatic cancer (T_3/T_4, M_0 or T_xM_+) with the DEPOT-ZOLADEX^R preparation. The initial 20 patients were treated by the LHRH-analogue alone while the next 14 patients received cyproterone acetate (ANDROCUR^R) 50 mg × 3 daily. The anti-androgen was given the day of the first injection of ZOLADEX^R and continued for 2 weeks.

In the first group, we did not observe serious adverse effect but 2 patients (10 %) reported an increase of lumbar pain, starting 2 or 3 days after the injection and lasting for about 1 week.

Moreover, in 3 patients with widespread metastases we observed a significant increase of acid and alkaline phosphatases 2 weeks and 4 weeks after the start of the treatment. In all these cases, the enzymes return to the initial values after 2 months and reach normal values after 3 to 9 months.

In the second group, we did not observe any complaint (except for the well-known side-effects of impotency and hot flushes) and we did not notice such an initial increase of alkaline and acid phosphatases.

D. Conclusion.

Although relatively uncommon, disease flare occurs in about 5-10 % of the patients with metastatic prostatic cancer treated with LHRH-analogue alone. It may sometimes be life-threatening and thus requires measures to block the initial and transient stimulation of androgen-dependent cancer cells in relation with the peak of plasma testosterone.

The administration of an estrogen (Diethylstilboestrol, 3×1.0 mg/day) or of an anti-androgen (cyproterone acetate, 3×50 mg/day) for 2 weeks, starting the day before or even the day of the first administration of LHRH-analogue proved to be a safe and useful mean to suppress this "flare-up" phenomenon.

Ch. BOUFFIOUX. Urological Department.
CHU Sart-Tilman. Liège (Belgium)

Bibliography.

1. D. RABIN, L.W. McNEIL. Pituitary and gonadal desensitization after continuous luteinizing hormone-releasing hormone infusion in normal females. J. Clin. Endocrinol. Metab. 51 : 873-876 (1980).

2. A.V. SCHALLY, T.W. REDDING and A.M. COMARU-SCHALLY. Potential use of analogs of luteinizing hormone-releasing hormones in the treatment of hormone-sensitive neoplasms. Cancer Treatm. Rep. 68 : 281-289 (1984).

3. F. LABRIE, A. DUPONT, A. BELANGER, Y. LACOURSIERE, J.P. RAYNAUD, J.M. HUSSON, J. GAREAU, A.T.A. FAZEKAS, J. SANDOW, G. MUNIFELIE, J.G. GIRARD, J. EMOND and J.G. HOULE. New approach in the treatment of prostate cancer : complete instead of partial withdrawal of androgens. The Prostate 4 : 579-594 (1983).

4. KAHAN A., DELRIEU F., AMOR B., CHICHE R., STEG A. Disease flare induced by D-Trp^6-LHRH-analogue in patients with metastatic prostatic cancer. Lancet, 1984, 971-972.

5. FAURE N., LEMAY A., LAROCHE B., ROBERT G., PLANTE R., JEAN C., THABET M., ROY R., FAZEKAS A.T. Preliminary results on the clinical efficacy and safety of androgen inhibition by an LHRH agonist alone or combined with an antiandrogen in the treatment of prostatic carcinoma. Prostate 1983, vol : 4 (6), p : 601-24.

6. DEBRUYNE F. et al. Clinical research with the Depot preparation ZOLADEX^R in prostate cancer. Abstract Book EORTC Symposium, Rotterdam 1986.

7. ROBINSON M. et al. Clinical and endocrinological results with a depot LHRH-analogue (ZOLADEX^R) in the management of advanced prostatic cancer. Personal communication, 1986.

Prostate Cancer, Part A: Research, Endocrine
Treatment, and Histopathology, pages 261–265
© 1987 Alan R. Liss, Inc.

THE VALUE OF REVERSIBLE ANDROGEN SUPPRESSION AS A DIAGNOSTIC
TEST

D.W.W. Newling F.R.C.S.

Consultant Urologist

Princess Royal Hospital, Saltshouse Road,
Hull, U.K.

Ninety per cent of prostatic cancer cells are apparently androgen dependent. (4) It would seem logical, therefore , that the primary treatment for metastatic prostatic
cancer should be androgen ablation by one means or another.
Since over 90% of the total androgen secretion in man eman-
ates from the testicles, orchidectomy is the logical first
treatment of choice in newly diagnosed prostatic cancer.(7)
There are, however, occasions when the permanent effects of
orchidectomy as a means of androgen suppression are not wan-
ted. Such occasions are when the following aims are to be
met:

1. To test for hormone responsiveness in a known carcinoma
of the prostate.
2. To test for hormone responsiveness in a metastatic tumour where the primary has not been diagnosed.
3. To avoid the side-effects of surgical orchidectomy when
there is no indication for continuing androgen ablation.

There are, in addition, a number of other advantages to
reversible orchidectomy which are a little more abstract and
arguable. Withdrawal of androgen blockade would enable the
effects of other therapies such as chemotherapy to be studied
in isolation. Withdrawal of androgens and their subsequent
reappearance on removal of the blockade is not a permanent
phenomenon and androgen depletion can always be reinstated,
if appropriate. There is also some recent evidence to suggest that the action of cytotoxic agents in carcinoma of the
prostate is enhanced by a normal level of serum testosterone
(5). It seems that testosterone enables more cells in the

cancer to be actively dividing and, therefore, susceptible
to the action of chemotherapeutic agents, particularly nuclear poisons, at any given time. If there is then a place
for reversible androgen ablation, there are a number of ways
this may be accomplished. An equivalent reduction in androgen levels to castration may be achieved by the use of Diethyl stilboestrol. We know from the VACURG studies (2,3)
that the greater effect of DES, 5 mg t.d.s. on prostatic
cancer compared to orchidectomy was offset by a prohibitive
incidence of cardiovascular deaths. Later, Byar and Blackard showed that 1 mg DES was as effective in diminishing
cancer deaths as a higher dose and was accompanied by fewer
cardiovascular side-effects. Whether it is relevant or not,
this dosage was not associated with a persistent level of
androgens in the castrate range. (3) In addition, DES has
other side-effects. (Table 1)

TABLE 1. Side-effects or toxicity of oestrogen therapy

    1. Excessive cardiovascular toxicity
    2. Hyperprolactinaemia
    3. Water and salt retention
    4. Hepatotoxicity
    5. Impotence
    6. Impairment of immune response

More recent alternatives to DES are the anti-androgens
cyproterone acetate and Flutamide. (8) In a recent EORTC
study, CPA was less effective than DES, 1 mg t.d.s., in
lengthening the time to progression but more effective than
Medroxy progesterone acetate. Flutamide is active but has
the disadvantage that a secondary rise in testosterone occurs since Flutamide acts only at the target organ in the
prostate. (9) In addition, both compounds have side-effects,
some severe. (Table 2)

TABLE 2. Side-effects of CPA and Flutamide

Side-effects of CPA	Side-effects of Flutamide
1. Fluid retention	1. Optical disturbances (? retinoid metabolism)
2. Impotence	2. Depression
3. C.V. side-effects	3. Methaemaglobinaemia
4. Gynaecomastia	4. ?? Testicular pathology

More recently, attention has focussed on LH-RH agonists as an alternative to orchidectomy. They would seem to be effective (1,6.9) in diminishing androgen production to castrate levels and their side-effects are mild. (Table 3)

TABLE 3. Comparison of the side-effects of Zoladex (LH-RH agonist) and orchidectomy

		Zoladex	Orchidectomy
1.	Impotence	61%	90%
2.	Hot flushes	48%	50%
3.	Fluid retention	0%	32%
4.	C.V. side-effects: Thrombo-embolism Angina Claudication	2%	12%

Being agonists there is, of course, an initial flare phenomenon which is reasonably controlled by a variety of anti-androgens. (6,11)

There are, therefore, a number of indications that there is a place for reversible androgen depletion and in the LH-RH agonists we probably have the most effective agents for achieving this. Apart from a number of advantages listed above, the principal use would seem to be in the diagnosis of the sensitivity, or otherwise, of a prostatic cancer to androgen blockade and a possible plan of action in this respect is outlined below. (Table 4)

In the primary treatment of metastatic prostatic cancer, if the tumour is seen to be hormone sensitive and there are good reasons for the patient not to have daily, weekly or monthly treatment, then an orchidectomy can obviously be carried out. If the response is not complete but partial, then the addition of an anti-androgen may make it more complete and, similarly, if there is initially no change, it is worth trying complete androgen blockade before abandoning primary hormonal therapy. If, however, progression occurs early, there is some indication that we should withdraw androgen blockade and treat the patient with a cytotoxic agent. The great advantage of reversible androgen ablation is that it is just that.

TABLE 4. Treatment plan for carcinoma of the prostate

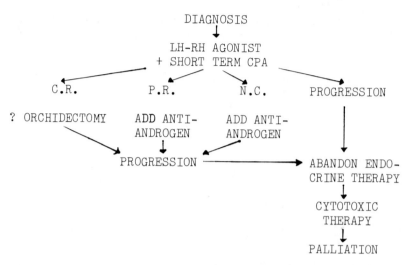

REFERENCES

1. Ahmed S R, Brooman P J C, Shalet S M, Howell A and Black-
    lock N J. (1983) Treatment of advanced prostatic can-
    cer with LH-RH analogue ICI 118630. Clinical response
    and hormonal mechanisms. Lancet 15, p.415
2. Byar D P, (1972) Treatment of Prostatic Cancer: Studies
    by the Veterans Administration Co-operative Urological
    Group. Bulletins of the New York Academy of Medicine.
    No. 48, p.751
3. Byar D P, (1976) The VACURG Experience on Treatment of
    Prostatic Cancer with oestrogens and orchidectomy in
    'The Tumours of G.U. Apparatus.' Ed.M.Pav.Macaluso,
    Pub. by Cofese, Palermo.
4. Coffey D, (1979) Physiological control of prostatic
    growth. U.I.C.C. Technical Report Series, Vol.48,P.4
5. Coffey D, and Isaacs J T, (1979) Experimental concepts
    in the design of new treatments for human prostatic
    cancer. U.I.C.C. workshop No. 9, Geneva 1979.
6. Debruyne F, Robinson M, Lungelmeyer G, Denis L, Newling
    D, Clinical Results of a Biodegradeable depot LH-RH
    analogue in the management of metastatic prostatic can-
    cer. (in press)
7. Huggins C and Hodges C V. (1941) Studies on Prostatic
    Cancer, Cancer Research 1, p.293

8. Jacobi G H, Altwein J E, Kurth K H, Basting R, Hohenfell-
    ner R. (1980) The Treatment of advanced prostatic
    cancer with parenteral CPA - Phase III randomised tri-
    al - Brit. Journ. Urol. No. 8, p.129
9. Neumann F, Jacobi G H. (1982) Antiandrogens in tumour
    therapy. Clin. Oncol. Vol. 1, No. 1, p.41
10. Robinson M R G and EORTC Data Centre (1986) Personal
    Communication.
11. Robinson M R G, Mahler C, Denis L, Lungelmeyer G, New-
    ling D, Debruyne F. Endocrine effects of a four-week-
    ly biodegradeable depot formulation of Zoladex - an
    LH-RH analogue. (in press)

Prostate Cancer, Part A: Research, Endocrine
Treatment, and Histopathology, pages 267–274
© 1987 Alan R. Liss, Inc.

CURRENT STATUS OF THE LHRH IMMUNIZATION APPROACH

Anne Hosmalin, André Morin and Louis Chedid

Immunothérapie Expérimentale, Institut Pasteur,
75015 Paris, France

I. INTRODUCTION

Arimura and Schally and the group of Fraser first reported in 1973 that immunological castration could be induced
by immunization against the hypothalamic hormone LHRH. These
authors, who were actually immunizing rabbits and rats with
the synthetic decapeptide hormone in order to produce LHRH
antisera suitable for radioimmunoassays, observed incident-
ally that the immunization caused a decrease in the LH
pituitary content associated with atrophy of the testes.
Immunological castration using LHRH immunization was subsequently induced in a variety of species including rats,
guinea pigs, dogs, cattle and monkeys, as reviewed by Fraser
(1980), Jeffcoate (1984) and Schanbacher (1984). These
findings were exploited from both a fundamental and clinical
standpoint. At the fundamental level, they prompted a number
of studies on the physiological role of LHRH (Fraser, 1984).
Such a procedure represents actually a selective pituitary
inhibition although the precise mechanisms involved are not
yet fully understood. At the clinical level, they provided
the rationale for developing veterinary and human LHRH
vaccines.

In veterinary practice, castration is usually achieved
by surgery. For a sake of convenience, the operation takes
place at about 3 months of age in cattle. This results in the
fact that the anabolizing effect of androgens is lost at an
early period of the animal growth. Developing alternative
procedures of castration which could be applied to older
animals would thus allow a substantial benefit in terms of

body weight increase. In pets, alternatives to surgical castration would also be most granted (Fraser, 1980). In humans,
the most obvious application of LHRH immunization is to
achieve an immunological castration in hormone-dependent neoplasia, particularly breast cancers and prostatic carcinoma.

An extensive review of the beneficial therapeutic effects
of LHRH agonists can be found in Schally (1984) and this book
presents the most recent data on this matter. As mentioned
there, this new interesting therapy is however associated
with problems such as long duration of treatment, raising
risk for the patient's compliance, and possible flare-up at
initiation of therapy. The use of LHRH antagonists represents
an alternative approach of chemical castration induced by
agonists. Along this line of antagonization LHRH immunization
is another approach which is theoretically easier to deal
with. It could be used either alone or in combination with
other drugs employed for inducing a chemical castration.

In most of the experimental studies of LHRH immunization
performed up to now the hypothalamic hormone was injected
either adsorbed on macromolecules or covalently linked to a
carrier in the presence of Freund's complete adjuvant (FCA).
FCA is a preparation comprised of killed whole Mycobacteria
in emulsion in a mineral oil. It represents the most efficient
adjuvant yet available for laboratory animals. However, it
can be responsible for undesirable reactions such as sensitization to tuberculin, granuloma formation, sensitization to
endotoxin shock and adjuvant arthritis (Chedid, 1978). For
these reasons, it cannot be used in human or veterinary
clinical practice (Robertson, 1979).

Largely as a result of Lederer's contribution, a detailed
study of the mycobacterial cell-wall structure was achieved
(Lederer, 1980). Successive fractionation of the cell-wall
led to the discovery that the minimal structure which could
replace whole Mycobacteria in FCA is rather simple. It is
comprised of a bacteria-specific sugar (N-acetylmuramic acid)
and 2 amino acids (L-alanine and D-isoglutamine). This structure was named MDP for muramyl dipeptide. Since this component had a simple structure, it could be produced synthetical-
ly (Ellouz, 1974; Merser, 1975; Kotani, 1975). Subsequently,
300 derivatives and analogs were synthesized and tested for
their biological activity in France, Japan, Switzerland, and
the United States (Chedid, 1978; Lederer, 1980; Lefrancier,
1981). These efforts provided an extensive study of the

relationships between chemical structure and biological activity, thus allowing the selection within the whole family of
certain groups of molecules endowed with a unique immunopharmacological profile. These groups are of interest from
two standpoints : fundamental as biological tools for dissect-
ing mechanisms involved in immune responses, clinical because
of a selective potential in various fields of pathology.
Indeed, muramyl peptides have been shown to be endowed with
adjuvant, anti-infectious and antitumoral activities. They
also possess anti-allergic, immunosuppressive and neuro-
pharmacological properties which might be clinically exploited (Leclerc, 1983; Audibert, 1985). At the present time, one
derivative called Murabutide has been administered to over
400 individuals. It has proven to be safe and adjuvant-active
vis-à-vis two different human vaccines, namely tetanus toxoid
and a streptococcal antigen derived from M24 protein (Telzak,
1986; Oberling, 1985). Muramyl peptides are able to enhance
humoral and cellular responses to many antigens when administered in oily emulsions such as Freund's incomplete adjuvant
(FIA), and to enhance the antibody response when administered
in aqueous solutions (Audibert, 1976; Chedid, 1976).

II. LHRH IMMUNIZATION USING LHRH DIRECTLY BOUND TO MDP-Lys

a) Immunogenicity and Castrative Effects of LHRH-Lys-MDP Compounds

LHRH immunization experiments were therefore performed
in which FCA was replaced by muramyl peptides. In 1982,
Carelli et al. observed that immunological castration could
be induced in male mice by immunization with the conjugate
LHRH-Lys-MDP(CDI). This conjugate was prepared by directly
coupling via carbodiimide (CDI) the decapeptide hormone to
MDP-Lys, an adjuvant derivative of MDP. A dose of conjugate
containing approximately 10 µg of LHRH and 5 µg of MDP-Lys
was injected sc in aqueous solution on days 0, 2, 4 and 30,
and animals were sacrificed one month after the last injection. As shown in Table 1, LHRH-Lys-MDP(CDI) induced LHRH
antibodies, decrease in testicular testosterone, and atrophy
of seminiferous tubules associated with a spermatogenesis
decrease (Carelli, 1982; Carelli, 1985; Hosmalin, submitted).

TABLE 1. Immunogenicity and castrative effects of 3 different LHRH-Lys-MDP compounds

Compounds[a]	LHRH antibody level (% binding)[b]	Testicular testosterone (ng/testis)	Histological features	
			Seminiferous tubules	Spermatogenesis
Controls (NaCl)	11 ± 3	170 ± 25	Normal 8/8	Normal 8/8
LHRH-Lys-MDP(CDI)	25 ± 2**	32 ± 13	Atrophy 10/10	Decrease 10/10
LHRH-Lys-MDP(s)	29 ± 3**	34 ± 16	Atrophy 7/7	Decrease 7/7
LHRH-LysNH$_2$-MDP	20 ± 8*	75 ± 44	Atrophy 4/9	Decrease 5/9

[a] CDI = carbodiimide coupling; s= total synthesis; LHRH-LysNH$_2$-MDP = amide analog of LHRH-Lys-MDP(s).

[b] Arithmetic mean and standard deviation of LHRH antibody levels measured by RIA in sera from individual mice.

* $p < 0.05$; ** $p < 0.001$ (Student's t test vs control group).

However, coupling by carbodiimide can induce oligomers
or isomers and lead to heterogenous preparations. In view of
possible clinical use it was necessary to have better defined
molecules. A linear monomeric molecule, LHRH-Lys-MDP(s), was
then obtained by total synthesis, and shown to be pure by
amino-acid analysis and high performance liquid chromatography
(Bernard, in preparation). This molecule was compared to
LHRH-Lys-MDP(CDI) and exhibited a similar degree of biological
activity in male mice (Table 1).

Since the synthesis yield was low, an analog containing
an amide residue was prepared (LHRH-LysNH$_2$-MDP). This latter
molecule was found not to be as active as the two former
ones (Table 1).

b) Absence of LHRH Agonistic Activity

In addition to their immunogenicity the hormonal activity
of MDP-linked LHRH compounds was studied. LHRH-Lys-MDP(CDI)
was found to have no significant LHRH agonistic activity in
a rat anterior pituitaries perifusion assay (Carelli, 1985).
LHRH-LysNH$_2$-MDP was tested in another *in vitro* assay measuring LH release in the supernatant of cultured rat anterior
pituitary cells. As shown in Table 2, the release of LH increased as a function of the LHRH concentrations added to the
cultures. In contrast, LHRH-LysNH$_2$-MDP had no significant
agonistic activity.

c) Absence of Pyrogenicity

It has been previously shown that MDP-Lys induced fever
in rabbits and that conjugation of MDP to macromolecules
greatly enhanced its pyrogenicity (Riveau, 1980; Carelli,
1985). At doses up to 10 µg/kg injected iv, LHRH-Lys-MDP(CDI)
and LHRH-Lys-MDP(s) did not induce a febrile reaction in
rabbits, nor did they by the more sensitive intracerebro-
ventricular route of administration. This lack of pyrogenicity
was specific of the covalent linkage of LHRH on MDP-Lys, since
both uncoupled molecules injected simultaneously induced
fever (Carelli, 1985).

CONCLUSIONS

The bulk of data presently available indicate that
immunological castration can be experimentally achieved by
LHRH immunization. However, the most consistent results have

TABLE 2. Absence of LHRH Agonistic Activity of
LHRH-LysNH$_2$-MDP.

Stimulation	LH release (ng/ml)
Control (culture medium)	30 ± 6
LHRH	
10^{-5}M (12 µg/ml)	170 ± 37
10^{-6}M (1.2 µg/ml)	189 ± 21
10^{-7}M (120 ng/ml)	159 ± 15
10^{-8}M (12 ng/ml)	166 ± 21
10^{-9}M (1.2 ng/ml)	151 ± 5
10^{-10}M (120 pg/ml)	117 ± 14
10^{-11}M (12 pg/ml)	84 ± 26
LHRH-LysNH$_2$-MDP	
10^{-5}M (18 µg/ml)	90 ± 8
10^{-6} (1.8 µg/ml)	49 ± 13
10^{-7} (180 ng/ml)	44 ± 5
10^{-8} (18 ng/ml)	30 ± 6

Cultured rat anterior pituitary cells were stimulated *in vitro* for 3 hr by various concentrations of LHRH or LHRH-LysNH$_2$-MDP. Each concentration was tested in triplicate. LH release in the supernatants was measured by RIA.

been obtained by administering in FCA the decapeptide hypothalamic hormone coupled to a carrier. Because of the undesirable reactions caused by FCA such an approach cannot be used neither for veterinary nor for human clinical purpose.

In 1982 our group achieved castration by immunizing male mice with a conjugate obtained by direct carbodiimide coupling of LHRH to the adjuvant glycopeptide MDP-Lys and administered in aqueous solution. In view of a potential clinical use, an analytically pure molecule, LHRH-Lys-MDP(s), was then prepared by total synthesis and shown to have a biological activity similar to that of the former compound. Since LHRH-Lys-MDP(s) had a poor synthesis yield, an amide analog was prepared which was found not to be as biologically active as its parent molecule in the same experimental conditions. Such totally synthesized molecules including a safe adjuvant make it possible to use LHRH immunization in clinical practice, especially in hormone-dependent cancers. Additional studies are therefore in progress in order to develop a clinically suitable vaccine.

REFERENCES

Arimura A, Sato H, Kumasaka T, Worobec RB, Debeljuk L, Dunn L, Dunn J, Schally AV (1973). Production of antiserum to LHRH associated with gonadal atrophy in rabbits : development of radioimmunoassays fo LHRH. Endocrinology 93:1092-1103.

Audibert F, Chedid L, Lefrancier P, Choay J (1976). Distinctive adjuvanticity of synthetic analogs of mycobacterial water-soluble components. Cell Immunol 21:243-249.

Audibert F, Leclerc C, Chedid L (1985). Muramyl peptides as immunopharmacological response modifiers. In Torrence PF (ed): "Biological Response Modifiers", Academic Press Inc. p 307.

Bernard JM, Gras-Masse H, Drobecq H, Tartar A, Lefrancier P, Hosmalin A, Carelli C, Audibert F, Chedid L. Improved synthesis of the conjugate between LHRH and MDP. A totally synthetic vaccine (in preparation).

Carelli C, Audibert F, Gaillard J, Chedid L (1982). Immunological castration of male mice by a totally synthetic vaccine administered in saline. Proc Natl Acad Sci USA 79: 5392-5395.

Carelli C, Ralamboranto L, Audibert F, Gaillard J, Briquelet N., Dray F, Fafeur V, Haour F, Chedid L (1985). Immunological castration by a totally synthetic vaccine : modification of biological properties of LHRH after conjugation to adjuvant-active muramyl peptide Int J Immunopharmac 7:215-224.

Chedid L, Audibert F, Lefrancier P, Choay J, Lederer E (1976). Modulation of the immune response by a synthetic adjuvant and analogs. Proc Natl Acad Sci USA 73:2472-2475.

Chedid L, Audibert F, Johnson AG (1978). Biological activities of muramyl dipeptide, a synthetic glycopeptide analogous to bacterial immunomodulating agents. Progr Allergy 25:63-105.

Ellouz F, Adam A, Ciorbaru R, Lederer E (1974). Minimal structural requirements for adjuvant activity of bacterial peptidoglycan derivatives. Biochem Biophys Res Com 59:1317-1325.

Fraser HM, Gunn A (1973). Effect of antibodies to LHRH in the male rabbit and on the rat oestrous cycle. Nature 244: 160-161.

Fraser HM (1980). Inhibition of reproductive function by antibodies to LHRH. In Hearn JP (ed): "Immunological Aspects of Reproduction and Fertility Control", Lancaster: MTP, p 143.

Fraser HM, McNeilly AS, Popkin RM (1984). Passive immunization against LHRH : elucidation of the role of LHRH in controlling LH and FSH secretion and LHRH receptors. In Crighton DB (ed): "Immunological Aspects of Reproduction in Mammals", Butterworths: p 399.

Hosmalin A, Carelli C, Gaillard J, Lefrancier P, Tartar A, Leclerc C, Audibert F, Chedid L.Structural requirements for the induction of immunological castration by linear monomeric LHRH-Lys-MDP administered in saline (submitted).

Jeffcoate IA, Keeling J (1984). Active immunization against LHRH in the female. In Crighton DB (ed): "Immunological Aspects of Reproduction in Mammals", Butterworths: p 363.

Kotani S, Watanabe Y, Shimono T, Narita T, Kato K, Stewart-Tull DES, Kinoshita F, Yokogawa K, Kawata S, Shiba T, Kusumoto S, Tarumi Y (1975). Immunoadjuvant activities of cell walls, their water-soluble fractions and peptidoglycan subunits, prepared from various gram-positive bacteria, and of synthetic N-acetylmuramyl peptides. Z Immun Forsch 149:302-319.

Leclerc C, Morin A, Chedid L (1983). Potential use of synthetic muramyl peptides as immunoregulating molecules. In Thompson RA, Rose NR (eds): "Recent Advances in Clinical Immunology", Edinburgh: Churchill Livingstone, 3:187.

Lederer E (1980). Synthetic immunostimulants derived from the bacterial cell wall. J Med Chem 23:819-825.

Lefrancier P, Lederer E (1981). Chemistry of synthetic immunomodulant muramyl peptides. Prog Chem Org Nat Prod 40:1-47.

Merser C, Sinay P, Adam A (1975). Total synthesis and adjuvant activity of bacterial peptidoglycan derivatives. Biochem Biophys Res Com 66:1316-1322.

Oberling F, Morin A, Duclos B, Lang JM, Beachey EH, Chedid L (1985). Enhancement of antibody response to a natural fragment of streptococcal M protein by Murabutide administered to healthy volunteers. Int J Immunopharmac 7:398.

Riveau G, Masek K, Parant M, Chedid L (1980). Central pyrogenic activity of muramyl dipeptides. J Exp Med 152:869-877.

Robertson IS, Wilson JC, Rowland AC, Fraser HM (1979). Immunological castration in male cattle. Vet Rec 105:556-557.

Schally AV, Comaru-Schally AM, Redding TW (1984). Antitumor effects of analogs of hypothalamic hormones in endocrine-dependent cancers. Proc Soc Exp Biol Med 175:259-281.

Schanbacher BD (1984). Active immunization against LHRH in the male. In Crighton DB (ed): "Immunological Aspects of Reproduction in Mammals", Butterworths: p 345.

Telzak E, Wolff SM, Dinarello CA, Conlon T, El Kholy A, Bahr GM, Choay JP, Morin A, Chedid L (1986). Clinical evaluation of the immunoadjuvant Murabutide, a derivative of MDP, administered with a tetanus toxoid vaccine. J Infect Dis 153:628-633.

Prostate Cancer, Part A: Research, Endocrine
Treatment, and Histopathology, pages 275–282
© 1987 Alan R. Liss, Inc.

AMINOGLUTETHIMIDE IN THE TREATMENT OF ADVANCED PROSTATIC
CANCER

Robin Murray and Paula Pitt

Cancer Institute, Melbourne, Australia

INTRODUCTION

The outlook for patients with advanced prostatic
cancer who have failed to benefit from, or relapsed after
orchidectomy or oestrogen treatment is grim. Their median
life expectancy is only six months (Johnson et al 1975) and
they face increasing pain and decreasing quality of life.
While several further hormonal manouevres are available as
treatment for these patients their efficacy is uncertain as
their use has often been haphazardly and unscientifically
investigated, and in many instances, response has not been
accurately determined. In this paper we demonstrate that
adrenal blockade with aminoglutethimide (A/G) is a useful
and non toxic second line treatment for patients with
advanced prostatic cancer, which not only prolongs survival
in some patients but also improves their quality of life.

MATERIALS AND METHODS

All patients had actively progressing advanced
prostatic cancer which was resistant to conventional
therapy. Prior to commencing treatment each patient had a
thorough history and examination including assessment of
performance status according to ECOG criteria. The
following tests were carried out: full blood examination,
measurement of urea and electrolytes, liver function tests
(alkaline phosphatase, gamma GT, AST bilirubin, albumin and
total proteins), serum calcium and prostatic phosphatase,
dehydroepiandrosterone and testosterone. All patients had

a bone scan and liver scan, while CT scanning was carried out if clinically indicated.

Treatment was started with cortisone acetate 25 mg a.m. 12.5 mg p.m., fludrocortisone 0.1 mg a.m. (unless the patient had hypertension or oedema) and aminoglutethimide 250 mg twice a day. After 3 - 5 days the dosage of A/G was increased to 250 mg three times a day unless the patient complained of drowsiness or lethargy, in which case the dose was left at the lower level until those symptoms disappeared.

Repeat clinical assessment and measurements of the biochemical, haematological and hormonal parameters were carried out at least monthly while the skeletal survey, bone scan and liver scan were repeated at 3 monthly intervals. Classification of response was by two observers according to the National Prostatic Cancer Project criteria. In patients who had not had an orchidectomy but had been treated with oestrogens, the latter drug was continued in the same dose.

RESULTS

One hundred and twenty six men were assessed for their response to A/G. Their pretreatment clinical character-istics are shown in Table 1.

Table 1

Pretreatment clinical characteristics of the patients

AGE (years) - median and range	70	49 - 84
	n	%
bony metastases	103	82
more than 1 tissue site involved	50	40
Prior Treatments		
Orchidectomy	106	84
Orchidectomy and oestrogens	72	57
Oestrogen only	20	16
Progesterone	17	13
Chemotherapy	5	4
X-ray therapy	92	73
1/2 body irradiation	24	19

Twenty two (17.5%) of the 126 patients had a partial
objective response to the treatment and a further 22 had
stabilization of disease. No patient had a mixed response
with regression of some lesions and progression of others.
The median duration of remission and stabilization is the
same for both groups and is approximately 9 months (Graph 1).

Graph 1

Duration of remission and stabilization in patients
responding to aminoglutethimide

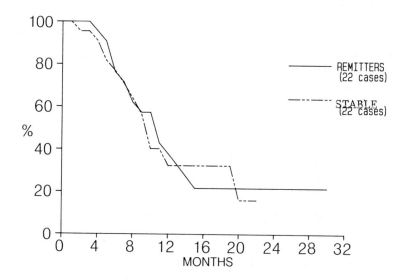

The performance status significantly improved in the
remitting and static groups (p < .001 and < .05 respectively)
and worsened in the non remitters (p < .001). This, together
with the clinical characteristics of the patients divided
according to their response to treatment is shown in
Table 2. There are no significant differences in their
clinical characteristics between the 3 groups of patients
with the exception that the static group had a significantly
greater percentage of patients (p < .01) with advanced
disease present at diagnosis than the group with
progressive disease.

Table 2

Clinical characteristics of the patients divided
according to their response to treatment

	Objective response (22)	Objectively stable (22)	Progressive disease 82
Median age (years)	70	73	68
Disease sites (% of patients)			
Bone	86	77	79
Viscera	9	14	16
1 site	23	9	22
Advanced disease present at diagnosis %	54	77	40
Pre-treatment performance status (mean)	2.1	2.0	2.3
On treatment performance status (mean)	1.6	1.9	2.5

When the effects of previous therapy were examined it
was found that in many instances the response could not be
accurately determined because of poor documentation,
inadequate investigation or concurrent treatment. However
in 52 instances the response to orchidectomy and in 28 the
response to oestrogen could be determined. Six out of 24
responders and 5 out of 28 non responders to orchidectomy
subsequently responded to A/G and 3 out of 18 responders
and 1 out of 10 non responders to oestrogen responded to
subsequent A/G. (Table 3).

Table 3

Response to aminoglutethimide of patients divided according
to their previous response to orchidectomy or oestrogen.
(R = response, S = stabilization, NR = no response)

		Aminoglutethimide	
Orchidectomy		R	S
R	24	6	3
NR	28	5	2
Oestrogens			
R	18	3	1
NR	10	1	4

The average duration between the time of diagnosis of
advanced disease and starting A/G was the same for both
remitting and non remitting patients. This is of particular
importance when survival is analysed as it can be seen that
the survival of the remitters (median 15.6 months) is
significantly longer (p $<$ .0001) than that of the non
remitters (median 5.5 months). Similarly the survival of
the static group (median 12.4 months) is significantly
longer (p = .0004) than that of the non remitters - Graph 2.

Aminoglutethimide was well tolerated and the drug was
stopped because of toxicity in only one instance - a patient
who developed exfoliative dermatitis. Fourteen percent of
patients developed a transient erythematous rash but in all
cases A/G was continued and the rash disappeared after about
1 week. Twenty six percent of patients with progressive
disease complained of lethargy but this appeared to be due
to their disease rather than the drug and was not a problem
in the remitting and static group. Five percent of patients
experienced minor giddiness but this responded to a decrease
in dose.

Graph 2

Survival of patients from commencement of treatment
classified according to their response to
aminoglutethimide

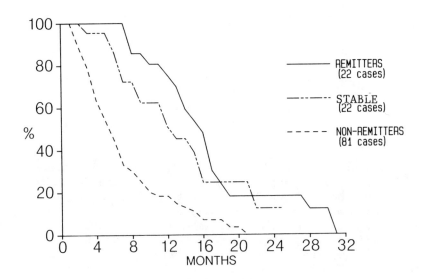

DISCUSSION

The treatment of choice in patients with prostatic
cancer who have relapsed following a remission to, or
failed to benefit from, orchidectomy or oestrogen treatment
is uncertain. Many patients are elderly, medically unfit
and poor candidates for surgical procedures (such as
adrenalectomy or hypophysectomy) or chemotherapy. Newer
hormones and antihormones such as progesterone derivatives,
cyproterone acetate and flutamide have been reported to be
of some benefit but their exact role has not yet been
clearly defined. (Geller and Albert 1983).

This study shows clearly that adrenal blockade with
aminoglutethimide and physiological steroid replacement is
an effective and safe treatment for patients with advanced

prostatic cancer who have failed orchidectomy and/or
oestrogen treatment. It confirms and enlarges our previous
report of the use of A/G in prostatic cancer (Murray and
Pitt 1985) and supports the findings of Worgul and
associates (1983) who reported a 47.8% response rate in
23 patients treated with A/G. In contrast to this Rostom
and associates (1982) failed to detect an objective
remission in any of 12 patients but noted a 75% subjective
improvement. In our study not only did performance status
significantly improve in the remitting and static groups,
but also survival was significantly longer in these groups
than in the patients who failed to respond. This appears
to have been due to the treatment as there was no
significant difference in the time from diagnosis of
advanced disease to starting A/G in the remitting and non
remitting groups. Similarly there was no significant
difference in the clinical characteristics of the groups
(with the one exception that the static group had a higher
percentage of patients with advanced disease present at
the time of initial diagnosis than the non remitting group).
It is of interest that some patients who had clearly failed
to respond to orchidectomy or oestrogen treatment
subsequently responded to aminoglutethimide, suggesting
that failure to respond should not preclude patients from
being given a second hormone treatment.

These patients had all been heavily pretreated and had
often had progressive disease for many months before
starting A/G. While it does not appear possible to select
patients likely to respond to A/G on a clinical basis, it
does appear logical to offer more patients earlier treatment. It is possible the response rate and survival may be
further improved if treatment is started before the tumour
burden is great and the health of the patient has already
been compromised by this and large amounts of radiotherapy.

Further studies are also necessary to compare the
effectiveness of A/G with other second line treatment such
as anti androgens and progestitional agents.

REFERENCES

1.   Geller J, Albert J D (1983). Comparison of various
      hormonal therapies of prostatic carcinoma. Semin
      Oncol 4: 34.

2.   Johnson D E, Faescher K E, Ayala A G (1975). Megestrol
      acetate for treatment of advanced carcinoma of the
      prostate. J Surg Oncol 7: 9.

3.   Murray R, Pitt P (1985). Treatment of advanced
      prostatic cancer, resistant to conventional therapy
      with aminoglutethimide. Eur J Clin Onc 4: 453.

4.   Rostom A Y, Folkes A, Lord C, Notley R G,
      Schweitzer F A W, White W F (1982). Aminoglutethimide
      therapy for advanced carcinoma of the prostate.
      Br J Urol 54: 552.

5.   Worgul T J, Santen R J, Samojlik E et al (1983).
      Clinical and biochemical effect of aminoglutethimide
      in the treatment of advanced prostatic carcinoma.
      J Urol 129: 51.

Prostate Cancer, Part A: Research, Endocrine
Treatment, and Histopathology, pages 283–289
© 1987 Alan R. Liss, Inc.

AMINOGLUTETHIMIDE IN METASTATIC ADENOCARCINOMA OF THE PROS-
TATE.

E. David Crawford, Frederick R. Ahmann, Marilyn
A. Davis, and Yvan J. Levasseur

Division of Urology, University of
Mississippi Medical Center, Jackson,
MS 39216, and Section of Hematology,
Veterans Administration Medical
Center, Tucson, Arizona 85723

INTRODUCTION

During 1986 there will be approximately 85,000 new
cases of adenocarcinoma of the prostate and 25,000 deaths
from the disease in the United States. This malignancy is
the second most common tumor found in men and the third
leading cause of cancer deaths. Unfortunately, 50–80% of
the patients present with advanced disease either to lymph
nodes or bone. The mainstay of treatment for metastatic
adenocarcinoma of the prostate gland remains endocrine
manipulation, either in the form of an orchiectomy or hormonal manipulation. In spite of the fact that more than
70% of men have a response to this therapy, the mean survival time remains 1.9 years. Once disease progression
occurs, the 6 month survival rate is less than 50%.

Treatment of disease refractory to endocrine manipulation remains controversial. A variety of regimens have
been proposed including chemotherapy, antiandrogens, hypophysectomy, adrenalectomy, transurethral resection, enzyme
inhibitors, high dose estrogen therapy and analgesics. Some
of these treatments are invasive and associated with significant patient morbidity.

Several studies in the past have documented not only
the production of testosterone from the adrenal gland, but
also the palliative value of adrenalectomy in advanced
disease. The development of a medical adrenalectomy through

the use of aminoglutethimide was, therefore, investigated.
Aminoglutethimide is derived from the hypnotic drug glute-
thimide. The addition of the amino group to the glutethi-
mide increases the anticonvulsant properties of the drug.
The drug was formerly used in the treatment of epilepsy,
but was found to be a potent inhibitor of adrenal steroidogenesis. Its effect is thought to be on the P-450 enzyme
conversion of cholesterol to pregnenolone. This is a reversible inhibition, which results in elevated ACTH levels
which can override the drug-induced blockade unless accompanied by concomitant glucocorticoid replacement. It has
also been found that the drug accelerates the metabolism of
dexamethasone.

By inhibiting the enzymatic conversion of cholesterol
to delta-5-pregnenolone, aminoglutethimide blocks adrenal
steroidogenesis thereby reducing the synthesis of gluco-
corticoids, mineralocorticoids, and sex steroids. This
block is achieved through competitive inhibition of the
mitrochondrial desmolase side chain splitting enzyme. The
compound also blocks the organification of iodine, resulting in a temporary reduction of thyroxine. This effect is
overcome by increased thyroid-stimulating hormone (TSH) production by the pituitary. Aminoglutethimide interferes with
the peripheral aromatization of androgens to estrogens.

METHODS:

This was a multi-institutional study organized to
evaluate the efficacy and safety of aminoglutethimide in
patients with hormone-refractory Stage D_2 prostate cancer.

ADMISSION CRITERIA

A. Inclusion Criteria
    1. Hospitalized or outpatient males capable of legal
        consent.
    2. Histological confirmation of prostatic carcinoma.
    3. Orchiectomy at least six weeks prior to entry into
        the study.
    4. Prior treatment with hormonal therapy, radiation
        therapy or chemotherapy with unresponsive or

progressive disease.
5. Measurable or evaluable disease.
6. Progressive disease at the time of entry into the study.
7. ECOG performance status of 0,1,2 or 3.

B. Exclusion Criteria
  1. Surgical adrenalectomy or hypophysectomy.
  2. CNS metastases unless brain and/or spinal lesions are treated; these sites are not to be included as evaluation sites.
  3. Chemotherapy or endocrine therapy within 1 week of entry into the study.
  4. Anticipated survival of less than 3 months.
  5. Bone marrow suppression defined as total white blood cell count less than 4,000/mm^3, platelet count less than 100,000/mm^3, hematocrit less than 25%, or hemoglobin less than 10 g/dl.
  6. Total bilirubin greater than or equal to 3 mg/dl, creatinine greater than or equal to 2 mg/dl.
  7. Concomitant antineoplastic surgery.
  8. Another type of neoplastic disease.
  9. ECOG performance status of 4.

STUDY MEDICATIONS:

A. Aminoglutethimide

Initially, during the first two weeks of the study, aminoglutethimide was administered at a dosage regimen of 250 mg (one tablet) twice daily orally. Thereafter, the dosage was increased to 1000 mg/day (250 mg q.i.d.) and maintained at that level for the remaining period of the study. If side effects (fever, rash, lethargy, nausea, ataxia, nystagmus and dizziness) occurred while the patient was on maintenance therapy, the daily dosage of aminoglutethimide was temporarily reduced until these signs and/or symptoms abated at which time the dosage was again increased to 1000 mg/day.

B. Hydrocortisone

Hydrocortisone was given in divided daily doses for glucocorticoid replacement. During the first two weeks of aminoglutethimide treatment, 100 mg/day was used (20 mg in the morning, 20 mg in the evening, and 60 mg just before sleep). The use of higher doses of hydrocortisone during the initial two weeks of aminoglutethimide treatment reduces the frequency of adverse drug reactions. The average maintenance daily dosage thereafter is 40 mg/day (10 mg in the morning, 10 mg in the evening, and 20 mg at bedtime), orally.

C. Mineralocorticoid Replacement

Fludrocortisone acetate (0.1 mg) was administered at the discretion of the investigator as indicated by the clinical condition of the patient.

TABLE I

TREATMENT EVALUATIONS

PHASE:	Pre-treatment Visit	Treatment Period					
Visit	1	2	3	4	5	6	7
Study Week	0	1	2	3	4	8	12
Medical History	X						
Complete Physical	X						X
Chest X-ray, PA Lateral	X						X
X-Ray Bone Survey	X					X	X
Bone Scan	X						X
Intravenous Pyelogram (if indicated)	X						X
Measurement Primary Tumor (if present)	X						X
Measurement Metastatic Lesion	X						X
Hematology	X	X	X	X	X	X	X
Blood Chemistry	X	X	X	X	X	X	X
Urinalysis	X	X	X	X	X	X	X
Hormone Assays	X	X	X	X	X	X	X
Performance Status	X	X	X	X	X	X	X
Pain Evaluation	X	X	X	X	X	X	X
Interim Report	X	X	X	X	X	X	X
NPCP Evaluation							X
Global Evaluation							X
Final Report							X

Patients demonstrating objective evidence of disease progression at 12 weeks were removed from the study and treated at the investigator's discretion. Those patients responding or exhibiting stable disease were offered the option of continuing on the study drugs.

RESULTS:

One hundred and twenty nine patients were enrolled on the study between February, 1983 and March, 1984. The mean age was 68 years; range 43-86 years. At the present time, 107 cases are deemed evaluable. Reasons for inevaluability included: intercurrent medical problems, 3; adverse drug reaction, 6; found not to meet study criteria, 2; therapy refusal, 4; failure to follow appointment schedule, 3; and other, 4. Table II outlines adverse drug reactions which were experienced by six patients.

TABLE II

DURATION OF THERAPY (DAYS)	ADVERSE DRUG REACTIONS
14	Lethargy, Somnolence
15	Agranulocytosis
66	Fever
24	Fever, Sedation
47	Fever
71	Neutropenia

Seven patients died before the completion of the study. All of the deaths were judged to be related to intercurrent medical problems rather than study drugs by the clinical investigators. Table III presents the duration of therapy for the early deaths.

TABLE III

EARLY DEATHS

PATIENT NUMBER	DURATION OF THERAPY (DAYS)
1	9
2	15
3	21
4	40
5	45
6	71
7	77

The side effects from the treatment were minimal. Table IV summarizes the most frequent adverse reactions, and Table V prior therapy.

TABLE IV

SIDE EFFECTS	INCIDENCE	PERCENT
Ankle edema	9	9.6%
Lethargy	7	7.4%
Weakness	5	5.3%
Thrombocytopenia	2	2.1%
Nausea	7	7.4%
Rash	4	4.2%
Fever	3	3.2%
Hyponatremia	1	1.1%
Hyperkalemia	2	2.1%

TABLE V

PRIOR TREATMENT

	NUMBER OF PATIENTS	PERCENT
Chemotherapy	30	23%
Radiation	86	67%
Estrogens	77	60%
Anti-androgens	4	3%
Corticosteroids	14	11%

NPCP criteria were used to evaluate objective responses at 3 months on the study and are as follows:

TABLE VI

	PATIENT NUMBER	PERCENT
Complete response	0	0%
Partial response	11	10%
Objectively stable	42	39%
Progression	54	50%

Subjective improvement was reported by 61% of the patients, no change by 19%, and deterioration by 20%.

Serum levels of dihydrotestosterone, testosterone, DHEA-S, and delta-4-androstendione levels were evaluated in all patients and will be the subject of another report.

DISCUSSION:

Results of treatment of hormone-refractory advanced prostate cancer are discouraging. A recent review by Eisenberger et al.,(1985), underscores the uniformly poor results obtained by chemotherapy.

Few patients with hormone-resistant prostate cancer experience any objective benefit from either single agent or combination chemotherapy. However some patients achieve subjective improvement. The objective responses of our group of patients treated with aminoglutethimide parallel those of many chemotherapy regimens, and subjective responses are superior.

Controversy exists regarding the role of adrenal androgens in the stimulation of prostate cancer growth. Yet surgical adrenalectomy and anti-androgens have been reported to have a salutary effect on patients with hormone refractory advanced prostate cancer. (Drago, et al., 1985)

Therapeutic action of aminoglutethimide in patients refractory to endocrine manipulation may result from (1) denervation hypersensitivity of the steroid receptor sites, similar to that described for neural tissues, (2) antiestrogen effect causing tumor regression, (3) the effect of the steroid administered with the drug. (Geller, et al., 1984)

We conclude that the combination of aminoglutethimide and hydrocortisone is an effective and well tolerated addition to our treatment armamentarium for the treatment of advanced hormone refractory prostate cancer.

REFERENCES
Drago, JR, Stanten, RJ, Lipson, A, et al. (1985). Clinical effect of aminoglutethimide, medical adrenalectomy, in the treatment of 43 patients with advanced prostatic carcinoma. Cancer, 53: 1447.
Eisenberger, M, Simon, R, O'Dwyer, P., et al. (1985). A reevaluation of nonhormonal cytotoxic chemotherapy in the treatment of prostatic carcinoma. J.Clin. Oncol. 3: 827-841
Geller, FL, de la Vega, DJ, Albert, JD, et al. (1984). Tissue dihydrotestosterone levels and clinical response to hormonal therapy in patients with advanced prostate cancer. J. Clin. Endocrinol. Metab. 58:36.

Prostate Cancer, Part A: Research, Endocrine
Treatment, and Histopathology, pages 291–297
© 1987 Alan R. Liss, Inc.

THE ENDOCRINE EFFECT OF KETOCONAZOLE HIGH DOSIS (KHD).

C. Mahler, L. Denis and R. De Coster*.
Depts. Endocrinology and Urology, A.Z.Middelheim,
Antwerp - Belgium. *Dept. Endocrinology, Research
Lab. Janssen Pharma, Beerse - Belgium.

Introduction :

Ketoconazole, known as an antimycotic agent, belongs
to the imidazolegroup. Effective at a single dose of 200
mg/day, it inhibits the cytochrome P-450 enzyme dependent
synthesis of ergosterol in fungi, thus leading to their
eventual destruction (Vanden Bossche H. et al 1986 - in
press).

EFFECTS OF KHD ON THE CYTOCHROME P-450 DEPENDENT TESTICULAR
TESTOSTERONE BIOSYNTHESIS.

In the testicles cholesterol is converted to pregnenolone by a side chain cleavage enzyme (20-22 desmolase).
Pregnenolone and progesterone, the precursors of the testicular androgens, are transformed by series of enzymatic
controlled steps, to dehydroepiandrosterone, androstenediol,
androstenedione and testosterone. Two enzymatic, cytochrome
P-450 dependent enzymes: the 17 α hydroxylase and the 17-20
lyase, catalyze this transformation. KHD inhibits the
action of both these enzymes (Vanden Bossche et al 1984,
Vanden Bossche H. et al 1985b, Vanden Bossche H. et al
1985c).
Several in vitro and in vivo studies demonstrated an
accumulation of 17 OH pregnenolone and 17 OH progesterone
with a concomitant decrease of the androgens (Vanden
Bossche et al 1985, Pont A. et al 1982, De Coster R. 1984).
In man within hours, testosterone values reach castration
levels (Pont A. et al 1982, Schürmeyer Th. and Nieschlag
1984).

As long as plasmatic K levels of more then 5 ng/ml are maintained this inhibition persists, leading to a compensatory increase of luteinizing hormone secretion (Pont et al 1982, Trachtenberg J. 1984b, Santen R.J. 1983 , De Coster R. and Denis L. 1985).

EFFECTS OF KHD ON THE CYTOCHROME P-450 DEPENDENT ADRENAL ANDROGENS.

In the adrenals the biosynthesis pathways of androgens allthough not identical are quite similar to those in the testes. Pregnenolone is partially converted to dehydroepiandrosterone and androstenedione. Here again in vitro and in vivo studies confirmed the decreased synthesis of androgens through blockade of the 17 α hydroxylase and the 17-20 lyase with increased values of the progestin precursors (Trachtenberg J. 1984b, Heyns W. et al 1985, De Coster R. et al 1985b).

EFFECTS OF KHD ON THE CYTOCHROME P-450 DEPENDENT ADRENAL MINERALO- AND GLYCOCORTICOID BIOSYNTHESIS.

The decreased androgen synthesis in the adrenals that results from KHD enzymatic blocking leads to an enhanced availability of pregnenolone and progesterone for the synthesis of 11 deoxycorticosterone and 11 deoxycortisol, precursors of aldosterone and cortisol (De Coster R. and Denis L. 1985).
The increased concentrations of these 2 precursors, noted in KHD treated patients, is also enhanced by the inhibition by KHD of the 11 β hydroxylase, responsible for the conversion of 11 deoxycortisol to cortisol and of 11 deoxycorticosterone to corticosterone (De Coster R. and Denis L. 1985).
This mechanism explains the decrease of free cortisol concentrations reported by several authors in vivo (Pont A. et al 1984, White M.C. and Kendall-Taylor P. 1985, Mahler C. et al 1985).
As a consequence of the impaired adrenal mineralocorticoid and glucocorticoid synthesis endogenous ACTH output increases in order to compensate for the diminished cortisol biosynthesis (Pont A. et al 1982b).
There is some in vitro evidence that the cholesterol side chain cleavage enzyme - a 20-22 desmolase - can be inhibited by KHD in high concentrations. As this enzyme catalyzes the transformation from cholesterol to pregnenolone,

blocking of this reaction might lead to a complete stop of adrenal steroidogenesis (Vanden Bossche H. et al 1986 in press).

Our own endocrine investigations in patients with advanced prostatic cancer confirm that KHD mainly inhibits the androgen biosynthesis pathways in testes and adrenals and that to a lesser extent it interferes with the glyco- and mineralocorticoids synthesis pathways in the adrenals. These effects, who are completely reversible after discontinuation of the treatment, are dose dependent and correlate with the plasma concentration of K (Mahler C. et al 1985, De Coster R. and Denis L. 1985).

As we have shown by challenging the adrenals under KHD therapy with ACTH intravenously, the inhibition of adrenal androgen production remains complete while the cortisol response is blunted (Figures 1 and 2).

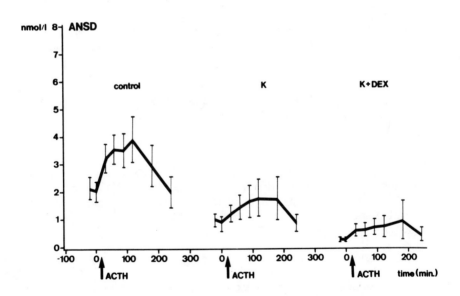

Fig. 1: Androstenedione levels challenged by ACTH before KDH treatment and after KHD and KHD combined with dexamethasone.

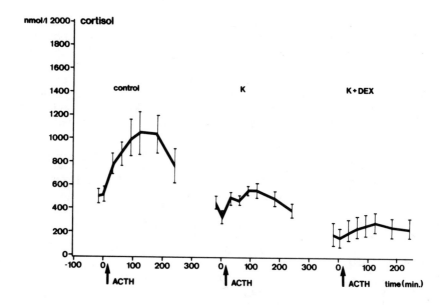

Fig. 2: Cortisol levels challenged by ACTH before KHD
         treatment and after KHD and KHD combined with
         dexamethasone.

This explains why in longterm KHD treated patients the
endogenous rise in ACTH does not affect the androgen production but might maintain plasma cortisol levels within
normal range (De Coster R. et al 1986, Denis L. et al
1986).

CONCLUSION

Evidence from the medical literature as well from our
own investigations shows that KHD has marked endocrine
effects through complete or partial inhibition of cytochrome P-450 dependent enzymatic systems responsible for
steroidogenesis in testes and adrenals. Its dose related
potency warrants extreme caution as the risk of precipi-
tating an Addisonian crisis in some patients is far from
negligible.

REFERENCES

De Coster, R. (1984): Effect of ketoconazole in testosterone biosynthesis in short term cultures of dispersed
rat testicular cells. Proc. 7th Int. Congress Endocrinology, July 1-7, Quebec p. 559 (abstract). Elsevier, Excerpta Medica, Amsterdam, Oxford, Princeton.
De Coster, R., Beerens, D., Dom, J., and Willemsens, G.
(1984): Endocrinological effects of single daily ketoconazole administration in male beagle dogs. Acta Endocrinologica 107, 275-281.
De Coster, R., and Denis, L. (1985): High dose ketoconazole
therapy blocks testosterone biosynthesis in patients
with advanced prostatic carcinoma: site of action.
Presented at XX Congress of the International Society
of Urology, Vienna, June 23-28, 1985.
De Coster, R., and Vanden Bossche, H. (1985): Ketoconazole:
mechanism of action. Presented at the symposium on
treatment of advanced prostatic cancer and the role of
LHRH-superagonists. Baden near Vienna, June 20-21, 1985.
De Coster, R., Caers, I., Haelterman, C., and Debroye, M.
(1985a): Effect of a single administration of ketoconaz-
zole in plasma total and physiologically free testosterone and 17 - estradiol levels in healthy male
volunteers. European Journal of Clinical Pharmacology
29, 489-493.
De Coster, R., Denis L., and Mahler, C. (1985b): Ketoconazole blocks both basal and stimulated androgen secretion
in castrated patients with prostatic cancer. Presented
at the 3rd International Forum of Andrology, Paris, June
17-18, 1985.
Denis, L., Mahler, C., and De Coster, R. (1986): Effects of
ketoconazole on adrenal steroidogenesis in orchidectomized prostatic cancer patients. Abstractbook AUA congress, May 1986, New York.
Heyns, W., Drochmans, A., van der Schueren, E., and Verhoeven, G. (1985): Endocrine effects of high dose ketoconazole therapy in advanced prostatic cancer. Acta
Endocrinologica 110: 276-283.
Mahler, C., Denis, L., and Chaban, M. (1985): Ketoconazole
in der Behandlung des Prostatakarzinoms. Abstractband
XXXVII Kongress der Deutschen Gesellschaft für Urologie,
Mainz, 2-5 Oktober 1985.
Pont, A., Williams, P.L., Azhar, A., Reitz, R.E., Bochra,
C., Smith, E.R., and Stevens, D.A. (1982a): Ketocona-
zole blocks testosterone synthesis. Archives of Inter-

nal Medicine 142, 2137-2140.

Pont, A., Williams, P.L., Loose, D.S., Feldman, D., Reitz, R.E., Bochra, C., and Stevens, D.A. (1982b): Ketoconazole blocks adrenal steroid synthesis. Annals of Internal Medicine 97, 370-372.

Pont, A., Graybill, J.R., Craven, P.C., Galgiani, J.M., Dismukes, W.E., Reitz, R.E., and Stevens, D.A. (1984): High-dose ketoconazole therapy and adrenal and testicular function in humans. Archives of Internal medicine 144, 2150-2153.

Santen, R.J., Vanden Bossche, H., Symoens, J., Brugmans, J., and De Coster, R. (1983): Site of action of low-dose ketoconazole on androgen biosynthesis in men. Journal of Clinical Endocrinology and Metabolism 57 (4), 732-736.

Schürmeyer, Th., and Nieschlag (1984): Effect of ketoconazole and other imidazole fungicides on testosterone biosynthesis. Acta Endocrinologica 105, 275-280.

Trachtenberg, J. (1983): Ketoconazole: a novel and rapid treatment for advanced prostatic cancer. The Journal of Urology 130, 152-153.

Trachtenberg, J. (1984a): The effects of ketoconazole on testosterone production and normal and malignant androgen dependent tissues on the adult rat. The Journal of Urology 132, 599-601.

Trachtenberg, J. (1984b): Ketoconazole therapy in advanced prostatic cancer. The Journal of Urology 132, 61-63.

Vanden Bossche, H. (1985): Biochemical targets for antifungal azole derivatives. Hypothesis on the mode of action. In: Current topics in medical mycology (Ed. M.R. McGinnis). Vol 1, pp. 313-351, Springer-Verlag, New York.

Vanden Bossche, H., Willemsens, G., Marichal, P., Cools, W., and Lauwers, W. (1984): The molecular basis for the antifungal activities of N-substituted azole derivatives. Foculs on R 51 211. In: Mode of action of antifungal agents (Eds. A.P.J. Trinci and J.F. Ryley), pp. 321-341. Cambridge University Press, Cambridge.

Vanden Bossche, H., Bellens, D., Gorrens, G., Marichal, P., Verhoeven, H., and Willemsens, G. (1985a): Yeast and plant cytochrome P-450 enzymes: Targets for azole derivatives. In: Cytochrome P-450, Biochemistry, Biophysics and Induction (Eds. L. Vereczkey and K. Magyar), pp. 423-429. Akademiai Kiodó-Budapest.

Vanden Bossche, H., Lauwers, W., Willemsens, G., and Cools, W. (1985b): The cytochrome P-450 dependent C_{17-20}-lyase in subcellular fractions of the rat testis: Differences in sensitivity to ketoconazole and itraconazole. In: Microsomes and Drug Oxidations (Eds. A.R. Boobis, J. Caldwell, F. de Matteis and C.R. Elcombe), pp. 63–73. Taylor and Francis, London.

Vanden Bossche, H., Lauwers, W., Willemsens, G., and Cools, W. (1985c): Ketoconazole, an inhibitor of the cytochrome P-450-dependent testosterone synthesis. In: EORTC Genitourinary Group, Monograph 2, Part A: Therapeutic principles in metastatic prostatic cancer. (Eds. F.H. Schröder, B. Richards), pp. 187–196. Alan R. Liss, New York.

Vanden Bossche, H., De Coster, R., and Amery, W.K. (1986): Pharmacology and clinical uses of ketoconazole. In press.

White, M.C., and Kendall-Taylor, R. (1985): Adrenal hypofunction in patients taking ketoconazole. The Lancet i, 44–45.

Prostate Cancer, Part A: Research, Endocrine
Treatment, and Histopathology, pages 299–300
© 1987 Alan R. Liss, Inc.

SIDE EFFECTS OF KETOCONAZOLE THERAPY IN ADVANCED CANCER OF THE PROSTATE. A CASE REPORT.

Svein Hassellund, Sten Sander, Nils Normann
Department of Surgery and Urology and Hormone Laboratory,
Aker Hospital, Oslo, Norway

Five previously untreated patients with advanced carcinoma of the prostate received Ketoconazole as sole therapy. Like other investigators, we found a rapid fall in serum testosterone and improvement in performance status. However, side effects illustrated by the following case report made four patients withdraw from the study. A 63 year old man with cancer of the prostate was admitted to the Urological Department of Aker Hospital, Oslo, Norway in July 1985. His performance status was subnormal due to pain from skeletal metastases. The patient refused orchiectomy. Ketoconazole was commenced at a dosage of 400 mg every 8 hours following clinical and hormonal evaluation. A rapid decrease in serum testosterone, prostatic acid phosphatase and adrenal androgen levels together with a fall in the erythrocyte sedimentation rate were recorded. After one week, the pain was reduced and the performance status was improved. However, after two weeks, the patient complained of weakness with difficulty walking, lethargy and loss of appetite. No changes were observed in liver function tests or in the serum cortisol levels.

The side effects increased and Ketoconazole was stopped after 7 weeks. Serum testosterone and prostatic acid phosphatase increased immediately. After one week, the patient was able to go for walks and work in his garden, but the pain increased and Ketoconazole was reintroduced at a dosage of 200 mg every 8 hours. This dosage was insufficient to reduce serum testosterone to castrate levels and no clinical improvement was noted. Although the side effects were now less pronounced, the patient decided to stop Ketoconazole therapy and orchiectomy was performed after 12 weeks. This procedure induced a sustained decrease in serum testosterone and the side effects disappeared.

No alteration in liver function has been observed in any of our five treated patients. Only minor gastrointestinal problems have been observed, but all patients have complained of varying degrees of weakness and fatigue. These side effects together with the fact that serum testosterone and serum prostatic acid phosphatase rose throughout treatment led us to stop Ketoconazole as sole therapy.

The rapid and striking clinical effects of Ketoconazole may possibly be used in combination with orchiectomy or LHRH agonist analogues.

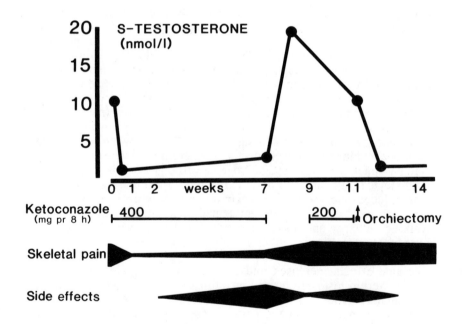

Prostate Cancer, Part A: Research, Endocrine
Treatment, and Histopathology, pages 301–313
© 1987 Alan R. Liss, Inc.

KETOCONAZOLE HIGH DOSE (H.D.) IN THE MANAGEMENT OF
HORMONALLY PRETREATED PATIENTS WITH PROGRESSIVE METASTATIC
PROSTATE CANCER

Frans M.J. Debruyne, Fred A. Witjes and the
Dutch South-Eastern Urological Coöperative
Group.
Department of Urology, St. Radboudhospital,
Cath. University, P.O. Box 9101, 6500 HB
Nijmegen, The Netherlands.

ABSTRACT

Ketoconazole high dose (H.D.) reduces effectively the
testosterone production in both adrenals and testes.
Its use in the management of (metastatic) prostate cancer
has been advocated. Even in relapsing patients after
previous hormonal therapy Ketoconazole H.D. could be of
value.

28 Relapsing patients, of whom 15 were evaluable at 3
months, have been treated with Ketoconazole H.D. As could
be expected, objective response was seen in only a small
number of patients followed up till 9 months.

Subjective improvement was however noticed in the
majority of symptomatic patients. The side effects and
toxicity of the therapy remains however a major limitation
for the use of Ketoconazole, be it as first line treatment
or as therapy for relapsing patients.

INTRODUCTION

Androgen suppression either by orchiectomy or by
estrogen therapy has remained most prominent in the
treatment of (metastatic) prostate cancer since its
proposal by Huggins and Hodges in 1941.

However, the duration of hormonal sensitivity of
prostate tumors is variable. Some tumors never respond,

whereas others, dispite initial response, show signs of reactivation in a considerable number within a year or two (Resnick and Grayhack, 1978).

The reason for hormonal escape remains unclear although it is suggested that increased androgen production from the adrenals might at least partly play a role in the progression of the disease during hormonal treatment (Labrie et al, 1982).

Ketoconazole, an orally administered antifungal drug, has been demonstrated to block the synthesis of adrenal and testicular androgen production, both in animal and man (Pont et al, 1982). Trachtenberg et al (1983) recently demonstrated that high dose ketoconazole could induce and maintain a remission in a patient with advanced prostatic cancer. Subsequently Trachtenberg published favourable results in a small series of previously untreated patients with metastatic prostate cancer (Trachtenberg et al, 1984).

Only a few cases on the use of ketoconazole H.D. in patients relapsing during hormonal treatment have been published so far (Allen et al, 1983; Williams et al, 1986). In view of the total androgen deprivation achieved with ketoconazole H.D., this therapeutic approach could however be of value in patients with progressive disease.

The present study deals with the management of such a group of patients with high dose of ketoconazole.

MATERIAL AND METHODS

28 Patients with relapsing prostatic cancer during hormonal treatment, as was noted by progression of their metastatic disease according to EORTC criteria (World Health Organisation, 1979), were included in this study. Seven patients had one, and 21 patients had several previous hormonal manipulations (table 1).

TABLE 1. Previous Hormonal Treatments

orchiectomy	21x
cyproteronacetate	12x
ethinylestradiol	8x
DES	8x
estracyt	5x
estradurine	2x
bromocryptine	1x
LHRH	1x

All patients had a histopathologically proven disseminated adenocarcinoma of the prostate, in general with a moderately or poorly differentiated tumor (19 out of 25). All patients had multiple skeletal metastases. The average age of the selected patients was 64.8 years (52-80 years). An expected survival time of at least three months was necessary for inclusion in this study.

Patients were randomized in two treatment programmes: 400 mg every 8 hours (n=17) or 600 mg every 12 hours (n=11) of a ketoconazole suspension (80 mg/ml) taken with milk or some food.

Assessments used in the follow-up were: performance status (score 0-4) and pain severity (score 0-5) according to WHO criteria (World Health Organisation, 1979); body weight; plasma testosterone and cortisol; serum acid phosphatases and/or prostate specific acid phosphatases; serum calcium, phosphorus, bilirubin and ketoconazole. These assessments were obtained before the treatment (except serum ketoconazole) on day 2 and 4 (serum cortisol only), on day 7 and 14, month 1, 2 and 3, and every 3 months thereafter. Before therapy and after every 6 months ECG and chest X-ray were controlled. Bone scans or X-ray findings were evaluated before therapy and every 3 or 6 months. Drug compliance, changes in concommitant treatments, side effects, and dosage changes were carefully monitored.

RESULTS

The period of follow-up was minimal six and maximal nine months.

Objective Response

Objective responses were judged according to the EORTC criteria (World Health Organisation, 1979).

An overview of the response is shown in table 2.

TABLE 2. Objective Response According To EORTC-Criteria

Period	0-3 m.	3m.	3-6m.	6m.	6-9m.	9m.
Number of patients	28	13	13	10	9	5
Unevaluable	1	-	-	-	-	-
Stop because of side eff.	7(4+)	-	-	-	-	-
Stop because of progress.	7(7+)	-	3(2+)	1	-	-
Progression	-	2	-	1	-	1
Stable Disease	-	7	-	7	-	4
"Clinically Stable"	-	4	-	1	-	-
No 9 months follow up yet					4	
Number of patients left.	13	13	10	9	5	5

Seven patients died within three months after starting the ketoconazole therapy and were in fact ineligible. The mortality reasons were metastases in four patients and not cancer related in three patients. One other patient was unevaluable and 7 patients dropped out due to drug related toxicity.

Thus at three months 13 patients were evaluable. Two patients were progressive, seven in an objective stable disease and four in a clinical stable disease (stable disease without radiological control).

At six months five patients were progressive. One patient was clinically stable and seven patients objectively stable.

Of the five patients, which are already in study for nine months, one is progressive and four patients were objectively stable. During the observation period 13 patients died of their metastatic disease.

Subjective Response

Subjective response, as judged by a pain severity score, was good. The pain score (score 0-5) reduced form an average of 2° to an average of 0.5°. This ment a significant reduction in the use of non-steroidal analgesics (fig. 1). In five patients the reduction was maintained until nine months of follow-up. The mean performance status improved also during the first two weeks of therapy.

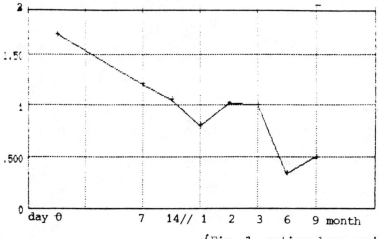

(Fig. 1 continued on next page)

Fig. 1. Mean pain score ("5 option pain score").
0= no pain; 2= continoous use of non steroidal
analgesics

Three patients experienced vanishing of gynaecomastia
and mastodynia due to previous estrogen therapy.

Endocrinological Findings

The timespan between bloodsampling and last dose of
ketoconazole was kept as long as possible (i.e. $\leq$ 8 hours
or $\leq$ 12 hours), in order to measure through plasma levels
of ketoconazole.

Testosterone, although already at castration level
(30 ng/100ml), was further reduced (halved) in all
patients within 2 days (no earlier assesments were done,
fig. 2). Cortisol levels were not significantly altered
(fig. 3).

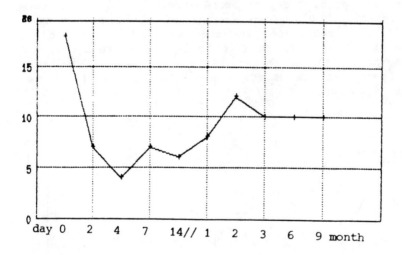

Fig. 2. Mean testosterone concentration (ng/dl)

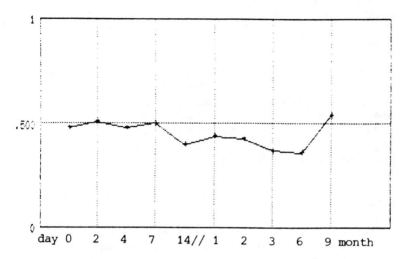

Fig. 3. Mean cortisol concentration (umol/l)

Biochemical Findings

Ketoconazole did not alter the level of calcium and phosphorus. The prostate specific acid phosphatases (PAP) are shown in fig. 4.

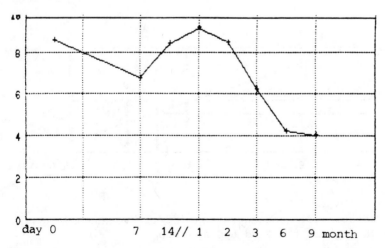

Fig. 4. Mean prostate specific acid phosphatases

Although normalisation (∠ 3 IU/l) was not to be expected in this group of patients, a further reduction of PAP was noted.

The serum ketoconazole concentration (which has to be at least 4 µg/ml to achieve testosterone concentration within the castrate range) showed a good correlation with the timespan between bloodsampling and last ketoconazole intake. After 7-8 (3 dd 400 mg group) or 11-12 (2 dd 600 mg group) hours the ketoconazole concentration is still sufficient, as shown in fig. 5 and 6.

Side Effects

Seven patients had to discontinue the therapy after an average period of 12 days (3-28) because of severe gastro-intestinal intolerance. Four of these patients died within 2 months (table 2). In three cases a temporary dose reduction, and once an antiemetic was sufficient to continue therapy.

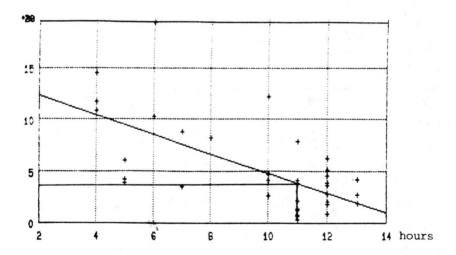

Fig. 5. Ketoconazole concentration (ug/ml) versus timespan (hours) in the 2 dd 600 mg group

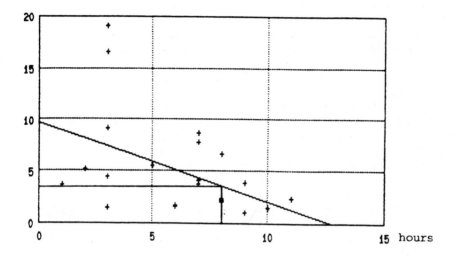

Fig. 6. Ketoconazole concentration (ug/ml) versus timespan
(hours) in the 3 dd 400 mg group

Other side effects were rare. Three times skin
symptoms occurred (itching, dry skin). Impotence was not
noted as a side effect because all patients were already
impotent as a result of previous therapy. No complications
resulting from the adrenal suppression were observed.

DISCUSSION

High oral dose of ketoconazole has been found to
block the synthesis of androgens in both the testes and
the adrenals, at the cytochrome P450 dependent step. The
predominant effect is an inhibition of 17, 20 lyase
converting 17α-OH progestrone or 17-OH pregnolone into
androstenedione, dihydroepiandrostenedione and
testosterone (Pont et al, 1982).

This mode of action explains why ketoconazole H.D.
can be used in patients with prostatic cancer.
Trachtenberg et al (1982, 1983) clearly demonstrated the
clinical efficacy of ketoconazole H.D. in patients with
metastatic prostatic carcinoma.

Our study shows that even in patients relapsing after

previous anti-androgen therapy, ketoconazole H.D. might be of some benefit. This can be explained by the theory postulated by Labrie et al (1982) that residual adrenal androgens may contribute to the emergence of hormonal resistant prostatic cancer. In our patients a clear beneficial subjective effect has been noted in a substantial part of the patients. Although 15 out of 28 patients could not be evaluated at 3 months (withdrawn from the study because of side effects or progression) a stabilisation was achieved in a number of patients who had a clearly progressive disease. In some cases this stabilisation lasted for a period of nine months or more.

Compared with other studies (Denis et al, 1985; Baert, 1985), the patients in this study had a bad prognosis since all patients were relapsing after previous hormonal therapy. For example, seven patients were in fact ineligible because they died within 3 months of follow-up. It is unrealistic to expect a significant prolonged survival in this group of patients. The clear subjective improvement in most of the patients, and objective stabilisation in some others underlines the possible role of ketoconazole H.D. in the management of patients with progressive metastatic disease. In this respect ketoconazole came up to our expectations.

The clinical, biochemical and endocrinological results in both therapeutic regimes (400 mg every 8 hours, 600 mg every 12 hours) were similar. The 3 dd 400 mg schedule however caused more often and more serious gastro- intestinal side effects. All "drop outs" occured in this group.

Absorption of ketoconazole H.D. in the stomach takes place quikly and the endocrinological response occurs within a few hours. However in some patients drug resorption can be hampered due to atrofic gastritis (v.d. Meer et al, 1980). This is easily overcome when an acid (e.g. 2-3 gr. Vit.C.) is added to the drug intake. This was necessary in four patients. In almost all patients sufficient serum levels of ketoconazole were observed indicating a reliable gastric resorption. In all patients an additional reduction in testosterone levels was obtained.

Gastric intolerance poses a major problem. As in

other studies (Williams, 1984; Denis et al, 1985) we too
encountered serious difficulties in this respect. Seven
patients, all in the 3 dd 400 mg group, had to be excluded
from further therapy due to severe gastro—intestinal side
effects such as gastric discomfort, loss of apetite and
vomiting. In such a group of seriously ill patients this
is not acceptable. Good instruction of the patient, as
well as the combination of ketoconazole H.D. with food or
fluid (e.g. milk) and the use of antiemetic drugs can
limit this side effect. There were no other side effects
interfering with the therapy.

In the literature an ideosyncratic hepatitis has been
discribed with ketocomazole. This serious adverse reaction
however is very rare (freq. $\angle$ 0.01%) and not dose
dependent (Janssen and Symoens, 1983; Lewis et al, 1984).
In our study no hepatic toxicity was seen. It is, however,
advisable to exclude patients with liver function
abnormalities (elevated bilirubine) from ketoconazole
H.D. therapy, except if due to metastatic liver disease.

Cortisol levels remained unchanged. There is a much
less apparent effect on the production of cortisol,
possibly as a result of a compensation by the increase of
ACTH levels (Pont et al, 1982; Kowal, 1983; Loose et al,
1983). Some authors however stress that the glucocorticoid
reserve might be affected (Pont et al, 1982), and even
life threathening situations in case of stress due to
fever or concomitant infections, might occur (Denis et al,
1985).

We did not observe such severe complications.
Patients at risk for infections should probably be
excluded from this therapy or at least be followed most
closely. Tests on glucocorticoid reserve were not
performed in our study.

The minor problems of a transient increase of
transaminases, and a transient decrease of blood levels of
calcium and phosphorus during the first weeks of therapy,
normally easily controlled, were not seen in our study.

From our study we can conclude that ketoconazol H.D.
offers a additive to the therapeutic possibilities for
prostatic cancer. Even in hormonally pretreated patients
this therapy may give a reduction in pain and an

improvement in the performance status. Major
inconveniences remain the gastro-intestinal intolerance
and possible hepatic toxicity. These serious side effects
limit substantially the use of ketoconazole H.D. on a
large scale. It is therefore mandatory that further
studies should be done to overcome these problems e.g. by
the development of a similarly effective but less toxic
formulation. Until such a formulation is available,to our
opinion, ketoconazole H.D. cannot be advised as first line
treatment for patients with metastatic prostate cancer.

REFERENCES

Allen JM, Kerle DJ, Ware H, Doble A, Williams G, Bloom SR
    (1983). Combined treatment with ketoconazole and
    luteinizing hormone releasing hormone analogue: a novel
    approach to resistant progressive prostatic cancer. Brit
    Med J 287: 1766.
Baert L (1985). Ketoconazole H.D. in the treatment of
    prostatic cancer. Absatract of the 20th int. congress of
    the urological society, Vienna, Austria.
Denis L, Chaban M and Mahler C (1985). Clinical
    application of ketoconazole in prostatic cancer.
    Prog Clin Biol Res 185A: 319.
Huggins C and Hodges CV (1941). Studies in prostatic
    cancer I. The effect of castration, of estrogen, and of
    androgen injection on serum phosphatases in metastatic
    carcinoma of the prostate. Cancer Res 1: 293.
Janssen PAJ and Symoens J (1983). Hepatic reaction during
    ketoconazole treatment. Am J Med 74 (1b): 80.
Kowal J (1983). The effect of ketoconazole on the steroid
    synthesis in cultured mouse adrenal cortex tumour
    cells. Endocrinology 112: 1541.
Labrie F, Dupont A, Belanger A, Cusam L, Lacourciere Y,
    Monfette G, Laberge JG, Emond JP, Fazekaz ATA,
    Raynaud JP and Husson JM (1982). New hormonal therapy in
    prostatic carcinoma: combined treatment with LHRH
    agonist and antiandrogen. Clin Invest Med 5: 267.
Lewis JH, Zimmerman HJ, Benson GD and Ishak KG (1984).
    Hepatic injury associated with ketoconazole therapy.
    Analysis of 33 cases. Gastroenterology 288: 188.
Loose DS, Kan PG, Hirst MA, Marcus RA and Feldman D
    (1983). Ketoconazole blocks adrenal steroidgenesis by
    inhibiting cytochrome P 450 enzymes. J. Clin. Invest.
    71, 1495.

Meer JWM vd, Keuning JJ, Scheijgrond HW, Heykants W, Cutsem J v and Brugman J (1980). The influence of gastric acidity on the bioavalability of ketoconazole. J Antimicr Chemoth 6(4): 552.

Pont A, Williams PL, Azhar S, Reitz RE, Bochra C, Smith ER and Stevens DA (1982). Ketoconazole blocks testosterone synthesis. Arch Intern Med 142: 2137.

Pont A, Williams PL, Loose DS, Feldman D, Reitz RE, Bohra C and Stevens DA (1982). Ketoconazole blocks adrenal steroidsynthesis. Ann Int Med 97: 370.

Resnick MI and Grayhack JT (1978). Treatment of stage IV carcinoma of the prostate. Urol Clin North Am 2: 141.

Trachtenberg J, Halpern N and Pont A (1983). Ketoconazole: a novel and rapid treatment for advanced prostate cancer. J Urol 130: 152.

Trachtenberg J (1984). Ketoconazole therapy in advanced prostatic cancer. J Urol 132: 61.

Williams G (1984). Ketoconazol for prostatic cancer. The Lancet II: 696.

Williams G, Kerle DJ, Ware H, Doble A, Dunlop H, Smith C, Allen J, Yeo T, Bloom SR (1986). Objective response to ketoconazole therapy in patients with relapsed progressive prostatic cancer. Brit J Urol 58: 45-51.

World Health Organisation: Handbook for reporting results of cancer treatment. Geneva 1979.

Prostate Cancer, Part A: Research, Endocrine
Treatment, and Histopathology, pages 315–340
© 1987 Alan R. Liss, Inc.

WHAT IS AN ANTIANDROGEN AND WHAT IS THE PHYSIOLOGICAL AND PHARMACOLOGICAL RATIONALE FOR COMBINED "CASTRATION" + "ANTI-ANDROGEN" THERAPY

M. Moguilewsky, M. Cotard, L. Proulx,
C. Tournemine, and J.P. Raynaud

Roussel-Uclaf
93230 Romainville, France.

INTRODUCTION

Since the discovery of Huggins and Hodges (1941) demonstrating the androgen dependence of most prostate cancers, treatments have been designed to suppress the stimulating effect of androgens. In man, the testes are the major source of androgens but the adrenals also secrete large quantities (Fiet et al., this volume), the importance of which has frequently been neglected owing to their low intrinsic activity. However, they are transformed in prostatic cells to testosterone and dihydrotestosterone, which are able to directly stimulate the growth of cancer cells, even in the absence of testicular androgens (Harper et al., 1974 ; Bhanalaph et al., 1974; Cowley et al., 1976; Geller et al., 1979). Rather than suppress the synthesis of both testicular (by orchiectomy, estrogens or LHRH agonists) and adrenal androgens (by adrenalectomy, aminogluthetimide or ketoconazole which suppress at the same time corticoid secretion, Walsh and Siiteri, 1975 ; Sanford et al., 1976 ; Trachtenberg et al., 1983), the most specific form of treatment would be to inhibit directly androgen action in their target cells. Antiandrogens are capable of blocking the trophic effect of all androgens on cancer cells, regardless of their site of origin, by inhibiting the binding of androgens to their specific receptor.

Because androgen receptors are present not only in the prostate, whether normal or cancerous, but also in other target tissues, such as the hypothalamus and pituitary, antiandrogens also act on these other sites. Thus antiandrogens block the negative feedback by which testicular androgens control their own secretion ; androgens decrease the sensitivity of the pituitary to LHRH decreasing the secretion of LH and, consequently, of testosterone (Drouin and Labrie, 1976). As antiandrogen treatment is continued, testosterone secretion increases to the extent that it could overcome the blocking effect of antiandrogens on the prostate (Neumann et al., 1977 ; Raynaud et al., 1979, 1984).

For an antiandrogen to have an optimum antiandrogenic effect on prostatic cells, it is advisable to prevent the increase in plasma testosterone by surgical or chemical castration. Thus, the combination treatment of an antiandrogen with castration will counteract the effect of the unsuppressed adrenal androgens resulting in a complete androgen blockade (Séguin et al., 1981 ; Lefebvre et al., 1982). In cases involving medical castration by LHRH analogs, the antiandrogen will have the added advantage of preventing the adverse effect of the testosterone surge that occurs in the first few days following treatment with the neuropeptide (Donnelly, 1984 ; Kerle et al., 1984 ; Debruyne et al., 1985).

An effective antiandrogen should be specific, i.e., interact with the androgen receptor only, be devoid of agonist or other hormonal activities and have minimal side-effects. Its pharmacokinetics should result in a continued and elevated concentration of compound at the receptor sites permanently blocking the binding of androgens with a single daily administration. Antiandrogens that are currently on the market or in clinical trials can be divided into two classes based on their chemical structure (steroid or non steroid).Among steroid antiandrogens which are also potent progestins, cyproterone acetate has been included in many oncology trials in Europe, alone or in association with castration (Neumann, 1977; Schroeder et al., 1984), and is marketed in several countries; megestrol acetate is prescribed in association with estrogen in North America (Geller et al., 1981 ; Geller and Albert, 1983); chlormadinone acetate is used in Japan (Nishimura and Shida, 1981); medroxyprogesterone acetate has been included in EORTC protocols (Pavone-Macaluso et al., 1980; Schroeder et al., 1984). Amongst non steroid antiandrogens, flutamide (Koch, 1984) is now on the market in some countries. Anandron[R] (Raynaud et al., 1977) is being tested in double-blind clinical trials in Europe, Canada and the US following the promising results obtained in an

open trial (Labrie et al., 1982, 1984). The interaction
of the above antiandrogens with steroid receptors as well
as their hormonal and antihormonal activities are reported
in this chapter. The pharmacokinetics of three of them are
reported elsewhere in this volume (Tremblay et al.).

While the interaction with steroid receptors can be
easily measured in vitro not only in animal tissues but
also in human prostate, the study of the inhibitory effect
of antiandrogens on the abnormal growth of the prostate
has been hampered by the lack of a suitable model system.
Prostate tumors rarely arise spontaneously in animals. In
addition, laboratory animals secrete only minimal amounts
of adrenal androgens compared to man (Moguilewsky et al,
1986). To overcome these drawbacks, we studied the effect
of a combined "antiandrogen plus castration" treatment in
normal rats that have been supplemented with adrenal androgens
to plasma levels similar to those recorded in man. The inhibition
of the effect of the transient rise in testosterone induced
by LHRH analogs was also studied (Moguilewsky et al, 1986).
Finally, the combined therapy was investigated in an experimental
animal carcinoma model, the Shionogi tumor, which, in spite
of its mammary origin, can mimic certain aspects of human
prostate cancer since it is androgen dependent (Minesita
and Yamaguchi, 1964 ; Sutherland et al., 1974 ; King et
al., 1976).

INTERACTION OF ANTIANDROGENS WITH CYTOSOL STEROID HORMONE RECEPTORS - HORMONAL AND ANTIHORMONAL ACTIVITIES

In order to induce its biological responses, a steroid
hormone binds to a specific receptor present in target cells.
The potential hormonal or antihormonal effects of a compound
can be established from its ability to interact with the
receptors of the different classes of steroid hormone although
mechanisms other than receptor interaction including inhibition
of hormone biosynthesis and modification of hormone metabolism
in responding cells can be responsible for antihormonal
activity.

The well-known interaction of steroid antiandrogens
with the progestin receptor and their related progestin
activity, as well as their binding to the androgen receptor,
correlated with androgenic and antiandrogenic activities,

are well documented (Neumann 1977, 1984; Bullock and Bardin 1977; Brown et al., 1979; Raynaud et al., 1980b, 1981). The interaction with the glucocorticoid receptor and the glucocorticoid and antiglucocorticoid activities of cyproterone acetate (Neumann 1977, 1984), medroxyprogesterone acetate (Duncan and Duncan 1979, Guthrie et al., 1980) and of other progestin antiandrogens (Raynaud et al., 1981) have been measured in several assays. The interaction of the non steroid antiandrogens, flutamide and Anandron, with the cytosol androgen receptor was observed in vitro (Liao et al., 1974; Mainwaring et al., 1974; Raynaud et al., 1978; Simard et al., 1986) after they were reported to inhibit the in vivo uptake of androgens in prostatic whole tissue or nuclei (Peets et al., 1974, Raynaud et al., 1977). Their hormonal and antihormonal activities have been measured in different tests (Neri et al., 1967; Neri and Peets 1975; Koch, 1984; Raynaud et al., 1980b, 1984).

In this chapter, we have systematically compared in the same assays the in vitro interaction of steroid and non steroid antiandrogens with the cytosol receptors of the five steroid hormone classes and their biological activities after repeated treatments by the oral route (which is the route of administration used in clinic) in the same target tissues as used for receptor assays.

In vitro Interaction with Cytosol Steroid Hormone Receptors

The interaction of a compound with a receptor can be measured in vitro by determining its relative binding affinity (RBA), i.e., its ability to compete for the binding of a tritiated (3H) hormone to its specific cytosol receptor in comparison with the natural hormone or a synthetic agonist. The competition can be measured under two sets of incubation conditions, chosen in relation to the kinetics of interaction of the endogenous hormone with the receptor, in order to evaluate the stability of the complex (Raynaud et al., 1980a).

■ As shown in Table 1, the RBA profiles of the steroid and nonsteroid antiandrogens for the cytosol receptor of the five steroid hormone classes are very different. Whereas nonsteroid antiandrogens competed only for (3H) testosterone binding to the androgen receptor (AR), steroid antiandrogens also inhibited the binding of (3H) promegestone to the progestin receptor (PR), of (3H) dexamethasone to the glucocorticoid receptor (GR) and of (3H) aldosterone to the mineralocorticoid receptor (MR). The RBAs of all compounds for AR decreased with incubation time indicating that the antiandrogen-AR complexes formed are more short-lived than the testosterone-receptor complex, as previously shown for other classes of antihormones (Raynaud et al., 1980a, 1980b).

TABLE 1. **RBAs of antiandrogens for the cytosol receptors of steroid hormones.**

	AR*		PR	GR	MR	ER
Incubation time at 0°C	30min	24h	2h	4h	1h	2h
Cyproterone acetate	20	8	60	5	1	<0.1
Megestrol acetate	36	5	152	50	3	<0.1
Medroxyprogesterone acetate	54	40	125	70	6	<0.1
Chlormadinone acetate	35	5	175	38	1	<0.1
Flutamide	0.3	<0.1	<0.1	<0.1	<0.1	<0.1
Hydroxyflutamide	4.5	0.5	<0.1	<0.1	<0.1	<0.1
Anandron	4.5	0.5	<0.1	<0.1	<0.1	<0.1

* AR, PR, GR, MR and ER : androgen (rat prostate), progestin (rabbit uterus), glucocorticoid (rat thymus), mineralocorticoid (rat kidney) and estrogen (mouse uterus) receptors, respectively. The RBAs were measured as described previously (Ojasoo and Raynaud, 1978). The RBAs of testosterone, progesterone, dexamethasone, aldosterone and estradiol for AR, PR, GR, MR and ER were taken to be equal to 100.

Amongst non steroid antiandrogens, flutamide had a very weak RBA for AR, while hydroxyflutamide interacted with the same affinity as Anandron. This could explain why flutamide is practically devoid of activity in vitro and needs to be converted into hydroxyflutamide in vivo to exert its antiandrogen effects (Katchen and Buxbaum, 1975 ; Neri et al., 1979).

■ The RBA of Anandron for the androgen receptor was measured in cytosols prepared from the prostate of different species (Table 2). Anandron competed much more effectively for (3H) testosterone binding to AR in the prostate of the castrated dog and hamster than in that of the rat. Its affinity for human prostate AR was also higher than for rat prostate AR.

TABLE 2 . **RBA of Anandron for AR in prostate cytosol from different species.**

	Rat	Hamster	Dog	Man
RBA*	1.4 ± 0.3	10 ± 1	24 ± 5	9 ± 3
(n=)	(10)	(2)	(5)	(4)

* The RBA of Anandron was measured after incubation of prostate cytosol for 2 hr at 0°C with (3H) testosterone (for rat, hamster and dog) or with (3H) RU 1881 (human BPH) in the presence or absence of increasing concentrations of testosterone or of Anandron. (3H) RU 1881 (in the presence of a 100-fold excess of triamcinolone acetonide) was used as androgen ligand in the human prostate cytosol since it is not trapped by sex binding protein which can be present at varying concentrations in the different human samples tested. The RBA of Anandron was compared to that of testosterone taken as the reference hormone whatever the radioligand used (RBA of testosterone = 100).

In vivo Dynamics of the Interaction of Anandron with the Androgen Receptor

The in vivo interaction of Anandron with the androgen receptor was determined by measuring the occupancy of the cytosol receptor after administration of Anandron to animals. Following an oral dose of 10 mg/kg to castrated rats, only 10-30% of the prostate androgen binding sites were unoccupied over the first 16 hr (Fig.1). The high and prolonged occupation level of cytosol AR **in vivo** can be explained by the high and prolonged plasma level of Anandron (Pottier et al., 1985 ; Raynaud et al., 1985).

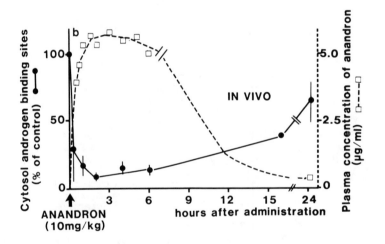

Figure 1. **In vivo interaction of Anandron with cytosol AR.** Castrated adult male rats received an oral administration of 10 mg/kg of Anandron or solvent (controls) and were killed at different time intervals after treatment. Cytosols from pooled prostates were prepared and free specific androgen binding sites were determined (Moguilewsky et al., 1986). The results are the means of 2-4 determinations (■———■). **Plasma kinetics.** Groups of adult male rats received an oral administration of 10 mg/kg of (14C) Anandron. Blood was drawn at different time intervals after treatment. The radio-activity associated with Anandron was determined in plasma after extraction and separation by TLC (■...■) (Pottier et al., 1985).

Androgen and Antiandrogen Activities

■ The ability of the different compounds to inhibit the binding of testosterone to the androgen receptor is related to an **inhibition of the effect of testosterone on its target cells**. After repeated treatment in castrated rats, all the compounds tested in vitro on the receptor (Table 1) inhibited the trophic effect of testosterone propionate on the prostate, at doses between 1 and 50 mg/kg (Fig.2). The most potent antiandrogens by the oral route were flutamide, cyproterone acetate and Anandron, then megestrol acetate, whereas chlormadinone acetate and medroxyprogesterone acetate had only a weak effect.

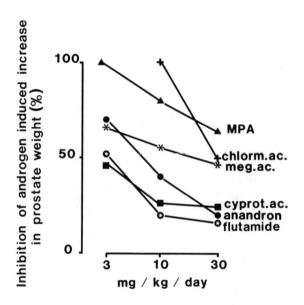

Figure 2. **Antiandrogen activity in the castrated male rat.** Groups of 5 male rats (100 g) castrated for 24 hr received a daily s.c. administration for 8 days of testosterone propionate (0.5 mg/kg/day) alone or in combination with increasing doses of different compounds. Control rats were injected with solvent only. The weight of ventral prostates was determined 24 hr after the last treatment. (cyprot. ac. = cyproterone acetate, meg. ac. = megestrol acetate, chlorm. ac. = chlormadinone acetate, MPA = medroxyprogesterone acetate).

■ The **inhibition of the trophic effect of testosterone propionate** by Anandron was also observed in the prostate of the castrated dog (Fig.3). The effective dose of Anandron was about 6 times lower in the castrated dog than in the castrated rat. The higher antiandrogen activity of Anandron in the dog could be related to its stronger interaction with dog prostate AR as observed in vitro (Table 2). A potent antiandrogen activity of Anandron was also observed in the castrated hamster : less than 1 mg/kg/day was sufficient to inhibit by 50% the trophic effect on the prostate of 1 mg/kg/day of testosterone propionate after a daily treatment for 8 days.

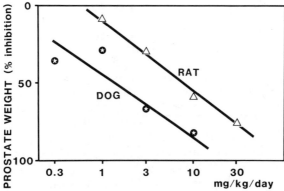

Figure 3. **Antiandrogen activity of Anandron in the castrated dog and rat.** Groups of adult dogs (n=3) or rats (n=5), castrated for 24 hr, received daily injections of testosterone propionate (0.5 mg/kg) alone or in combination with an oral administration of Anandron for 13 days (dog) or 8 days (rat). Controls were injected with solvent only. Prostates were weighed 24 hr after the last treatment.

■ The **androgen activity** of the compounds was assessed by measuring their ability to increase prostate weight after 8-day treatments (30 and 100 mg/kg) in castrated rats. Only medroxyprogesterone acetate was able to significantly increase (62 and 66% increases at respectively 30 and 100 mg/kg/day) prostate weight and thus possessed intrinsic androgen activity (Tausk and de Visser, 1973; Bullock and Bardin, 1977). The other antiandrogens had no significant trophic effect by the oral route in contrast to the weak trophic effect of steroid antiandrogens observed after sc administration (Raynaud et al., 1980b; Poyet and Labrie 1985).

Other Hormonal and Antihormonal Activities

The non steroid antiandrogen Anandron, like flutamide (Neri et al., 1975), was totally devoid of progestin (and antiprogestin) activity by the oral route up to 30 mg/kg/day, as measured in a Clauberg test (Clauberg, 1930) by the absence of endometrial proliferation in the estrogen-primed immature female rabbit. On the other hand, all steroid antiandrogens presently used in the clinic showed potent progestin activity related to their strong interaction with the progestin receptor (Table 1) : they were able to induce maximal endometrial proliferation at oral doses as low as 3-10 µg/kg/day as reported with sc treatments (Raynaud et al., 1980b; Neumann 1984). Antiestrogenic effects of steroid antiandrogens, related to their progestin activity, have also been observed (Neumann, 1984; Raynaud, 1980b).

Since, like all known progestins (Raynaud et al., 1980), steroid antiandrogens interact with the glucocorticoid receptor, the glucocorticoid activity of the compounds was assessed by their ability to decrease thymus weight after a 4-day treatment in the rat (Fig.4). Steroid antiandrogens decreased thymus weight at antiandrogenic doses while Anandron had no thymolytic activity up to the dose of 30 mg/kg/day.

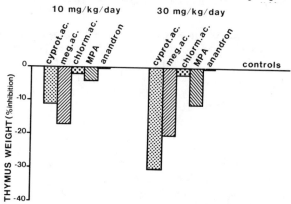

Figure 4. **Determination of the glucocorticoid activity of antiandrogens.** Groups of 5 male rats (100 g) received a daily oral administration of antiandrogens for 4 days. Thymus weight was measured 24 hr after the last treatment (cyprot.ac. = cyproterone acetate ; meg.ac. = megestrol acetate ; chlorm.ac. = chlormadinone acetate ; MPA = medroxy-progesterone acetate).

PHARMACOLOGICAL RATIONALE FOR COMBINED "CASTRATION + ANTI-ANDROGEN" THERAPY

Anandron Inhibits the Trophic Effect of Adrenal Androgens on the Prostate of the "Castrated" Rat

As illustrated in Fig. 5, the plasma concentrations of androgens of adrenal origin are totally different in humans and in rats. Human adrenals secrete very high levels of androgen precursors, especially dehydroepiandrosterone sulfate (DHAs), whereas, in rat plasma, adrenal androgens are very low or even undetectable.

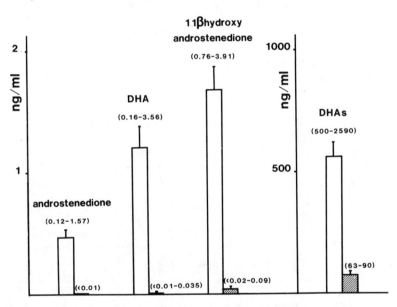

Figure 5. **Plasma concentrations of adrenal androgens in the human and in the rat.** Δ4-androstenedione, 11β-hydroxyandrostenedione and DHA were measured simultaneously by radioimmunoassay after celite chromatography (Fiet et al, 1980) in the plasma of orchiectomized prostate cancer patients (aged between 46 and 70, n=30; ☐) and of orchiectomized adult male rats (n=5 ;▨). DHAs was determined in the same plasmas by radioimmunoassay using a DHA-3CMO-BSA antiserum (Kit ER-660).Means ± s.e.m. and ranges are represented.

To measure the antiandrogenic effect of Anandron against adrenal androgens in an experimental model closer to the human, rats were implanted with osmotic minipumps containing the four adrenal androgens (Fig. 6). Controlled doses were released over a period of 15 days to obtain circulating levels (0.7 ± 0.1, 1.3 ± 0.2, 3.7 ± 0.6, 684 ± 55 ng/ml, respectively for androstenedione, 11β-hydroxyandrostenedione, DHA and DHAs) in the same range as those recorded in orchiectomized men (Fig. 5). As shown in Fig.6, when intact rats receiving adrenal androgens had their testicular source of androgens suppressed either by orchiectomy or by DES treatment, prostate weight levelled off at 28% (for orchiectomized rats) and 63% (for DES-treated rats) of control due to the trophic effect of adrenal androgens transformed into active androgens.

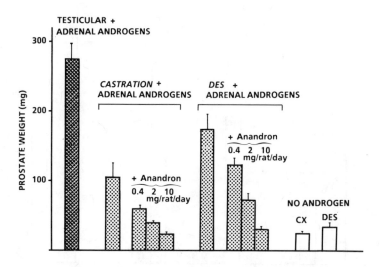

Figure 6. **Inhibition by Anandron of the trophic effect of adrenal androgens on the "castrated" rat prostate.** Groups of 5 adult male rats were continuously administered adrenal androgens by minipumps for 15 days. One group was left intact, while the others had their testosterone secretion suppressed either by orchiectomy or by daily DES treatment (10 μg/rat/day) from the first day of adrenal androgen administration. Each "castrated" group was treated simultaneously with solvent or increasing doses of Anandron. Two groups of rats were castrated by orchiectomy or DES treatment but had no adrenal androgen supplementation. Prostate weights were determined on the 16th day.

When Anandron was administered to orchiectomized or DES-treated rats (Fig.6), the effect of adrenal androgens was totally counteracted and prostate weight was similar to that of androgen-deprived rats (orchiectomy or DES treatment in the absence of adrenal androgen supplementation).

Although DES treatment led to a decrease in prostate weight comparable to orchiectomy in the absence of adrenal androgen supplementation, indicating that testicular secretion had been totally suppressed by estrogens, the trophic effect of adrenal androgens was greater in estrogen-treated rats. This could be due to AR induction in the prostate by estrogen treatment (Bouton et al., 1981; Raynaud et al., 1985), hence enhancing the androgen sensitivity of the organ. In this experiment, the AR concentration in DES-treated rat prostate was 4.4 pmol/g tissue while AR concentration in orchiectomized rat prostate was only 1.8 pmol/g tissue.

In the rat, testosterone secretion was less effectively suppressed by daily s.c. injections of the LHRH analog buserelin (250 ng) than by other types of castration, since these injections act principally on the testes (desensitization of LH receptors) rather than on the pituitary as in

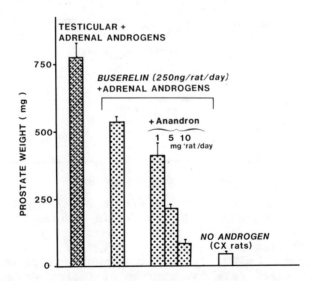

Figure 7. **Inhibition by Anandron of the trophic effect of adrenal androgens and of residual testicular androgens on the prostate of buserelin-treated rats.**

the human. Pituitary receptor down-regulation can only be maintained in the rat by continuous administration by infusion or implants (Sandow, 1983; Sandow and Beier, 1985). This may explain why prostate weight was only decreased to 69% of control in adrenal androgen-supplemented rats treated with buserelin (Fig.7). Combining Anandron with buserelin led to a decline in prostate weight almost identical to that of androgen-deprived rats.

Anandron Inhibits the Trophic Effect on Prostate Due to the Rise in Testosterone Induced by LHRH Analogs

When intact rats (unsupplemented with adrenal androgens) received daily s.c. injections of buserelin (1 µg/kg/day) (Fig.8), their prostate weights were increased during the first few days of treatment. The castrating effect of the peptide started only after 6 or 7 days in contrast to the immediate atrophic effect of orchiectomy. When Anandron

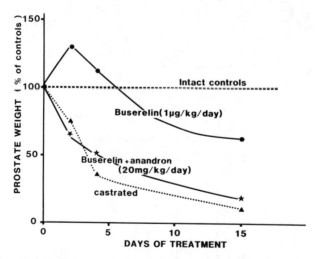

Figure 8. **Inhibition of the effect of the initial rise in testosterone induced by buserelin treatment in the rat.** Groups of 5 adult male rats received daily for 15 days a s.c. injection of buserelin (1 µg/kg/day) alone or combined with an oral administration of Anandron (20 mg/kg/day). Control intact rats and a group of castrated rats received solvent only. The rats were killed after 2, 4 or 15 days of treatment or 2, 4 or 15 days after castration. Prostates were weighed.

(20 mg/kg/day) was administered together with buserelin, the "flare-up" effect of buserelin was totally inhibited and the onset of the castrating effect of the combination was very similar to that achieved by orchiectomy.

Anandron Potentiates the Castrating Effect of Buserelin

When buserelin (0.04 - 25 µg/kg/day) was administered s.c. daily for 15 days to male rats, prostate weight decreased in a dose-dependent manner but the inhibition was never as great as that produced by orchiectomy since testosterone was never totally suppressed by this mode of treatment in the rat (Fig.9). The combination of Anandron (20 mg/kg/day) with low doses of buserelin led to a total decrease in prostate weight. This might be considered as an additivity of effects, Anandron impeding the action on the prostate of residual testosterone unsuppressed by buserelin, and buserelin preventing the rebound testosterone increase

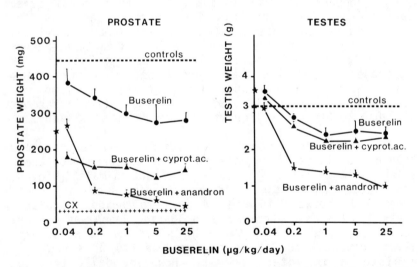

Figure 9. **Potentiation by antiandrogens of the "castrating" effect of buserelin in the rat.** Groups of 5 adult male rats received daily for 15 days a s.c. injection of buserelin, an oral administration of Anandron or cyproterone acetate (20 mg/kg/day) or both treatments. Control intact rats and castrated rats received solvent only.The rats were killed 24 hr after the last treatment and the prostates and testes were weighed.

induced by Anandron. However, whereas Anandron alone had a weak trophic effect on the testes (related to LH increase) and buserelin a weak atrophic effect (related to testicular desensitization), the combination of both compounds led to a marked decrease in testicular weight more characteristic of a synergistic than an additive effect.

The combination of a steroid antiandrogen cyproterone acetate (20 mg/kg/day) with buserelin did not potentiate the castrating effect of the peptide on the testis and was less effective on prostate weight than the combination treatment Anandron + buserelin.

ANTITUMORAL EFFECT OF ANANDRON IN THE EXPERIMENTAL SHIONOGI CARCINOMA MODEL

The ideal animal model for prostatic cancer does not exist but the Shionogi carcinoma 115 (SC 115) offers an excellent opportunity for examining the antitumoral effect of an antiandrogen since this mouse mammary carcinoma cell line, first established by Minesita and Yamaguchi (1964), is responsive to androgens in vivo and in cell culture (Sutherland et al., 1974; King et al., 1976). The stimulating effect of androgens on SC 115 tumor growth has been shown to be mediated by a classical androgen receptor (Matsumoto et al., 1972; Stanley et al., 1977) and other steroid hormones are unable to affect cell growth (Kitamura et al., 1980).

When castration was performed two days before the inoculation of SC 115 cells in male mice, the appearance of tumors was delayed by 15 days (as compared to intact animals) (Fig.10). In the intact group, the incidence of animals bearing tumors reached 100% between 10 and 14 days following inoculation whereas, in the castrated group, a 30% incidence was observed after 25 days and 100% of the animals had tumors at 66 days. Daily treatment with 0.5 mg of Anandron had no effect when administered in intact animals. However, daily treatment with 0.2 mg of Anandron started the day of castration led to an incidence of 22% of animals having tumors at day 25 with a maximum of 56% 120 days after inoculation. The 0.5 mg dose further delayed the appearance of tumors and reduced the incidence to 11% at day 42 with a maximal 44% at day

120. However, measurements of tumor area indicated that the maximal size of the individual tumors present was not different in the various groups.

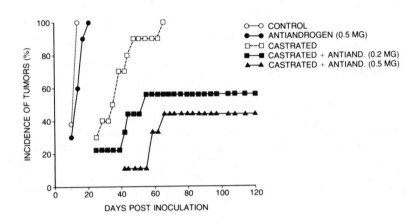

Figure 10. **Effect of orchiectomy or Anandron treatment alone or in combination on the percentage of male Shionogi mice having tumors** (incidence of tumors) at different time intervals after the inoculation of 10^6 tumor cells up to 120 days. Orchiectomy was performed two days before the inoculation of tumor cells and/or Anandron treatment was started on the same day (10 animals/group).

DISCUSSION

Amongst antiandrogens at present under clinical study or on the market, non steroids (flutamide and Anandron) offer an advantage over steroids (megestrol, cyproterone, chlormadinone acetates) in that they interact only with AR and not with other steroid hormone receptors. They are thus devoid of other hormonal or anti-hormonal activities unlike steroid antiandrogens which have potent progestin and modest glucocorticoid activities that could lead to side-effects in long-term clinical use. Moreover, the structural similarity of steroid antiandrogens and natural hormones implies better recognition by AR than for nonsteroids. Their higher RBAs for AR can, under certain experimental conditions, be related to a weak androgenic effect, as previously reported for cyproterone acetate and megestrol acetate (Neri et al., 1967 ; Tisell and Salander, 1975 ; Poyet and Labrie, 1985). Because of its antigonadotrophic activity, medroxyprogesterone acetate has been included in different clinical assays, but its well-known intrinsic androgen activity (Tausk and de Visser, 1972; Bullock and Bardin, 1977) could compensate for its testosterone suppressing effect and directly activate the growth of the androgen-dependent cancer cell. In contrast, non steroid antiandrogens can be considered to be "pure" antiandrogens devoid of androgen activity.

Anandron interacted with the androgen receptor present in the prostate of different species; its RBA was higher in dog, hamster and human prostate than in rat prostate. This might explain why its antiandrogen activity is higher in the dog and hamster than in the rat. We can thus speculate that the active Anandron dose might be lower in man than in the rat, although RBA values were somewhat different from one prostate sample to the next.

Antiandrogens are active on all target cells containing AR and thus inhibit the negative feedback of androgens at the pituitary level giving rise, in the case of non steroids, to an increase in testicular secretion (Neumann et al., 1977, Raynaud et al., 1979, 1984). Since steroid antian- drogens are progestational, their antigonadotropic activity compensates for their antiandrogen activity on the pituitary for a time, but their hypothalamic antiandrogen action leads to an increase in LHRH which enhances LH and testosterone secretion during treatment (Geller et al., 1981). Therefore, all these antiandrogens are more effective on prostate cells when the compensatory increase in testosterone secretion is suppressed by chemical or surgical castration. This combina- tion therapy is now currently under investigation in clinical trials.

Unlike flutamide which needs to be converted into its hydroxy metabolite to interact with AR (Neri et al., 1979), Anandron is not a prodrug but is an antiandrogen per se (Raynaud et al., 1985). Its slow disappearance rate from plasma maintains a permanently high level of unchanged compound in the vicinity of the target cell which can reassociate with the receptor as and when dissociation occurs. Anandron thus impedes the binding of any androgen to AR and consequently their action.

Anandron can therefore be used as an adjuvant therapy to chemical or surgical castration to counteract the effect of adrenal androgens in prostate cancer patients. Since the rat secretes very low levels of adrenal androgens, the advantage offered by an antiandrogen over castration alone cannot be demonstrated unless adrenal androgens are added in circulating amounts equivalent to those recorded in humans. In this way, we have shown that the activity of adrenal androgens is far from negligible since they have at least 30% of the trophic activity of total androgens on the prostate and that Anandron can totally block their activity. Anandron can thus offer a real improvement upon classical treatments.

Anandron would also be effective in patients castrated by estrogens but, according to our animal experiments, higher doses might be required here to counteract the greater activity of adrenal androgens resulting from higher AR concentrations in the prostate. The estrogen inducibility of androgen binding sites (Bouton et al., 1981 ; Raynaud et al., 1985) has also been demonstrated in the Dunning rat tumor model (Mobbs and Johnson, 1984), the androgen-dependent Shionogi carcinoma (Noguchi et al., 1984) and in DES-treated prostate cancer patients (Mobbs et al., 1983). This method of castration should be progressively replaced by other types of castration not only because of its known cardiovascular side effects (Byar, 1973 ; Hedlung et al., 1980) but also because it increases the sensitivity of prostatic cells to androgens.

When combined with castration by an LHRH analog, Anandron inhibits not only the activity of adrenal androgens but also any temporary increase in androgen secretion during the predesensitization phase of the LHRH analog treatment. In rats whose prostate weights were temporarily increased by buserelin treatment, Anandron was able to counteract this increase.

We have shown that, in the rat, antiandrogens poten-tiated the castrating effect of an LHRH analog. Daily s.c. injections of the LHRH agonist for 15 days did not totally suppress testicular secretion, unlike continuous adminis-tration which can lower testosterone to castration levels (Sandow and Beier, 1985 ; Redding and Schally, 1985). Antian-drogens counteracted the effect of this residual testosterone on the prostate. However, whereas the combination buserelin + cyproterone acetate never totally atrophied rat prostates, low s.c. doses of buserelin were sufficient to decrease prostate weight to castrate levels in the presence of Anandron. The addition of Anandron, but not of cyproterone acetate, to buserelin also greatly decreased testes weight. Thus, potentiation of LHRH analog effects by Anandron might occur not only in the prostate but also directly in the testes, where the LHRH analog also exerts a castrating action in the rat, or in the pituitary whose sensitivity to LHRH administration has been shown to be increased by Anandron in cell culture experiments (Raynaud et al., 1979). On the contrary, the antigonadotropic activity of cyproterone acetate and of other progestin antiandrogens decreases pituitary sensitivity to LHRH. LHRH receptors have also been identified in rat Leydig cells (Sharpe and Fraser, 1980) and are thought to mediate inhibition of Leydig cell function by LHRH agonists, resulting in a decrease in testosterone secretion. Anandron might increase the sensitivity of LHRH receptors to LHRH agonists in the testes as well as in the pituitary. This could lead either to a faster castrating action of buserelin or to an action of lower buserelin doses in the presence of Anandron. Whether such an action of Anandron also exists in the human is under investigation; if it does occur, lower doses of LHRH analogs may be required for chemical castration.

Finally, we have shown in an experimental androgen-dependent tumor model, the Shionogi carcinoma model, that the addition of Anandron to castration was able not only to delay the appearance of mammary tumors in mice inoculated with carcinoma cells, but also to decrease the incidence of these tumors. However, in the few animals bearing tumors in the Anandron-treated group, the maximal size of tumors was the same as in the other groups. These data suggest that either androgen-dependent cells had become autonomous after a time of total androgen deprivation, as previously shown in culture (Stanley et al., 1977 ; Yates and King, 1978), or that an androgen-independent subpopulation might exist within the total tumor subpopulations and start growing after disappearence of androgen-dependent cells. Whether androgen-independent cancer cells will also appear in the human prostate, even under complete androgen blockade, will be apparent from the double-blind clinical trials in progress (Brisset et al.; Béland et al.; Navratil et al., this volume).

REFERENCES

Bhanalaph T, Varkarakis MJ, Murphy GP (1974). Current status of bilateral adrenalectomy of advanced prostatic carcinoma. Ann Surg 179 : 17-23.

Bouton MM, Pornin C, Grandadam JA (1981). Estrogen regulation of rat prostate androgen receptor. J steroid Biochem 15 : 403-408.

Brown TR, Bullock L and Bardin CW (1979). In vitro and in vivo binding of progestins to the androgen receptor of mouse kidney : correlation with biological activities. Endocrinology 105 : 1281-1287.

Bullock LP, Bardin CW (1977). Androgenic, synandrogenic and antiandrogenic actions of progestins. Ann NY Acad Sci 286 : 321-330.

Byar DP (1973). The Veterans Administration Cooperative Urological Research Group's studies of cancer of the prostate. Cancer 32 : 1126-1130.

Clauberg C (1930). Zur Physiologie und Pathologie der Sexual-hormone ins besondere des Hormons des Corpus luteum. I. Der biologische Test für das Luteohormon an infantilen Kaninchen. Zbl Gynäcol 54 : 2457-2470.

Cowley IH, Brownsey BG, Harper ME, Peeling WB, Griffiths KO (1976). The effect of ACTH on plasma testosterone and androstenedione concentrations in patients with prostatic carcinoma. Acta Endocr Copenh 81 : 310-320.

Debruyne FMJ, Karthaus HFM, Schröder FH, De Voogt HJ, De Jong FH, Klijn JGM (1985). Results of a Dutch phase II trial with the LHRH agonist Buserelin in patients with prostatic cancer. In Schröder FH, Richards B (eds) EORTC Genitourinary Group Monograph 2, Part A : Therapeutic Principles in Metastatic Prostatic Cancer, New York : Liss, p 251.

Donnelly RJ (1984). Continuous subcutaneous administration of "Zoladex" (ICI 118, 630 and LHRH analogue) to patients with advanced prostatic cancer. J steroid Biochem 20 : 1375.

Drouin J, Labrie F (1976). Selective effect of androgens on LH and FSH release in anterior pituitary cells in culture. Endocrinology 98 : 1528-1534.

Duncan MR, Duncan GR (1979). An in vivo study of the action of antiglucocorticoids on thymus weight ratio, antibody titre and the adrenal pituitary-hypothalamus axis. J steroid Biochem 10 : 245-259.

Fiet J, Gourmel B, Vilette JM, Brerault JL, Julien R, Cathelineau G, Dreux C (1980). Simultaneous radioimmunoassay of androstenedione, dehydroepiandrosterone and 11β-hydroxyandrostenedione in plasma. Horm Res 13 : 133-149.

Geller J, Albert JD (1983). Comparison of various hormonal therapies for prostatic carcinoma. Semin Oncol 10 : 34-41.

Geller J, Albert J, Loza D (1979). Steroid levels in cancer of the prostate - markers of tumour differentiation and adequacy of anti-androgen therapy. J steroid Biochem 11 : 631-636.

Geller J, Albert J, Yen SSC, Geller S, Loza D (1981). Medical castration of males with megestrol acetate and small doses of diethylstilbestrol. J Clin Endocr Metab 52 : 576-580.

Guthrie GP, John WJ (1980). The in vivo glucocorticoid and antiglucocorticoid actions of medroxyprogesterone acetate. Endocrinology 13 : 1393-1396.

Harper ME, Pike A, Peeling WB, Griffiths K (1984). Steroids of adrenal origin metabolized by human prostatic tissue both in vivo and in vitro. J Endocr 60 : 117-125.

Hedlung PO, Gustafsson H, Sjögren S (1980). Cardiovascular complications to treatment of prostate cancer with estramustine phosphate (Estracyt*) or conventional estrogen. A follow-up of 212 randomized patients. Scand J Urol Nephrol (Suppl.) 55 : 103-105.

Huggins C, Hodges CV (1941). Studies of prostatic cancer. I. Effect of castration, estrogen and androgen injections on serum phosphatases in metastatic carcinoma of the prostate. Cancer Res 1 : 293-297.

Katchen B, Buxbaum S (1975). Disposition of a new non-steroid, anti-androgen α,α,α-trifluoro-2-methyl-4'-nitro-m-propionotoluidide (flutamide), in men following a single oral 200 mg dose. J Clin Endocr Metab 41 : 373-379.

Kerle D, Williams G, Ware H , Bloom SR (1984). Failure of long-term luteinising hormone releasing hormone treatment for prostatic cancer to suppress serum luteinising hormone and testosterone. Br Med J 289 : 468-469.

King RJB, Cambray GD , Robinson JH (1976). The role of receptors in the steroidal regulation of tumour cell proliferation. J steroid Biochem 7 : 869-873.

Kitamura Y, Uchida N, Odaguchi K, Yamaguchi K, Okamoto S, Matsumoto K (1980). Insignificance of pituitary for growth of androgen-dependent mouse mammary tumor. J steroid Biochem 13 : 333-337.

Koch H (1984). Flutamide, a new non-steroidal antiandrogen. Drugs Today 20 : 561-574.

Labrie F, Dupont A, Bélanger A, Cusan L, Lacourcière Y, Monfette G, Laberge JG, Emond JP, Fazekas ATA, Raynaud JP, Husson JM (1982). New hormonal therapy in prostatic carcinoma : combined treatment with LHRH agonist and an antiandrogen. Clin Invest Med 5 : 267-275.

Labrie F, Dupont A, Bélanger A, Labrie C, Lacourcière Y, Raynaud JP, Husson JM, Emond J, Houle JG, Girard JG, Monfette G, Paquet JP, Vallières A, Bosse C , Delisle R (1984). Combined antihormonal treatment in prostate cancer, a new approach using an LHRH agonist or castration and an antiandrogen. In Bresciani F, King RJB, Lippman ME, Namer M, Raynaud JP (eds) : Hormones and Cancer 2: "Progress in Cancer Research and Therapy" New York : Raven Press, p 533.

Lefebvre FA, Seguin C, Bélanger A, Caron S, Sairam MR, Raynaud JP, Labrie F (1982). Combined long-term treatment with an LHRH agonist and a pure antiandrogen blocks androgenic influence in the rat. Prostate 3 : 569-578.

Liao S, Howell DK, Chang TM (1974). Action of a non-steroidal antiandrogen, flutamide, on the receptor binding and nuclear retention of 5α-dihydrotestosterone in rat ventral prostate. Endocrinology 9 : 1205-1209.

Mainwaring WIP, Mangan FR, Feherty PA, Freifeld M (1974). An investigation into the anti-androgenic properties of the non steroidal compound, SCH 13521 (4'-nitro-3'-trifluoromethylisobutyrylanilide). Mol cell endocr 1 : 113-128.

Matsumoto K, Kotoh K, Kasai H, Minesita T, Yamaguchi K (1972). Subcellular localization of radioactive steroids following administration of testosterone ^{3}H in the androgen dependent mouse tumor, Shionogi carcinoma 115. Steroids 20 : 311-320.

Minesita T, Yamaguchi K (1964). An androgen-dependent tumor derived from a hormone-independent spontaneous tumor of a female mouse. Steroids 4 : 815-830.

Mobbs BG, Johnson IE, Connolly JG ,Thompson J (1983). Concentration and cellular distribution of androgen receptor in human prostatic neoplasia : can estrogen treatment increase androgen receptor content ? J steroid Biochem 19 : 1279-1290.

Mobbs BG, Johnson IE (1984). Increased androgen binding capacity in experimental prostatic carcinomas treated with estrogen. In Bresciani F et al (eds): "Hormones and Cancer 2 : Progress in Cancer Research and Therapy" New York : Raven Press, p 467.

Moguilewsky M, Fiet J, Tournemine C, Raynaud JP (1986). Pharmacology of an antiandrogen, Anandron, used as an adjuvant therapy in the treatment of prostate cancer. J steroid Biochem 24 : 139-146.

Neri RO, Monahan MD, Meyer JG, Afonso BA ,Tabacnick JA (1967). Biological studies of an antiandrogen (SH 714). Eur J Pharmac 1 : 438-444.

Neri RO, Peets EA (1975). Biological aspects of antiandrogens. J steroid Biochem 6 : 815-819.

Neri R, Peets E , Watnick A (1979). Antiandrogenicity of flutamide and its metabolite Sch 16423. Biochem Soc Trans 7 : 565-569.

Neumann F (1977). Pharmacology and potential use of cyproterone acetate. Horm Metab Res 9 : 1-13.

Neumann F (1984). Experimental basis for the clinical use of antiandrogens. In Bruchovsky N, Chapdelaine A, Neumann F (eds) : "Regulation of androgen action " Berlin : Congressdmak R. Brückner, p 43.

Neumann F, Gräf KJ, Hasan SH, Schenck B , Steinbeck H (1977). Central actions of anti-androgens. In Martini L, Motta M (eds) "Androgens and Antiandrogens" New York: Raven Press, p 163.

Nishimura R, Shida K (1981). Antiandrogenic therapy for the treatment of early stage prostatic cancer . Prostate Suppl 1 : 27-34.

Noguchi S, Kitamura Y, Uchida N, Yamaguchi K, Sato B, Matsumoto K (1984). Growth-stimulative effect of estrogen on androgen-dependent Shionogi carcinoma. Cancer Res 44: 5644-5649.

Ojasoo T, Raynaud JP (1978). Unique steroid congeners for receptor studies. Cancer Res 38 : 4186-4198.

Pavone-Macaluso M, Lund F, Mulder JH, Smith PH, De Paw M, Sylvester R, EORTC Urological Group (1980). EORTC protocols in prostatic cancer. Scand J Urol Nephrol Suppl. 55 : 163-168.

Peets EA, Heusen MF, Neri R (1974). On the mechanism of the anti-androgenic action of flutamide (α-α-α-trifluoro-2-methyl-4'-nitro-m-propionotoluidide) in the rat. Endocrinology 94 : 532-540.

Pottier J, Coussedière D, Raynaud JP (1985). Pharmacokinetics of a non steroid anti-androgen (RU 23908) in rats and dogs. In Abstracts, 67th Annual Meeting of the Endocrine Society, Baltimore, Md : 239 : Abstr 954.

Poyet P, Labrie F (1985). Comparison of the antiandrogenic/androgenic activities of flutamide, cyproterone acetate acetate and megestrol acetate. Mol cell endocr 42 : 283-288.

Raynaud JP, (1978). The mechanism of action of anti-hormones. In Jacob J (ed) : Advances in Pharmacology and Therapeutics, vol. 1 "Receptors" Oxford : Pergamon Press, p 259.

Raynaud JP, Azadian-Boulanger G, Bonne C, Perronnet J, Sakiz E (1977). In Martini L, Motta M (eds) : "Androgens and Antiandrogens" New York : Raven Press, p 281.

Raynaud JP, Bonne C, Bouton MM, Lagacé L, Labrie F (1979). Action of a non steroid androgen, RU 23908 in peripheral and central tissues. J steroid Biochem 11 : 93-99.

Raynaud JP, Bouton MM, Ojasoo T (1980a). The use of interaction kinetics to distinguish potential antagonists from agonists. TIPS 1 : 324-327.

Raynaud JP, Bouton MM, Moguilewsky M, Ojasoo T, Philibert D, Beck G, Labrie F, Mornon JP (1980b). Steroid hormone receptors and pharmacology 12 : 143-157.

Raynaud JP, Ojasoo T, Labrie F (1981). Steroid hormone agonists and antagonists. In Lewis GP, Ginsbourg M (eds): "Mechanisms of steroid action" : MacMillan Publishers LTD, p 148.

Raynaud JP, Bonne C, Moguilewsky M, Lefebvre FA, Bélanger A, Labrie F (1984). The pure antiandrogen RU 23908 (Anandron*), a candidate of choice for the combined antihormonal treatment of prostatic cancer : a review. Prostate 5 : 299-311.

Raynaud JP, Moguilewsky M, Tournemine C, Coussedière D, Salmon J, Husson JM, Bertagna C, Tremblay R, Pendyala L, Brisset JM, Vallancien C, Serment G, Navratil H, Dupont A, Labrie F (1985). Pharmacology and clinical studies with Anandron. In Schröeder FM, Richards B (eds) EORTC Genitourinary Group Monograph 2, Part A : "Therapeutic Principles in Metastatic Prostatic Cancer" New York: Alan R. Liss, p 99.

Redding TW, Schally AV (1985). Investigation of the combination of the agonist D-Trp-6-LH-RH and the antiandrogen flutamide in the treatment of Dunning R 3327 H prostate cancer model. Prostate 6 : 219-232.

Sandow J (1983). The regulation of LHRH action at the pituitary and gonadal receptor level : a review. Psychoneuroendocrinology 8 : 277-297.

Sandow J, Beier B (1985). LHRH agonists mechanism of action and effect on target tissues. In Schröder FM, Richards B (eds) : EORTC Genitourinary Group Monograph 2, Part A : "Therapeutic Principles in Metastatic Prostatic Cancer" New York : Alan R. Liss, p 121.

Sanford EJ, Drago JR, Rohner TJ, Santen R , Lipton A (1976). Aminoglutethimide medical adrenalectomy for advanced prostatic carcinoma. J Urol 115 : 170-174.

Schröder FH, EORTC Urological Group (1984). Treatment of prostatic cancer : the EORTC experience - preliminary results of prostatic carcinoma trials. Prostate 5 : 193-198.

Seguin C, Cusan L, Bélanger A, Kelly PA, Labrie F, Raynaud JP (1981). Additive inhibitory effects of treatment with an LHRH agonist and an antiandrogen in androgen-dependent tissues in the rat. Mol Cell Endocr 21 : 37-41.

Sharpe RM, Fraser HM (1980). Leydig cell receptors for luteinizing hormone-releasing hormone and its agonists and their modulation by administration or deprivation of the releasing hormone. Biochem Biophys Res Commun 95: 256-262.

Simard J, Luthy I, Guay J, Bélanger A, Labrie F (1986). Characteristics of interaction of the antiandrogen flutamide with the androgen receptor in various target tissues. Mol Cell Endocr 44 : 261-270.

Stanley ER, Palmer RE, Sohn U (1977). Development of methods for quantitative in vitro analysis of androgen-dependent and autonomous Shionogi carcinoma 115 cells. Cell 10:35.

Sutherland DJA, Meakin JW, Robins EC (1974). Effects of androgen on Shionogi carcinoma 115 cells in vitro. J Natl Cancer Inst 52 : 37.

Tausk M, de Visser J (1972). Pharmacology of orally active progestational compounds : animal studies. In Tausk M (ed) : "Pharmacology of the endocrine system and related drugs : progesterone, progestational drugs and anti-fertility agents" Oxford : Pergamon, p 35.

Tisell LE, Salander H (1975). Androgenic properties and adrenal depressant activity of megestrol acetate observed in castrated male rats. Acta Endocr Copenh 78 : 316-324.

Trachtenberg J, Halpern N, Pont A (1983). Ketoconazole : a novel and rapid treatment for advanced prostatic cancer. J Urol 130 : 152-153.

Walsh PC, Siiteri PK (1975). Suppression of plasma androgen by spironolactone in castrated men with carcinoma of the prostate. J Urol 114 : 254-255.

Yates J, King RJB (1978). Multiple sensitivities of mammary tumor cells in culture. Cancer Res 38 : 4135-4141.

Prostate Cancer, Part A: Research, Endocrine
Treatment, and Histopathology, pages 341–350
© 1987 Alan R. Liss, Inc.

THE KINETICS OF ANTIANDROGENS IN HUMANS

D. Tremblay, A. Dupront, B.H. Meyer and J. Pottier

Roussel-Uclaf, 93230 Romainville, France
Orange Free State University (B.H.M.), South Africa

INTRODUCTION

The study of kinetics has become an essential part of
drug investigation with immediate relevance to therapy :
for instance, it is of importance in assessing and, if possible, quantifying absorption, in choosing the delivery
system, and in optimising dose. The final dose is established on the basis of the results of clinical trials.

In the present chapter, we shall review published kinetic results on two known antiandrogens, cyproterone acetate
and flutamide, and compare them to more recently available
data on a new antiandrogen, Anandron, in order to rationa-
lise the chosen administration forms and schedules in the
clinic.

Cyproterone acetate (CPA) is a steroid progestin with
glucocorticoid, antiestrogenic and antiandrogenic properties (Neri et al., 1967 ; Neumann, 1977). Flutamide is a
nonsteroid antiandrogen devoid of other endocrine activities but whose antiandrogenic activity is largely due to
its hydroxylated metabolite (Koch, 1984). Anandron is a
nonsteroid antiandrogen also devoid of other hormonal properties but active per se (Raynaud et al., 1977, 1979). Its
kinetics and metabolism in the rat and dog have been
briefly reported (Pottier et al., 1985 ; Raynaud et al.,
1985). Its kinetics in human volunteers are reported for
the first time in the present chapter and can be compared
to its kinetics in prostate cancer patients described elsewhere (Pendyala et al., 1985, 1986 ; Creaven et al., this
volume).

CYPROTERONE ACETATE (CPA)

Studies in Healthy Volunteers

Two studies have been published on ^{3}H- and ^{14}C-labelled CPA administered orally or i.m. to separate groups of male subjects (Gerhards et al., 1973 ; Speck et al., 1976). A first group of two subjects (42-58 yrs) received a 100 mg capsule, a second group of four subjects (19-29 yrs) a 50 mg tablet and a third group of three subjects 10 mg of an oily solution i.m.. Total radioactivity was measured in the urine and feces over 8 or 10 days. The results, expressed as a percentage of the dose administered, are given in Table 1.

TABLE 1. Percent radioactivity excreted after administration of cyproterone acetate to healthy volunteers

	ORAL		I.M.
Dose (mg)	100 a)	50 b)	10 b)
Label	^{3}H	^{14}C	^{14}C
Form	capsule	tablet	oily sol'n
N° subjects	2	4	3
Urine	5	33	34
Feces	90	60	57
Total	95	93	91

a) Gerhards et al., 1973 ; b) Speck et al., 1976

Recovery was, in each case, above 90 %. An i.m. oily solution or a tablet of CPA was totally absorbed giving the same distribution of radioactivity between urine and feces. However, urinary elimination was lower with the capsule indicating decreased absorption of CPA from this administration form. Since the areas under the plasma curves (AUCs) of CPA, isolated by TLC and expressed as a percent of the dose per unit time, did not differ for the oral and i.m. routes (Gerhards et al., 1973), CPA does not undergo a first-pass effect and its availability after oral administration of tablets can be considered total. However, these conclusions are drawn from parallel groups of small numbers of cases and, since the doses are not the same, it is necessary to suppose that the kinetics of CPA is independent of dose.

Intact CPA was assayed in the plasma of the subjects receiving the tablets and accounted for about half the total radioactivity ; its half-life was 38.5 h (Table 2). In another study in five healthy volunteers (25-32 yrs) receiving the marketed 50 mg tablet, CPA was assayed in the plasma by RIA (Hümpel et al., 1978). The results are in agreement with those obtained by radioactivity determinations (Table 2).

TABLE 2. Kinetic parameters of cyproterone acetate after a single oral 50 mg dose to healthy volunteers

| | Total radioactivity n=4 a) | Cyproterone acetate ^{14}C n=4 a) | RIA n=5 b) |
	m	m	m ± S.E.M.
Tmax (h)	4	4	3.4 ± 0.2
Cmax (mg/1)	0.40	0.22	0.28 ± 0.01
AUC (mg/1 h)	7.7	4.1	4.5 ± 0.3
t 1/2 (h)	45	39	38 ± 2

a) Speck et al., 1976 ; b) Hümpel et al., 1978

Studies in Patients

CPA was assayed in patients with prostate cancer during long-term treatment (Becker et al., 1980). Assays were performed by RIA in two groups of five patients (48-82 yrs) receiving either 100 mg orally per day (2 tablets) or 300 mg every two weeks as an i.m. oily injection. Blood samples were drawn during treatment between two administrations (Table 3). Plasma concentrations before administration (Cmin) did not differ ; the steady-state had thus been attained. The ratio of the AUCs is the same as the dose ratio. However, the AUC ratio after oral administration of 100 mg to patients (Table 3) compared to 50 mg to healthy volunteers (Table 2) is nearly 3, i.e. higher than the dose ratio. The clearance of CPA is thus lower in patients than in healthy volunteers.

TABLE 3. Kinetic parameters of cyproterone acetate during
         repeated dosing in patients with prostatic carci-
         noma. Assay by RIA (from Becker et al., 1980)

	ORAL	I.M.
Dose (mg)	100 q̧ 1 day	300 q̧ 14 days
Form	tablet	oily soln
N° patients	5	5
Cmin (mg/1)		
. before a dose	0.3 ± 0.1	0.07 ± 0.03
. before next dose	0.45 ± 0.07	0.07 ± 0.02
Cmax (mg/1)	0.8 ± 0.1	0.22 ± 0.01
AUC (mg/1.h)		
between 2 doses	12 ± 2	34 ± 5

mean ± S.E.M.

The time required to reach the steady state can be estimated from two other studies, one in hyperandrogenic women, the other in prostate cancer patients. Ten women received 100 mg of CPA in tablet form once a day for 10 days
(Hammerstein et al., 1983). Plasma concentrations increased
during treatment and reached the steady state after 9 to 10
days. Cmax was about 0.3 mg/1 after the first dose and
0.6 mg/1 on the 10th administration. The concentration just
before a dose was stable and around 0.3 mg/1. Five prostate
cancer patients received 300 mg of CPA i.m. in an oily solution once a week (Rost et al., 1981). The steady state
did not seem to be reached after the 5th injection. The
Cmax was ca. 0.3 mg/1 after the first dose and ca. 0.4 mg/1
after the 5th dose. One week after the 5th dose, the concentration was ca. 0.2 mg/1.

CPA is quickly and completely absorbed from tablets.
Its long half-life justifies once daily administration. The
steady state is reached in 9 to 10 days. The usual doses
are 100 to 400 mg/day. By the i.m. route, it takes longer
to reach the steady state probably because of the slow
diffusion of the compound from the site of injection. The
i.m. doses in use, 300 mg every one or two weeks, are lower
than the oral doses but this is without any pharmacokinetic
basis since the quantities of active principle reaching the
organism are the same by both routes.

FLUTAMIDE

There are very few published studies on the kinetics of flutamide. A single paper describes results in healthy volunteers where an oral dose of 200 mg of ^{3}H-labelled flutamide was administered in capsule form to three subjects (Katchen and Buxbaum, 1975). Radioactivity eliminated in the feces over 120 h accounted for only 4.7 % of the dose administered : the absorption of flutamide is therefore practically total. In the urine, 51.1 % of the dose was eliminated over 120 h, partly as tritiated water formed during metabolism. Residual radioactivity was eliminated with a half-life close to that of tritiated water. The calculation of the quantity of tritiated water formed gave a total radioactivity recovery of 100 %. Total radioactivity and that of metabolites after chromatography was measured on samples pooled for each time-point.

Kinetic parameters are given in Table 4. Although the maximum plasma flutamide concentration was attained rapidly (1 h), it was low whereas total radioactivity was high. The AUC represented only 1 % of total radioactivity. Flutamide was thus very rapidly metabolized. Amongst the metabolites formed, hydroxyflutamide is the most abundant and is pharmacologically active (Koch, 1984). The activity of this metabolite could be responsible for that of the parent compound, but its half-life is also short (5.2 h).

TABLE 4. Kinetic parameters of flutamide after a single oral 200 mg dose to three healthy volunteers (from Katchen and Buxbaum, 1975)

	Total radioactivity	Flutamide	Hydroxylated flutamide
Tmax (h)	3	1	4
Cmax (mg/l)	3.1	0.05	0.6
AUC (mg/l.$^{-1}$h) 0-8h	21	0.2	3.0
t 1/2 (h)	–	5.2	5.2

Flutamide is presently prescribed at a total dose of 750 to 1500 mg taken 3 times a day. The short half-lives of flutamide and of hydroxylated flutamide prevent a reduction in the number of daily intakes.

ANANDRON

Two studies have been performed on the kinetics of Anandron, each in 12 healthy volunteers (18-25 yrs). One was on the relative bioavailibility of different delivery forms, the other on the linearity of plasma concentrations according to dose. The study design was a randomized cross-over protocol with a two-week interval period. Anandron was assayed in the plasma by HPLC.

The aim of the first study was to compare two adminis-tration forms, tablet and capsule, to a reference aqueous suspension. The results in Table 5 show that the kinetic parameters describing availability (Tmax, Cmax, AUC) are similar for the tablet and capsule but better than for the suspension. Thus these bioequivalent delivery forms improve the bioavailability of Anandron and can be used indifferen-tly in therapy.

TABLE 5. Kinetic parameters of Anandron after a single oral 100 mg dose to 12 healthy volunteers in a randomi-zed cross-over trial

	Suspension	Tablet	Capsule
Tmax (h)	2.6 ± 0.4	1.9 ± 0.4	1.9 ± 0.4
Cmax (mg/1)	0.45 ± 0.04	0.84 ± 0.05	0.8 ± 0.1
AUC (mg/1 h)	16 ± 2	26 ± 3	26 ± 3
t 1/2 (h)	41 ± 5	43 ± 4	49 ± 5

mean ± S.E.M.

The aim of the second study was to establish that the kinetics of Anandron are not dose dependent. The results in Table 6 show that Tmax and t 1/2 are independent of dose and that Cmax and the AUC are proportional to dose. The kinetics of Anandron after administration of increasing single doses is therefore linear (Fig. 1) and, in practice, the plasma concentrations obtained during treatment will be proportional to the dose administered.

TABLE 6. Kinetic parameters of Anandron after a single oral dose to 12 healthy volunteers in a randomized cross-over trial

	100 mg	200 mg	300 mg
Tmax (h)	1.8 ± 0.4	1.5 ± 0.3	1.5 ± 0.3
Cmax (mg/l)	0.8 ± 0.1	1.6 ± 0.1	2.3 ± 0.2
AUC (mg/l h)	25 ± 3	56 ± 5	84 ± 7
t 1/2 (h)	43 ± 3	45 ± 4	49 ± 4

mean ± S.E.M.

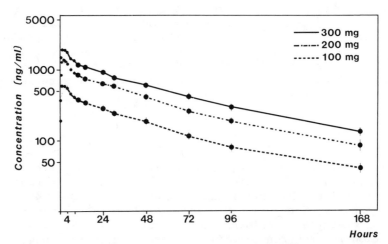

Figure 1. Plasma anandron in healthy volunteers

Doses presently given to prostate cancer patients are 150 and 300 mg daily. Initially the dose was taken tid but the results of the kinetic studies indicate that Anandron can be administered once daily since its half-life, as determined in healthy volunteers, is about 45 h.

DISCUSSION AND CONCLUSION

All three antiandrogens, cyproterone acetate, flutamide and Anandron, are well absorbed but their other kinetic parameters differ. The greatest differences are recorded between the chemically most similar compounds, i.e. between the nonsteroids flutamide and Anandron, whereas the steroid cyproterone acetate is closer to Anandron. Flutamide does not compete for the uptake of testosterone in vitro by human prostate unlike its principal metabolite, hydroxyfluta- mide, and unlike cyproterone acetate (Symes et al., 1978 ; Symes and Milroy, 1980). In this respect, flutamide can be considered a prodrug that needs to be converted to hydroxy- flutamide for activity. It is rapidly metabolized but both flutamide and hydroxyflutamide give low plasma concentra- tions of intact substance with a short half-life. In clini- cal practice, this means that the drug has to be adminis- tered at short intervals in order to maintain plasma con- centrations. On the other hand, the steady state is reached fairly quickly. Cyproterone acetate and Anandron give rise to high plasma concentrations with long half-lives which enable once daily administration. Of the latter products, it is Anandron which gives the highest concentrations with the longer half-life. Thus very stable levels are attained during treatment and should lead to permanent saturation of androgen receptors.

REFERENCES

Becker H, Düstenberg B, Klostcrhalfen H (1980). Bioverfüg- barkeit von Cyproteronacetat nach oraler und intramusku- lärer Applikation bei Männern. Urol Int 35:381-385.

Gerhards E, Gutsche H, Riemann J (1973). Biodynamik von 1,2αMethylen-6-chlor-pregna-4,6-dien-17α-acetoxy-3,20- dion (Cyproteron-acetat) nach oraler Verabreichung beim Menschen. Arzneim-Forsch (Drug Res) 23:1550-1555.

Hammerstein J, Moltz L, Schwartz U (1983). Antiandrogens in the treatment of acne and hirsutism. J steroid Biochem 19:591-597.

Hümpel M, Dogs G, Wendt H, Speck U (1978). Plasmaspiegel und Pharmacokinetic von Cyproteronacetat nach oraler Applikation als 50 mg Tablette bei 5 Männern. Arzneim Forsch (Drug Res) 28:319-322.

Katchen B, Buxbaum S (1975). Disposition of a new, non ste- roid, antiandrogen, α,α,α-trifluoro-2methyl-4'-nitro-m- propionotoluidide (Flutamide) in men following a single oral 200 mg dose. J Clin Endocrinol Metab 41:373-379.

Koch H (1984). Flutamide - a new non-steroidal anti-andro- gen. Drugs of Today 20:561-574.

Neri RO, Monahan MD, Meyer JG, Afonso BA, Tabachnik IA (1967). Biological studies on an antiandrogen (SH 714). Eur J Pharmacol 1:438–444.

Neumann F (1977). Pharmacology and potential use of cyproterone acetate. Horm Metab Res 9:1–13.

Pendyala L, Creaven PJ, Huben R, Madajewicz S, Plager J, Tremblay D, Bertagna C. Pharmacokinetics of Anandron in patients with carcinoma of the prostate. In: Abstracts, Basic and Clinical Issues in Endocrinology and Malignancy, Rome, April 1986.

Pendyala L, Madajewicz S, Creaven P (1985). Pharmacokinetics of anandron (RU 23908, 5,5-dimethyl 3-(4-nitro 3 (trifluoromethyl)-phenyl)2,4-imidazolidine-dione) in man. Proc Am Assoc Cancer Res 26:626.

Pottier J, Coussedière D, Dupront A, Meyer BH, Salmon J, Tremblay D, Deraedt R (in press). Plasma kinetics of the antiandrogen Anandron in the rat, dog and human. In: Abstracts, VII Intl Congress on Hormonal Steroids, Madrid, Sept 1986.

Pottier J, Coussedière D, Raynaud JP. Pharmacokinetics of a non-steroid antiandrogen (RU 23908) in rats and dogs. In: Abstracts, 67th Annual Meeting of the Endocrine Society, Baltimore n°954:239, June 1985.

Raynaud JP, Azadian-Boulanger G, Bonne C, Perronnet J, Sakiz E (1977). Present trends in antiandrogen research. In Martini L, Motta M (eds): "Androgens and Antiandrogens". New York: Raven Press, pp.281–293.

Raynaud JP, Bonne C, Bouton MM, Lagacé L, Labrie F (1979). Action of a non-steroid antiandrogen, RU 23908, in peripheral and central tissues. J steroid Biochem 11:93–99.

Raynaud JP, Moguilewsky M, Tournemine C, Pottier J, Coussedière D, Salmon J, Husson JM, Bertagna C, Tremblay D, Pendyala L, Brisset JM, Vallancien G, Serment G, Navratil H, Dupont A, Labrie F (1985). Pharmacology and clinical studies with RU 23908 (Anandron[R]). In: Schröder FH, Richards B (eds) "EORTC Genitourinary Group Monograph 2, Part A. Therapeutical Principles in the Management of Metastatic Prostatic Cancer" New York:Alan Liss, pp.99–120.

Rost A, Schmidt-Gollwitzer M, Hantelmann W, Brosig W (1981). Cyproterone acetate, testosterone, LH, FSH and prolactin levels in plasma after intramuscular application of cyproterone acetate in patients with prostatic cancer. The Prostate 2:315–322.

Speck U, Jentsch D, Kühne G, Schulze PE, Wendt H (1976). Bioverfügbarkeit und Pharmacokinetik von 14 C-Cyproteron acetat nach Applikation als 50 mg Tablette. Arzneim Forsch (Drug Res) 26:1717-1720.

Symes EK, Milroy E (1980). Studies on the effects of various antiandrogenic substances on the human prostate in vitro. Excerpta Medica ICS 494:182-189.

Symes EK, Milroy EJG, Mainwaring WIP (1978). The nuclear uptake of androgen by human benign prostate in vitro: Action of antiandrogens. J Urol 120:180-183.

Prostate Cancer, Part A: Research, Endocrine
Treatment, and Histopathology, pages 351-363
© 1987 Alan R. Liss, Inc.

CLINICAL PHARMACOKINETICS OF A NEW ANTIANDROGEN ANANDRON (RU 23908)

Lakshmi Pendyala, Patrick J. Creaven, Robert Huben,
Dominique Tremblay, Michel Mouren, Christine
Bertagna.

Roswell Park Memorial Institute (LP, PJC, RH),
Buffalo, New York, USA and Institut Roussel Uclaf
(DT, MM, CB), Paris, France.

INTRODUCTION

Anandron (RU 23908, 5,5-dimethyl-3[4-nitro-3-(triflu-oromethyl)phenyl-2,4-imidazolidinedione]) is a non-steroid antiandrogen (Raynaud et al., 1979, 1985) undergoing clinical trials for the treatment of carcinoma of the prostate. The drug is given orally and currently a twice or three times daily dosage schedule is employed. Studies in the rat indicated that the terminal phase half-life of Anandron is 7 h (Raynaud et al., 1985 ; Pottier et al., 1985) while that in the dog is 11.6 h (Pottier et al., 1985). The most recent study in humans using normal volunteers has indicated a longer half-life for the drug in humans compared to animals, namely 46 h (Tremblay et al., this volume ; Pottier et al., 1986). No data were available, however, on the pharmacokinetics of the drug in patients with prostatic carcinoma, on the disposition of [^{14}C] Anandron in man, on the accumulation of the drug on repetitive dosing in man, or on the effect of repetitive dosing on the disposition of the drug. We have, therefore, undertaken pharmacokinetic and drug monitoring studies of Anandron in patients with advanced carcinoma of the prostate who received daily oral dosing of the drug to gain information on these factors. We report here an initial brief account of the results of these studies.

MATERIALS AND METHODS

Drug Administration and Sampling - Pharmacokinetic Study

Anandron was supplied by Roussel Uclaf (France) as 50 mg tablets. Radiolabeled drug was supplied as tablets containing 40 µCi of [^{14}C] Anandron in 50 mg. The structure is shown in Figure 1, the asterisk indicating the position of the label.

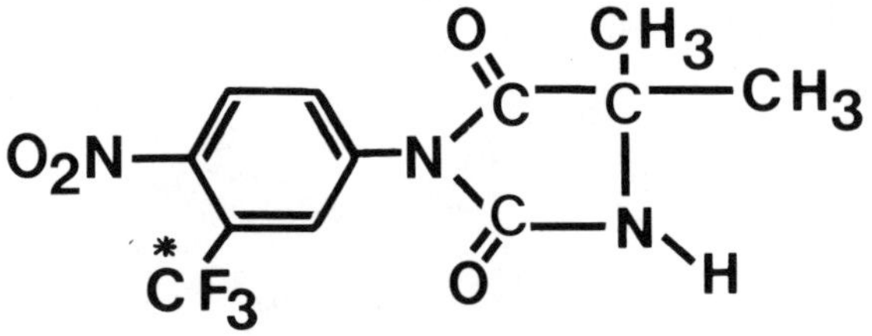

Figure 1. Structure of Anandron

The drug was administered orally to 12 patients with a microscopically confirmed diagnosis of Stage D carcinoma of the prostate. All patients were hospitalized and were fasting for 10 h before and 4 h after receiving a 120 µCi dose of [^{14}C] Anandron in 150 mg (2 patients received 160 µCi in 200 mg) on day 1. Single dose pharmacokinetics of radioactivity and of the unchanged drug were studied. Starting on day 4 in 8 patients and on day 8 in 3 patients, 150 mg of non-radioactive drug (200 mg in one patient) was given twice daily for 2-7 weeks. The plasma pharmacokinetics of the drug were studied during this period to establish the steady state levels and time to achieve steady state. With those patients who were on the multiple dose study for more than 3 weeks, sampling was carried out every 12 h prior to the drug intake when patients were still in the hospital and, subsequent to this, on a 1 to 2 week outpatient basis. At the end of this period, patients were again hospitalized and received another dose of [^{14}C] Anandron followed by a continuation of twice daily dosing of non-radioactive Anandron for another week. Plasma and urine samples were collected after the second radioactive dosing so that the plasma pharmacokinetics and urinary excretion of radioactivity could be compared to those after the first radioactive dosing.

Drug Administration and Sampling - Drug Monitoring Study

Blood samples were obtained from 184 orchiectomized patients with stage D prostate cancer, enrolled in the clinical trials on Anandron in France (Brisset et al., this volume). Anandron was administered by the oral route at two doses : either 150 mg daily, i.e., one 50 mg capsule three times a day, or 300 mg daily, i.e., one 100 mg capsule or two 50 mg tablets three times a day. The blood samples were drawn one month (25 to 40 days), three months (80 to 104 days), six months (160 to 200 days), and/or twelve months (345 to 405 days) after initiation of treatment.

Analytical Methodology - Pharmacokinetic Study

Unchanged Anandron in plasma and urine was measured by a high performance liquid chromatography (HPLC) method developed for this purpose. The HPLC system consisted of an M6000A pump, an automatic sample injector (WISP), and a 441 UV absorbance detector (Waters Associates, Milford, MA). One volume of plasma or urine is extracted with 2 volumes of chloroform, a measured volume of the chloroform extract is evaporated and reconstituted in an appropriate volume of mobile phase and injected into HPLC. The HPLC procedure is an isocratic, reverse-phase method using an IBM C-18 column, with 70 % methanol as the mobile phase at 1.2 ml/min flow rate. The method is specific for Anandron with a retention time of approximately 4.5 min and a detection limit of 50 ng/ml. Total radioactivity in plasma and urine was measured by liquid scintillation counting (Searle Mark III, DesPlaines, Ill), using an external standard method for quench correction. Radioactivity in feces was measured in 3 patients also by liquid scintillation counting, using an internal standard method.

Analytical Methodology - Drug Monitoring Study

Anandron was assayed in plasma by a radioimmunological method. The antibody was raised in rabbits receiving an antigen prepared by conjugation of the propanoic derivative (on the N3 of the hydantoin moiety) of Anandron with BSA. Tritiated Anandron, reference solution or diluted plasma, antiserum and anti-rabbit-γ-globulin antiserum raised in sheep, were incubated together for 16 h at 4°C. After centrifugation, the radioactivity in the pellet was measured by liquid scintillation. Each measurement was performed in triplicate. The sensitivity of the assay is 0.3 ng/ml. The specificity of the Anandron antibody towards endogenous substances is such that no extraction procedure is required. The cross-reactions with two metabolites that have been identified in rat plasma (products of NO_2 reduction into NH_2 or NHOH, Pottier et al., 1985) are less than 0.4 %.

Data Analysis

A non-compartmental analysis of the plasma data was carried out using the computer program Lagran (Rocci and Jusko, 1983) for both unchanged drug and radioactivity. The pharmacokinetic parameters, AUC (area under the concentration x time curve) and the terminal phase half-life ($t_{1/2}$), were calculated. Comparison of parameters was carried out using a paired t-test with the software package "Epistat" on a microcomputer (Sperry-PC, Blue Bell, PA).

The mean plasma concentrations recorded during the clinical trial were compared : between groups for each time point and between different times within each group using Student's t test.

RESULTS

Single Dose Plasma Pharmacokinetics

Plasma radioactivity consisted of both unchanged drug and metabolites. The plasma concentration profile of unchanged drug after the initial single dose of [^{14}C] Anandron was similar in all patients, with distinct absorp-

tion, distribution and elimination phases (Figure 2). Total
radioactivity showed two patterns, 3 patients demonstrated
a distribution phase while the remainder did not.

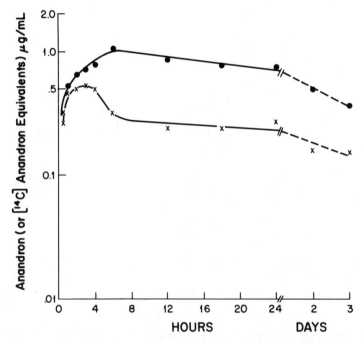

Figure 2. Plasma decay profiles of total radioactivity (-o-)
and unchanged Anandron (-x-) in a patient after
[^{14}C] Anandron (150 mg) administration

The mean (±S.D.) and the ranges for the pharmacokinetic
parameters for total radioactivity and unchanged Anandron
after a single dose are shown in Table 1. The mean C_{max}
(maximum plasma concentration) of unchanged Anandron was
0.9 μg.ml^{-1} and that of radioactivity was 1.29 μg.ml^{-1}
Anandron equivalents. Thus the mean C_{max} of unchanged
drug represents 70 % of the mean C_{max} of the total radioactivity. Calculated for each individual patient the C_{max}
of Anandron was 49-90 % of the C_{max} of radioactivity. The
mean AUC for unchanged Anandron represents 30 % of the
mean AUC for radioactivity. Calculated for each individual
patient it ranged from 23-38 %. The observed t_{max} (time to
achieve maximum concentration) was 1-4 h for unchanged drug
and 2-12 h for radioactivity.

TABLE 1. Pharmacokinetic parameters of radioactivity and Anandron after the first [^{14}C] Anandron dosing

	Total Radioactivity		Unchanged Anandron	
	Mean (±S.D.)	Range	Mean (±S.D.)	Range
C_{max} [a,c] ($\mu g \cdot ml^{-1}$)	1.29 (±0.24)	1.03– 1.76	0.90 (±0.20)	0.52– 1.20
AUC [a] ($\mu g \cdot ml^{-1} \cdot h$)	136.00 (±21.00)	103.2– 169.4	38.62 (±8.35)	23.30– 87.20
t_{max} [b,c] (h)	5.80 (±3.68)	2.00– 12.00	2.80 (±1.14)	1.00– 4.00
$t1/2$ [b] (h)	86.90 (±27.11)	34.5– 137.3	56.25 (±18.78)	23.30– 87.20

a: n = 10, patients receiving 150 mg dose
b: n = 12, all patients
c: the C_{max} and t_{max} are observed values

The mean $t_{1/2}$ for Anandron was approximately 2.5 days (range: 1-4 days) and that for radioactivity was approximately 3.5 days (range: 1.5-6 days). The plasma decay of radioactivity was measurable for 6 or more days after a single dose. Multiple dosing with non-radioactive drug starting on days 4-8 did not affect the slope of the plasma decay curve.

All pharmacokinetic parameters showed large patient to patient variability as reflected by the ranges and standard deviations in Table 1.

Urinary excretion

Figure 3 shows the urinary excretion of radioactivity and unchanged drug up to 5 days after the initial dose of [^{14}C] Anandron. It can be seen that radioactivity is still being excreted at 5 days. This was true of all patients studied. In 10 patients 49-78 % of the administered radio-activity was found in the urine in 120 h (Table 2). Only minor amounts of unchanged Anandron are excreted in the urine (about 1 % of the dose) (Table 2). The bulk of the urinary radioactivity is not extractable with chloroform and presumably represents hydrophilic metabolites.

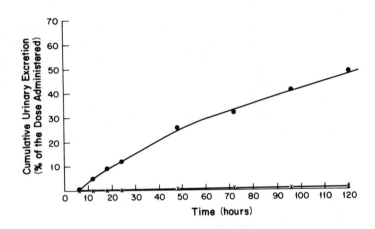

Figure 3. Cumulative urinary excretion of radioactivity (-o-) and unchanged Anandron (-x-) in a patient after [^{14}C] Anandron (150 mg) administration

TABLE 2. Cumulative urinary excretion of radioactivity and Anandron[a]

	% of Dose Excreted	
	Total Radioactivity (at 120 h)	Unchanged Anandron (at 72 h)
Mean	61.49	0.81
(±S.D.)	9.92	0.38
Range	48.6 – 77.9	0.14 – 1.32

a: n = 10

Fecal Elimination

The fecal elimination of radioactivity measured in 3 patients represented 1.4, 1.6 and 6.9 % of the total dose administered.

Accumulation Kinetics

The accumulation of Anandron during twice daily dosing for 6 weeks for one of the patients is shown in Figure 4. This is typical of the pattern observed in the six patients studied for 6-7 weeks. The steady state levels were attained in approximately 2 weeks from the initiation of the multiple dosing regimen and the levels (at a dose of 150 mg every 12 hours) ranged from 4.4 to 8.5 μg/ml.

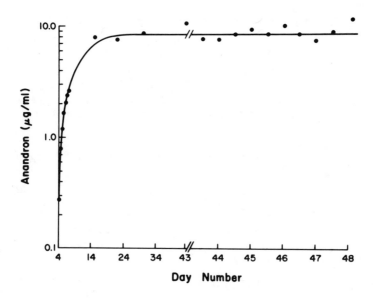

Figure 4. Accumulation of unchanged Anandron in plasma of a patient receiving twice daily doses of Anandron (150 mg) for 6 weeks

Plasma kinetics of Radioactivity and Anandron after the Second Radioactive Dose

At 38 to 51 days from the initiation of multiple dosing, when patients had achieved steady state plasma levels of drug, six patients received a second dose of [^{14}C] Anandron. Repeated sampling was carried out in the following 12 h period so that the pharmacokinetic parameters of the unchanged drug ($AUC_{0-12\ h}$ and $t_{1/2}$) could be derived during this dosing interval. The pharmacokinetic parameters for radioactivity ($AUC_{0-\infty}$, $t_{1/2}$) on the other hand were calculated based on the entire period the plasma radioactivity was measurable, since the dosing with non-radioactive drug did not affect the plasma decay of radioactivity. In Table 3, are shown the mean, standard deviation and range of AUC and $t_{1/2}$ for radioactivity and unchanged Anandron after the first single dose and during the steady state. A comparison of the AUC and $t_{1/2}$ after the first dose with those seen during the steady state reveals that the $AUC_{0-12\ h}$ of unchanged Anandron at steady state is significantly higher than the $AUC_{0-\infty}$ after the first dosing (p < 0.0001).

TABLE 3. Plasma kinetics[a] of radioactivity and Anandron after the first dose and during steady state

	First dose		Steady state	
	$AUC^b_{0-\infty}$	$t1/2^c$	$AUC^b_{0-\infty}$	$t1/2^c$
	($\mu g \cdot ml^{-1} \cdot h$)	(h)	($\mu g \cdot ml^{-1} \cdot h$)	(h)
Total radioactivity	131.94 (±24.14)	75.50 (±28.53)	139.70 (±46.94)	91.75 (±29.59)
Unchanged Anandron	38.70^d (±10.78)	53.37 (±25.16)	89.76^{d,e} (±13.38)	38.70 (±9.27)

a: values reported are means and standard deviations in parentheses
b: n = 5 patients
c: n = 6 patients
d: differences are highly significant (P = 7 x 10^{-5})
e: $AUC_{0-12\ h}$

Plasma Anandron Concentrations in Patients Participating in a Clinical Trial (Drug Monitoring Study)

The mean recorded Anandron concentrations in patients participating in a multicentric clinical trial are given in Table 4. A comparison between time points reveals no significant difference $(0.35 \geqslant p \geqslant 0.11)$ between the Anandron tablets and capsules when administered at a daily dose of 300 mg and no significant difference $(0.95 \geqslant p \geqslant 0.50)$ between the concentrations obtained with the 300 and 150 mg doses, administered in the form of capsules, once these have been divided by dose. The comparison between the concentrations obtained at different times with the capsule and tablet (300 mg/day) does not reveal any significant difference either $(0.95 \geqslant p \geqslant 0.58)$.

TABLE 4. Plasma Anandron concentrations $(ug.ml^{-1})$ during long-term treatment of patients

Months		Tablet 300 mg tid	Capsule 300 mg tid	Capsule 150 mg tid	Ratio $\dfrac{300 \text{ mg}}{150 \text{ mg}}$
1	m	6.44	7.24	3.38	
	S.D.	2.58	3.65	1.12	2.14
	n	57	33	26	
3	m	6.45	7.30	3.58	
	S.D.	3.14	3.95	1.23	2.04
	n	44	31	32	
6	m	6.17	7.42	3.73	
	S.D.	2.84	2.71	1.70	1.99
	n	25	27	28	
12	m	6.05	7.04	3.83	
	S.D.	1.97	2.69	0.92	1.84
	n	10	12	14	

m = mean ; S.D. = standard deviation ; n = number of patients

DISCUSSION

The lack of availability of a parenteral form of Anandron for administration to humans precluded the determination of bioavailability in the present study. However, from the negligible excretion of radioactivity in feces and from the levels of radioactivity recovered in the urine, it appears that Anandron is well absorbed from the GI tract, which agrees with the observations made in experimental animals (Pottier et al., 1985). After a dose of [^{14}C] Anandron, plasma radioactivity consisted of unchanged drug and metabolites, unchanged drug representing about 30 % of the total radioactivity, based on AUC comparisons. The radioactivity and the unchanged drug profiles in the first two hours after drug administration, however, were quite similar, the unchanged drug accounting for about 79 % of total radioactivity at 2 h, but declining from then on to about 32 % at 72 h. The high proportion of unchanged drug at very early times in humans is similar to that reported in rats where 70–95 % of radioactivity was associated with unchanged drug in the first 6 h (Raynaud et al., 1985). However, the terminal phase half-life found for Anandron in the present study is extremely long compared to those observed in the rat and dog (7 and 11.6 h respectively) (Raynaud et al., 1985 ; Pottier et al., 1985). These differences cannot be attributed to differences in protein binding because, at concentrations achieved in vivo, both animal species showed 80 % protein binding of the drug. From studies in vitro we estimate an 85 % binding in human plasma (data not reported in this paper). The reported half-life of 46 h in studies of human volunteers (Tremblay et al., this volume ; Pottier et al., 1986) falls into the range of half-lives in our patients (23–87 h). The C_{max} values reported by Tremblay et al. after doses of 100 mg and 200 mg were 0.81 and 1.58 $\mu g.ml^{-1}$ respectively. The AUCs in the same study were 27.8 and 63.4 $\mu g.ml^{-1}h$ respectively. Our mean C_{max} and AUC values for Anandron after 150 mg were 0.9 $ug.ml^{-1}$ and 38.8 $\mu g.ml^{-1}h$ which fall in the general range of expected values based on the above study, for a drug with linear kinetics. The two patients who received a single dose of 200 mg in our study had C_{max} values of 1.4 and 2.0 $\mu g.ml^{-1}$ respectively and AUC of 73.6 and 37.4 $\mu g.ml^{-1}h$. We observed a large interpatient variability for the pharmacokinetic parameters in our study which is usual with this patient population and can be attributed to the presence of many confounding variables which include administration of other medications, variability in vital organ function, and alteration in plasma protein binding. However, in general, the results of our study in cancer patients are similar to those obtained in healthy individuals.

After repeated dosing, the AUC of Anandron between two doses was higher than expected whereas the AUC for total radioactivity was unchanged. Therefore, if we assume that bioavailability is constant, the total clearance of Anandron decreased on initiating treatment with repeated doses. On the other hand, the time required to reach the steady state, about two weeks, was 4 to 5 half-lives, as expected. Since the half-life remained unchanged, the decrease in clearance would appear to have been due to an increase in the volume of distribution.

When results are obtained in patients partaking in a clinical trial, the time that has elapsed between drug intake and blood sampling is not known with precision. In the case of Anandron, this is not a major obstacle. Since the half-life of Anandron is much longer than the 8 h-interval between two intakes, any fluctuation in steady state levels is negligible. Moreover, since the real time intervals between administration and sampling are distributed randomly around a mean time, no bias is introduced even though the power of the statistical analysis may be reduced. The plasma concentrations can therefore be considered to be given by the mean concentrations between two doses. On these premisses, the steady state in these patients is not modified over 1 year of treatment. The total clearance, reduced at the onset of treatment, remains constant thereafter and is independent of dose since the ratio of the levels reached with 150 and 300 mg/day is the same as the dose ratio. Results in these patients also confirm the bioequivalence of the capsules and tablets already reported in the studies in healthy volunteers (Tremblay et al., this volume).

To summarize, Anandron in patients with advanced cancer appears to be well absorbed, whatever the drug delivery form, has a prolonged half-life and is extensively metabolized to largely hydrophilic metabolites which are excreted in the urine. At a dose of 150 mg twice daily, steady state plasma levels are reached in approximately two weeks.

Repeated dosing reduces the total clearance during the first two weeks which thereafter remains constant when the steady state is attained. The observed plasma concentrations are stable during at least one year and proportional to the administered dose.

Based on the data obtained in these studies we recommend evaluation of a once daily drug administration.

REFERENCES

Pottier J, Coussedière D, Raynaud JP (1985). Pharmacokinetics of a non-steroid anti-androgen (RU 23908) in rats and dogs. Proc Endocrine Society, Baltimore, Maryland, Abst #954, p. 239.

Pottier J, Coussedière D, Dupront A, Meyer BH, Salmon J, Tremblay D, Deraedt R (1986). Plasma kinetics of the antiandrogen anandron in the rat, dog and human. Proc VII International Congress on Hormonal Steroids. Madrid, Spain, in press.

Raynaud JP, Bonne C, Bouton MM, Lagacé L, Labrie F (1979). Action of a non steroid androgen, RU 23908, in peripheral and central tissues. J steroid Biochem 11:93–99.

Raynaud JP, Moguilewsky M, Tournemine C, Pottier J, Coussedière D, Salmon J, Husson JM, Bertagna C, Tremblay D, Pendyala L, Brisset JM, Vallancien G, Serment G, Navratil N, Dupront A, Labrie F (1985). Pharmacology and clinical studies with RU 23908 (Anandron[R]). In Schroeder FH, Richards B (eds): "EORTC Genitourinary Group Monograph 2, Part A: Therapeutic Principles in Metastatic Prostate Cancer", New York: Alan R Liss, Inc pp. 99–120.

Rocci ML, Jusko WJ (1983). Lagran program for area and moments in pharmacokinetic analysis. Computer Programs in Biomedicine. 16:203–216.

Prostate Cancer, Part A: Research, Endocrine
Treatment, and Histopathology, pages 365–368
© 1987 Alan R. Liss, Inc.

CLINICAL EXPERIENCE WITH CYPROTERONE ACETATE IN A
RANDOMISED AND IN AN OPEN TRIAL

Tunn, U.W., Weiglein, W., Saborowski, J., &
Senge, Th.
Department of Urology, Städtische Kliniken,
D-6050 Offenbach/Main.
Department of Urology, University of Bochum,
D-4690 Herne 1

From experimental data it can be concluded that Cyproterone Acetate (CPA) in a dosage high enough reduces the
dihydrotestosterone (DHT) content in the prostate about
90% and consequently induces a total withdrawal of
androgen effect at the target cell level (1). The
therapeutic efficacy can only be determind by clinical
trials.

In this paper we shall present some clinical experience
with CPA in one randomised and in one open trial in
previously untreated patients with advanced prostatic
cancer:

First the results of a prospective phase III trial of CPA
monotherapy versus a standard estrogen treatment.

Design of the study: Patients with advanced virginal
prostatic cancer were randomized in two treatment groups:
one group received cyproterone acetate (CPA), the other
estradiolundecylate (E) as a standard regimen. The dosage
was 300 mg CPA weekly, resp. 100 mg E monthly. In the
multicentre short-term phase clinical effects and toxicty
of a 6 months treatment with CPA and E were compared in
191 patients. These results are already published in
detail in cooperation with Jacobi and Senge (2). Briefly,
CPA was as effective as the standard estrogen regimen,
but was associated with fewer side effects.

39 patients, primarily from the department of Urology of the University of Bochum, were maintained on the intitial treatment, until there was evidence of tumor progression. The observation was done for 5 years.

The overall survival curves of these patients reveal no significant difference in both treatment groups. After a follow-up of 5 years only 30% of all patients were still alive.

Comparing exclusively the patients without distant metastases (M_0) at the entry of the study, CPA appeared to exhibit an improved effect of 5-year survival. The 5-year survival rate in M_0-patients was nearly 60% in the CPA group compared to 45% in the E-group.

Secondly we shall present some clinical experience of an open study of treatment with castration plus CPA.

51 patients with advanced virginal prostatic cancer were treated by combination of castration and CPA in a dosage of 50 mg daily. After 6 months the patients were evaluated by transrectal ultrasonography, computer-tomography, bone scan, serum prostatic acid phosphatase, and non specific criteria. Since treatment response criteria are differently defined by NPCP and EORTC (3) both response criteria systems were used in the evaluation of these patients.

The response rates ar summarized in this table 1. Complete remission occured in none of the patients, partial remission occured in 29% according to NPCP, resp. 25% according to EORTC, stable desease in 55%, resp. 59%. 16% were rated as progressing.

Since stable desease is not considered as an objective response according to EORTC, the results of responses in the two evaluation systems are significantly different using the so-called positive objective response as a parameter. These data are summarized in table 2. Using NPCP criteria positive response is rated in 97% of M_0 patients and in 65% of M_1 patients in contrast to 35% of M_0 patients and 10% of M_1 patients using EORTC criteria.

	Response criteria	
	NPCP	EORTC
Complete response (CR)	0 (0%)	0 (0%)
Partial response (PR)	15 (29%)	13 (25%)
Stable (S) No Change (NC)	28 (55%)	30 (59%)
Progression (P)	8 (16%)	8 (16%)

Table 2
Positive response rates of 51 patients using NPCP and EORTC response criteria

M-stage	n	Response criteria	
		NPCP	EORTC
M_0	31	97%	35%
M_1	20	65%	10%
Total	51	84%	25%

In summary these results of evaluation demonstrate that partial remission occured in 25% of all patients and progression in 16%. The first group is considered to have a good prognosis, the last group a poor one. The prognosis of the remaining 59% of patients in the stable category seems not to be predictable by using clinical parameters. Both trials with CPA, the randomised and the open one, demonstrate the heterogeneity of agressiveness of advanced prostatic cancer.

Table 1
Response rates of 51 patients with advanded prostatic cancer after 6 months treatment with complete androgen withdrawal (castration plus CPA).

REFERENCES

1. Neumann, F., Hümpel, M., Senge, Th., Schenck, B., Tunn, U.W. (1982). In: Prostate Cancer. Ed.: Jacobi, G.H., Hohenfellner, R., Williams & Wilkins, Baltimore, London, 269-302
2. Jacobi, G.H., Tunn, U.W., Senge, Th.: Clinical experience with cyproterone acetate for palliation of inoperable prostatic cancer (1982). In: Prostate Cancer. Ed.: Jacobi, G.H., Hohenfellner, R., Williams & Wilkins, Baltimore, London, 305-319
3. Schroeder, F.H. 1984. Treatment response criteria for prostatic cancer. In: Prostate 5, 181-191

Prostate Cancer, Part A: Research, Endocrine
Treatment, and Histopathology, pages 369–377
© 1987 Alan R. Liss, Inc.

TREATMENT OF PROSTATIC CANCER WITH CYPROTERONE ACETATE AS MONOTHERAPY

D. Beurton, J. Grall, Ph. Davody, J. Cukier
Clinique Urologique, Hôpital Necker, Paris

Cyproterone acetate (ANDROCUR), synthesised in 1961 by F. NEUMANN (9), is a steroidal anti-androgen catabolised by the liver. Animal pharmacology studies have demonstrated a triple action for the product : 1. potent progestagen, 2. competitive anti-androgen by blocking the transport of the DHT-cytoplasmic protein complex on the nuclear receptors of the target organs, in particular the prostate, 3. anti-gonadotrophic by saturation of the hypophyseal androgen receptors.

It has low toxicity at the doses used (50 to 100 mg/24 hr). Following oral absorption, the peak plasma level is obtained within 3 to 4 hours. The half-life is 38 ± 5 hours. The serum testosterone is decreased to 2/3 of its initial value within two weeks.

The inhibitory action of cyproterone acetate on the target organs is reflected by decreased libido, decreased activity of the sebaceous glands and hair growth, atrophy of the prostate and seminal vesicles and arrest of spermatogenesis and puberty. Clinically, apart from prostatic cancer, this drug is used in transexuals and hypersexuals, for the treatment of acne and hirsutism, to inhibit precocious puberty and as a contraceptive in women.

Its anti-androgenic and anti-gonadotrophic activity led some authors to use this drug in the treatment of prostatic cancer in preference to oestrogens because of its low toxicity, especially cardiovascular toxicity. W.W. SCOTT (10) reported the first application in human prostatic cancer in 1966. Subsequently, J. GELLER in 1968 (2), A. WEIN in 1973 (12) and U. BRACCI in 1979 (1) reported small series in which ANDROCUR, administered as monotherapy at high doses, varying between 200 and 250 mg per day, induced more than 80 % objective responses with a mean duration of remission of 17 months.

In 1980, L. GIULIANI (3) compared two groups of patients with stage C and D cancer, treated by a combination of oestrogens and castration in one group and by castration and ANDROCUR in the other group, but the action of this combination was found to be more effective for earlier stages and lower grades.

In 1980 and 1983, two randomised studies, one conducted by G. JACOBI (6) and the other by V. TUNN (11), compared the effects of ANDROCUR and an oestrogen, both administered as monotherapy either parenterally or orally. These studies demonstrated comparable efficacy of the two treatments after six months, but a less marked decrease in the serum testosterone levels with ANDROCUR. The incidence of side effects was much lower with ANDROCUR : gynaecomastia, oedema and venous thrombosis were reported in 94 % of the patients treated with oestrogen compared with only 37 % with the anti-androgen.

More recently, in 1984, L. LABRIE (7) stressed the value of simultaneously using an LHRH agonist and a pure anti-androgen in order to minimise the development of hormone-resistant cells and to prolong the duration of remission.

MATERIAL AND METHODS

Population : Between 1976 and 1985, 112 patients between the ages of 50 and 88 years (mean of 72.3 years) were treated with a daily oral dose of 100 mg of Cyproterone acetate (CPA). The maximal duration of continuous single-agent treatment in the same patient is currently 102 months. 54 patients, including 39 patients with cardiovascular contraindications to oestrogens, received ANDROCUR as strict monotherapy ; 58 patients received one or several other treatments either previously or concomitantly to the administration of the anti-androgen (46 cases of radical prostatectomy, 14 cases of castration, 13 cases of oestrogen therapy, 6 cases of radiotherapy and 5 miscellaneous surgical procedures).

Classification of the tumours

Staging procedures classified the prostatic tumours as follows :

- 28 cases of Stage B

- 35 cases of Stage C and D1
- 49 cases of Stage D2

75 % of the cancers treated therefore corresponded to advanced stages. However, it should be noted that the classification of Stage B in 28 cases was purely based on the findings of the rectal examination in elderly patients, in whom curative treatment was considered to be excessive and in whom, therefore, a more precise staging was unnecessary.

Histological examination revealed 60 well differentiated tumours, 5 moderately well differentiated tumours, 31 poorly differentiated tumours and the grade was not defined in 16 cases (obvious diagnosis of advanced stage which did not require histological confirmation). Overall, 37.5 % of the tumours studied presented high histological grades.

Criteria of evaluation and duration of treatment

The efficacy of treatment was evaluated on the basis of subjective and objective criteria : improvement in the general condition, modification in micturition (clinical and urodynamic evaluation), resolution of bone pain, decreased prostatic volume on rectal examination, improved condition of the urinary tract evaluated by intravenous pyelography and ultrasonography, variations in plasma creatinine, prostatic phosphatases and testosterone and, lastly, full blood count, erythrocyte sedimentation rate and cytobacteriological examination of the urine.

The patients were reviewed after 1 month, 3 months, 6 months and then every year by the clinician. In addition, every 6 months, between 2 annual visits, the patient sent, by the post, the results of follow-up laboratory tests : full blood count, erythrocyte sedimentation rate, prostatic phosphatases, creatinine and cytobacteriological examination of the urine.

56 of the 112 patients treated have been followed regularly over a period of between 1 and 102 months with a mean follow-up of 34 months.
56 patients have been lost to follow-up between 1 and 65 months (mean : 17.6 months) after starting treatment. A large percentage of these patients have probably died, but no information is available to confirm this.

RESULTS

1. Overall results

97 patients are evaluable, with a follow-up of between 7 and 102 months (mean : 25.8 months).

81 patients (83.5 %) obtained an objective remission after one month of treatment. This remission has been maintained for 102 months in the longest survivor in our series. 36 patients (44.5 %) presented a secondary escape from ANDROCUR control between 3 and 78 months (mean : 20.5 months) after starting treatment, which was initially very active. 19 patients developed metastases (19.6 %).

20 patients have died (20.65 %, 17 from their cancer and 3 from a complication of treatment : 1 myocardial infarction and 1 cerebral haemorrhage in 2 patients treated with oestrogens after escape from CPA and 1 case of pulmonary embolism with CPA.

At the present time, 45 of the patients still being followed are in complete remission, i.e. 46.6 %. The actuarial survival of the 56 patients not lost to follow-up during the period of the study (Fig. 1), regardless of the stage, is 68.6 % at three years and 51.5 % at 5 years.

2. Results in terms of stage and grade (Table I)

The objective response rate was higher (92.3 %) in the lower stages (B) than in the higher stages (C-D1-D2) (80 %).

Table 1. Results according to stage and grade

	Objective response	Secondary escape
B = 28 patients	92,3 %	29,2 %
C + D1 = 35 patients	80 %	45,5 %
D2 = 49 patients	80 %	54,5 %
Well differentiated = 60 patients	92,1 %	40,4 %
Poor or moderately differentiated = 60 patients	71 %	59 %
Unspecified =	80 %	33,3 %

The incidence of secondary escape increased in parallel with the stage : 29% for stage B, 45.5 % for stage C and D1 and 54.5 % for stage D2. A similar difference was observed in relation to the grade of the tumour : 92 % objective responses and 40.5 % secondary escapes for well differentiated tumours ; 71 % remissions and 59 % escapes for poor or moderately well differentiated tumours.

3. Comparison between monotherapy and combination treatment (Table II)

50 evaluable patients were only treated with ANDROCUR. 47 evaluable patients received hormonal treatment, castration or radiotherapy previously or radical prostatectomy either previously or concomitantly to the administration of CPA. No significant difference in the remission rate or recurrence rate was observed between these two groups.

Table II. Monotherapy versus combined therapy

	Objective response	Secondary response
Mono-therapy 50 evaluable	82 %	41,5 %
Combined therapy 47 evaluable	85,1 %	47,5 %

4. Cyproterone acetate prescribed as salvage therapy (Table III).

8 patients received CPA after escaping from oestrogen control : 4 initially responded and then 2 of them subsequently escaped. In the 6 castrated patients with tumour progression, ANDROCUR controlled this progression in 2 patients, one of whom subsequently relapsed. Finally, one patient treated with radiotherapy responded temporarily to treatment with the anti- androgen and then rapidly escaped.

Table III. Salvage CPA

	Objective response	Secondary escape
Estrogens : 8 patients	50 %	50 %
Castration : 6 patients	33,3 %	50 %
Radiotherapy : 1 patients	+	+

5. Side effects of treatment with ANDROCUR (Table IV)

Thirteen complications were observed in 10 patients, i.e. 10.3 % of the 97 evaluable patients. Only one complication was responsible for death due to pulmonary embolism (1 %). Treatment had to be stopped in one case of very severe diarrhoea. Thrombo-embolic complications were reported in 3 % of cases. Oedema and gynaecomastia (5.2 %) were rare in comparison with their incidence with oestrogens (11).

The effects on sexuality were difficult to evaluate. However, in the 18 patients in whom they could be evaluated, libido was decreased in every case, while 6 patients reported occasional erections.

Table IV. Morbidity

Side effects :	13 in 10 patients	: 10,3%	
	Gastrointestinal		
	disorders	: 3	Stop Androcur : 1
	Mental aberration	: 1	
	Phlebitis	: 2	3 %
	Pulmonary		
	embolism	: 1	3 %
	Oedema	: 1	
	Gynecomastia	: 5	5,2 %
Sexuality :	18 patients		
	Potency preserved	: 6	
	Impotence	: 12	

DISCUSSION

The results of treatment with Cyproterone acetate in 112 cases of prostatic cancer, 3/4 of which were advanced, corroborate those reported in the literature (1, 2, 6, 8, 11, 12). CPA, administered as monotherapy, has an immediate action as potent as that of oestrogens on all stages of the tumour, provided it is hormone-dependent. Its anti-gonadotrophic action is certainly less intense than that of oestrogens, but it is completed by its predominant anti-androgenic action. The fact that the reduction is plasma testosterone is less dramatic with CPA than with oestrogens is not, however, a sign of its inefficacy, as it has an anti-androgenic action on the receptors. The advantage of CPA over oestrogen therapy is that it induces far fewer side effects, in particular gynaecomastia and water retention (11). Its cardiovascular toxicity is also much less, at least at moderate doses (100 mg per 24 hours), which are still largely sufficient to ensure complete efficacy. THis advantage is counter-balanced by the more rapid escape from treatment than with oestrogens, occurring an average of 20 months after starting treatment (however, some patients are still in complete remission after more than 5 years of monotherapy with ANDROCUR). This is due to the development of hormone-resistant cells and to the progressive exhaustion of the anti-androgenic effect and, consequently, the anti-gonadotrophic action of CPA, while oestrogens present a combination of a potent and prolonged anti-gonadotrophic action (hypophyseal suppression and increased TeBG) and a direct toxic action on the tumour cell (4). Conversely, remissions have been obtained with Cyproterone acetate following escape of the tumour from oestrogen treatment and, to a lesser extent, after castration.

These findings seem to suggest that escape of a prostatic cancer depends on 2 different mechanisms which may be involved to varying degrees (5) : firstly, the development of a separate cellular contingent which adapts to the low doses of androgen which continue to circulate (this explains the positive action of an anti-androgen after escape from oestrogens or castration). Secondly, the progressive development of a hormone-resistant cellular contingent which becomes predominant in relation to the hormone-sensitive cells (this explains the positive action of high dose oestrogens after escape from ANDROCUR or castration).

It is obvious that each therapeutic modality used in the palliative treatment of prostatic cancer has its advantages and disadvantages : oestrogen therapy is still the most effective but also the most toxic treatment. Castration is the simplest, least dangerous and least expensive modality and is almost as effective as oestrogens, but it may be poorly accepted by the patient ; it does not suppress all of the androgens, it does not increase the TeBG which reduces free testosterone and, unlike oestrogens, it does not have a direct action on the tumour cells.

Cyproterone acetate is more effective than castration as it neutralises all androgenic activity, but is is associated with a few vascular risks and its duration of action is limited in time.

At the present time, if one wishes to avoid using oestrogens as first line treatment because of their side effects or castration because of its irreversible nature, it is reasonable to propose Cyproterone acetate which has an immediate action as potent as that of the other two modalities. The plasma testosterone levels should be monitored regularly. When they start to increase, after remaining at a low plateau level for a long period of time, escape is probable and castration should be proposed before the appearance of clinical signs. It appears to be useful to continue ANDROCUR, but at lower doses, of the order of 25 to 50 mg per day (11), which is sufficient to neutralise the remaining circulating androgens, without exposing the patient to cardiovascular risks. Some authors recommend a combination of castration and anti-androgen as initial treatment in order to delay the appearance of hormone-resistant cells (3, 7) ; however, it has not been demonstrated whether this objective is actually achieved. Oestrogen therapy is then used as the last resort in an attempt to rescue an escape from castration or Cyproterone acetate, if the cancer cells are still sensitive to the direct toxic action of oestrogens.

CONCLUSION

Cyproterone acetate is an excellent alternative to oestrogen therapy or castration in the treatment of prostatic cancer. The choice of this treatment in preference to another modality is guided by the patient's age and cardiovascular status, the stage and the grade of the tumour and the patient's acceptance or refusal of castration. Its combination with castration, either immediately or at the time of escape, is apparently logical, but randomised studies must be conducted in order to confirm its value.

REFERENCES

1 - GRACCI U. - Antiandrogens in the treatment of prostatic cancer. Eur. Urol., 1979, 5, 303-306.
2 - GELLER J. et al. - The effect of cyproterone acetate on advanced carcinoma of the prostate. Surgery, Gynecol. Obst., 1968, 123, 748-758.
3 - GIULANI L. et al. - Treatment of advanced prostatic carcinoma with cyproterone acetate and orchiectomy. 5 years follow-up. Eur. Urol., 1980, 6, 145-148.
4 - HUDSON R. - The effects of androgens and oestrogens on human prostatic cells in culture. J. Physiol. Pharmacol., 1981, 59, 949.
5 - ISAACS J. - The timing of androgen ablation therapy and/or chemotherapy in the treatment of prostatic cancer. Prostate, 1984, 5, 1.

6 - JACOBI G.H. - Treatment of advanced prostatic cancer with parenteral cyproterone acetate : a phase III randomised trial. Brit. J. Urol., 1980, 52, 208-215.

7 - LABRIE F. - A new approach in the hormonal treatment of prostate cancer : complete instead of partial blockade of androgens. Int. J. Androl., 1984, 7, 1-4.

8 - LE GUILLOU et al. - Cancers de prostate traités par Androcur. A propos de 198 cas. J. d'Urol., Paris, 1984, 90, 636.

9 - NEUMANN F. et al. - Antiandrogens and prostatic tumours (experimental base and clinical use). Prog. Clin. Biol. res., 1976, 6, 169-185.

10 - SCOTT W.W. et al. - A new oral progestational steroid effective in treating prostatic cancer. Trans. Ame. Ass. Genito-Urin. Surg., 1966, 58, 54-62.

11 - TUNN U. et coll. - Clinical experience with cyproterone acetate as monotherapy in inoperable carcinoma of the prostate in the therapy of advanced carcinoma. In Worshops for urologists. Berlin 1983. Edit. by H. Klostoshaffen-SHERING-AG-WEST GERMANY, 67-75.

12 - WEIN A.J., MURPHY J.J. - Experience in the treatment of prostatic carcinoma with cyproterone acetate. J. Urol., 1973, 109, 68-70.

Prostate Cancer, Part A: Research, Endocrine
Treatment, and Histopathology, pages 379–382
© 1987 Alan R. Liss, Inc.

CYPROTERONE ACETATE VERSUS MEDROXYPROGESTERONE ACETATE VER-
SUS DIETHYLSTILBESTROL IN THE TREATMENT OF PROSTATE CANCER:
RESULTS FROM EORTC STUDY 30761

M. Pavone-Macaluso (1), G.B. Ingargiola (1), H.
de Voogt (2), G. Viggiano (3), E. Barasolo (4),
B. Lardennois (5), M. De Pauw (6) and R. Sylvester (6)

(1) Institute of Urology, University of Palermo, Italy
(2) Free University, Amsterdam, The Netherlands
(3) Ospedale Civile Umberto 1, Mestre, Italy
(4) Ospedale S. Andrea, Vercelli, Italy
(5) Hopitale de la Maison Blanche, Reims, France
(6) EORTC Data Center, Brussels, Belgium

INTRODUCTION

In 1976 the EORTC Urological Group was established in
its present form. It was felt imperative to implement
randomized trial to compare new forms of hormonal treatment
of prostate cancer with the classical oestrogenic therapy.
As new progestational agents had been investigated and found
to be effective and less toxic than DES, a prospective study
was activated (protocol 30761). The general outline of the
study is as follows: patients with previously untreated
prostatic cancer of category T2–T4 Mo, or with M1 disease,
were randomly allocated to cyproterone acetate (CPA) 250 mg
per day; medroxyprogesterone acetate (MPA) loading dose
500 mg l.m., 3 times weekly for 8 weeks, then 100 mg orally
twice daily; or diethylstilbestrol (DES) 1 mg t.i.d.

Of 236 patients entered from February 1977 to April 1981
by 18 institutions, 210 were assessed. Almost half (41%) of
the patients were entered by 8 Italian Institutions. The
following investigators participated in this study: Italy:

G. Viggiano and A. Nasta (Mestre), R. Zolfanelli and E.
Barasolo (Vercelli), M. Pavone-Macaluso and G.B. Ingargiola
(Palermo), C. Bondavalli (Mantova), F. Merlo (Biella),
M. Porena (Teramo), M. Laudi (Torino), V. Nadalini (Genova);
The Netherlands: H. de Voogt (Leiden), J. Alexieva-Figusch
(Rotterdam); France: B. Lardennois (Reims), P. Fargeot
(Dijon); England: B. Richards (York), M. Robinson (Castle-
ford), D. Newling (Hull); Spain: J.A. Martinez-Pineiro
(Madrid); Belgium: C. Bouffioux (Liege); Portugal: F.
Calais da Silva (Lisbon).

Preliminary results were previously reported (De Pauw
et al., 1983). Patients characteristic at entry on study,
eligibility criteria, investigations performed before and
during the study, response criteria and statistical techniques were reported in detail in the original paper. It
should be mentioned, however, that only 56% of the patients
had distant metastases before starting the treatment. The
remaining patients had category T3 or T4 prostatic cancer
without detectable metastases.

In this communication we shall present the results of
an analysis performed approximately 4 years after the last
patient had entered. The full report has been submitted to
the Journal of Urology and accepted for publication (Pavone-
Macaluso et al., 1986).

RESULTS

Out of 210 patients, the best local response achieved
during treatment could be evaluated in 175 patients. Of 60
evaluable patients treated with CPA, 9 (15%) showed a
complete response, 15 (25%) had a partial response, 28 (47%)
were stable, 8 (13%) progressed and 15 were not evaluable.
The corresponding figures were 1 (2%), 14 (24%), 32 (55%),
11 (19%) and 13 for 58 evaluable patients treated with MPA
and 9 (6%), 22 (39%), 24 (42%), 2 (3%) and 7 for the 57
evaluable patients treated with DES. If complete and partial
responses are added together, local objective responses were
seen in 40% of the patients on CPA, 26% on MPA and 55% on
DES. There is a highly significant difference in the local
response rate between MPA and DES, whereas the difference
between DES and CPA and between CPA and MPA were not
significant.

Distant response could be evaluated in 101 of the 118

patients with bony metastases. DES was marginally better
than MPA (P = 0.11) but the difference is not significant.
No differences were observed between CPA and DES and between
CPA and MPA. There were very few complete responses, 2 in
the CPA and 1 in the DES group. Even the number of total
"objective"responses" (CR + PR) was rather small (11 out of
101 patients in all treatment groups). It is of interest
that the overall "objective response" rate in M1 patients
was 11% for the distant metastases (13% on CPA, 3% on MPA
and 18% on DES) but 32% for the primary tumor.

Of 210 eligible patients, 117 (=56%) showed progression
during treatment. More distant than local progression was
reported in all treatment groups, although some patients
progressed both locally and at distant sites.

The time to first progression (either local or distant)
was analyzed in 208 patients. The time to first progression
was significantly shorter on MPA than on either DES or CPA.

With regard to survival, 89 of 210 patients entered are
still alive having been followed for a median of 3 years
while 121 (58%) are dead. Among the patients who died, the
data suggest that patients treated with DES died less frequently from prostate cancer than those in the two other
treatment groups. In all patients with follow-up, irrespective of the metastatic status, the overall duration of survival was significantly shorter on MPA than on either CPA or
DES.

Palliative responses were observed in all treatment
groups.

With regard to cardiovascular toxicity, patients treated
with DES tended to develop C.V. side effects more often (34%)
than those treated with MPA (18%) or CPA (10%), independently
of whether or not a patient had a previous history of C.V.
disease (De Voogt et al., 1986).

However, 16 patients died due to cardiovascular disease:
10 on CPA, 5 on MPA and 4 on DES. Cardiovascular mortality
in DES-treated patients was much lower in this study than in
parallel trial 30762, comparing an identical dose of DES with
estramustine phosphate. Dietary or ethnical differences may
be responsible for this discrepancy. The other forms of

toxicity were of minor importance.

Our results clearly suggest that patients treated with MPA achieved inferior results concerning all the parameters of efficacy that are analyzed, namely objective response of local tumor and osseous metastases, progression rate, time to progression and survival.

This may be due either to the fact that the dose of MPA was too low to adequately suppress LH and testosterone procuction, or to a minor androgenic effect of this compound. In either case, a lower androgen-deprivation effect may be obtained in patients treated with MPA than in those treated with either DES or CPA.

Our results confirm that patients who show an objective response after an active hormonal treatment have a reduced propensity to progress. Furthermore, patients receiving active forms of hormonal treatment showed a significantly improved survival compared with those treated with MPA. Unless it can be demonstrated that survival is unfavorably influenced by undefined toxic effects produced by MPA, it appears that effective hormonal treatment not only induces objective tumor regression and delays progression, but may also improve survival.

REFERENCES

De Pauw M, Suciu S, Sylvester R, Smith PH, Pavone-Macaluso M and participants in the EORTC Genito-Urinary Tract Cooperative Group (1983). Preliminary results of two EORTC randomized trials in previously untreated patients with advanced T3-T4 prostatic cancer. In: Pavone-Macaluso M and Smith PH (Eds.): Cancer of the Prostate and Kidney. P. 433-447, Plenum Press, New York and London.

De Voogt HJ, Smith PH, Pavone-Macaluso M, de Pauw M, Suciu S and members of the EORTC (European Organization for Research on Treatment of Cancer) Urological Group (1986). Cardiovascular side effects of diethylstilbestrol, cyproterone acetate, medroxyprogesterone acetate and estramustine phosphate, used for the treatment of advanced prostatic cancer. Results from EORTC trials 30761 and 30762. J Urol 135:303-307.

Pavone-Macaluso M, de Voogt HJ, Viggiano G, Barasolo E, Lardennois B, de Pauw M, Sylvester R (1986). Comparison of diethylstilbestrol, cyproterone acetate and medroxyprogesterone acetate in the treatment of advanced prostatic cancer: final analysis of a randomized phase III trial of the EORTC Urological Group. J Urol in press.

Prostate Cancer, Part A: Research, Endocrine
Treatment, and Histopathology, pages 383–390
© 1987 Alan R. Liss, Inc.

COMPLETE ANDROGEN BLOCKADE: THE EORTC EXPERIENCE COMPARING
ORCHIDECTOMY VERSUS ORCHIDECTOMY PLUS CYPROTERONE ACETATE
VERSUS LOW-DOSE STILBOESTROL IN THE TREATMENT OF METASTATIC
CARCINOMA OF THE PROSTATE

M. R. G. Robinson, F.R.C.S.

Pontefract General Infirmary, Friarwood Lane,
Pontefract, West Yorkshire WF8 1PL,
England, U.K.

INTRODUCTION

     The rationale for the endocrine treatment of carcinoma
of the prostate was established by Huggins and Hodges in
1941 and depends upon the concept that malignant prostatic
cells, like normal prostatic cells are stimulated by
circulating androgens. For a variable period of time many,
if not all, of them depend upon this stimulation for growth
and reproduction. Castration removes, and oestrogen therapy
suppresses, the production of the principal androgen,
testosterone, produced by the testes. There are, however,
other androgens such as androstenedione and dehydroepiandrosterone which are produced by the adrenal gland and
may continue, having been converted peripherally to
testosterone, to stimulate prostatic cancer cells during
conventional hormonal therapy. For this reason, secondary
endocrine therapy by bilateral adrenalectomy was introduced
in 1945 by Huggins and Scott to treat patients whose
disease had relapsed after orchidectomy or oestrogen
treatment. Since then, it has been shown that as an
alternative to adrenalectomy, which is a very traumatic
procedure for elderly men with advanced metastatic disease,
hypophysectomy (Fergusson and Phillips 1962) or medical
adrenalectomy with Aminoglutethimide (Robinson et al 1974)
may produce relief of symptoms.

     More recently it has been claimed that primary
hormonal therapy of carcinoma of the prostate which
produces complete androgen blockade of the malignant cells
is superior to conventional hormonal therapy (Bracci 1977,

Labrie et al 1985). In 1981 the Genito-urinary Group of
the European Organisation for Research on the Treatment of
Cancer (EORTC-GU Group), began a randomised study in which
one treatment arm combined orchidectomy plus the antiandrogen
and progestational drug cyproterone acetate (CPA) in order
to produce complete androgen blockade of the prostatic
carcinoma. This paper reports the preliminary results of
that study.

PROTOCOL DESIGN

     The EORTC Protocol 30805 is a randomised study of
orchidectomy plus CPA 50 mg three times a day versus
Stilboestrol 1 mg daily. The scheme for the study is
shown in Table 1.

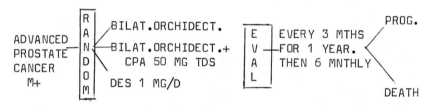

     Only patients with metastatic disease have been
entered. The objective of the study is to determine if any
of the three treatment regimes is superior in delaying time
to progression and increasing the length of survival.
Treatment toxicity, especially with respect to cardiovascular
complications of Stilboestrol 1 mg daily, is also being
analysed. Patients and their disease are being evaluated
every 3 months during the first year of the study and then
every 6 months until progression or death.

PATIENT RECRUITMENT

     A total of 350 patients have been entered into this
study between April 1981 and March 1986 from 16
Institutions within Europe. Eleven patients (3%) are
ineligible.

     Table 2 gives the on-study T category, distribution
of metastases and performance status for 262 patients
who have been analysed for these factors in the
different study arms.

TABLE 2

The On-study T Category, Distribution of Metastases
and Performance Status.

		Orchidectomy	Orchidectomy + CPA	DES
No of Patients		90	86	86
T Category-	(T0	0(0)	1(1.2)	0(0)
	(T1	1(1.1)	1(1.2)	2(2.3)
	(T2	9(10.0)	8(9.3)	8(9.3)
	(T3	49(54.6)	46(53.5)	43(50.0)
	(T4	31(34.4)	30(34.9)	33(38.4)
Bone Metastases	(None	0(0)	2(2.3)	2(2.3)
	(Confirmed	90(100)	84(97.7)	83(96.5)
	(Suspicious	0(0)	0(0)	1(1.2)
Visceral Metastases	(None	80(88.9)	80(93.9)	81(94.2)
	(Confirmed	8(8.9)	5(5.8)	1(1.2)
	(Suspicious	2(2.2)	1(1.2)	3(3.5)
	(Inknown	0(0)	0(0)	1(1.2)
Soft Tissue Metastases	(None	88(97.8)	83(96.5)	81(94.2)
	(Confirmed	1(1.1)	2(2.3)	5(5.8)
	(Suspicious	1(1.1)	1(1.2)	0(0)
Performance Status	(WHO* 0	23(25.6)	25(29.1)	36(41.1)
	(1	39(48.3)	34(39.5)	27(31.4)
	(2	25(27.8)	26(30.2)	23(26.7)
	(3	3(3.3)	0(0)	0(0)
	(4	0(0)	1(1.2)	0(0)

Figures in ( ) = percentages.

* 0 = Able to carry out all normal activity without
       restriction.
  1 = Restricted in physically strenuous activity but
       ambulatory and able to carry out light work.
  2 = Ambulatory and capable of self-care but unable to
       carry out any work; up and about more than 50%
       of the waking hours.
  3 = Only capable of limited self-care; confined to

bed or chair more than 50% of waking hours.
4 = Completely disabled; cannot carry out any self-care; totally confined to bed or chair.

The reasons for patients going off-study are given in Table 3.

TABLE 3

REASONS FOR PATIENTS GOING OFF STUDY

	Orchidectomy	Orchidectomy + CPA	DES
No of patients off study	44	48	52
Death before the confirmation of progression	3(6.8)	3(6.3)	9(17.3)
Lost to follow-up	1(2.3)	2(4.2)	2(3.8)
Treatment Refused	1(2.3)	4(8.3)	2(3.8)
Treatment Toxicity	1(2.3)	0(0)	5(9.6)
Progression, including death with progression	34(77.3)	38(79.2)	33(63.5)
Protocol Violation	2(4.5)	0(0)	0(0)
Other Causes	2(4.5)	1(2.1)	1(1.9)

Figures in () = percentages.

Six patients have gone off-study because of treatment toxicity. Four of these, receiving DES, developed cardiovascular disease and the treatment was changed. One, who had an orchidectomy was taken off study because he had severe hot flushes which required additional oestrogen therapy. The responsible clinician did not change treatment when cardiovascular disease developed following orchidectomy or orchidectomy + CPA and so far the death rate for cardiovascular toxicity is 4 patients who had orchidectomy and 4 patients who had DES. Only one patient died from cardiovascular toxicity on the ordhicectomy + CPA treatment.

For 241 patients the time to progression and length of

survival has been analysed. These are illustrated in
figures 1 and 2. For both end points there is, at the
present time, no significant difference between the
three methods of treatment.

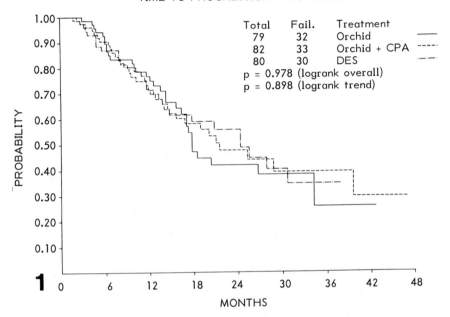

TIME TO PROGRESSION PROTOCOL 30805

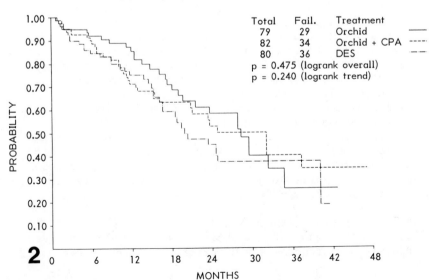

DURATION OF SURVIVAL PROTOCOL 30805

DISCUSSION

   The first two EORTC-GU Phase III trials in Prostatic
Cancer, Protocol 30761 and Protocol 30762, compared DES
1 mg three times a day with Medroxyprogesterone Acetate
(MPA) and CPA and the same dose of DES with Estramustine
Phosphate (Estracyt). The final analysis of these two
trials are shortly to be published (Pavone Macaluso
1986; Smith 1986). There was no difference in the time
to progression and survival between CPA and DES and
DES and Estramustine Phosphate. The results were inferior
for MPA but the doseage used in Protocol 30761 was lower
than that currently used to treat prostatic cancer.

   DES 1 mg three times a day caused more cardiovascular
toxicity than any of the other treatment regimes. Therefore
in the current EORTC Study, Protocol 30805, it was decided
to randomise between orchidectomy, orchidectomy plus CPA
and DES 1 mg daily to determine if there was any advantage
in combining orchidectomy with an antiandrogen and to see
if the reduced dose of DES, as reported by Byar (1980) was
active with less cardiovascular toxicity.

   The preliminary results in a large number of patients
well-matched for T category, distribution of metastases
and performance status, at the time of randomisation does
not demonstrate any benefit for orchidectomy plus CPA
over the other two treatment regimes. This does not
support the results of Bracci (1977), which suggested
that orchidectomy plus a slightly higher dose of CPA,
200 mgs per day, was more effective than orchidectomy
alone. Some of his patients did, however, receive
higher doses of CPA by intramuscular injection together
with Vitamin D, calcium and calcitonin. More recently,
Labrie (1985), has claimed improved results using an
LH-RH analogue with a pure antiandrogen Flutamide or its
analogue Anandron. He does not consider Cyproterone
Acetate a good antiandrogen to use for complete androgen
blockade because it has progestational activity and since
human prostate contains progesterone receptors, as well
as having an antiandrogen effect, it may possibly also
have a stimulatory effect.

   In our study, there has not been a very long
follow-up for many of the patients and detailed analyses
of subjective responses and toxicity for the different

treatment regimes have not yet been made. Since the quality of life as well as the time to progression and length of survival is very important to the patient, it is too soon to decide which of the three treatments is best. At the present time, however, the combination that we have used of Orchidectomy plus CPA, does not appear to give superior results to those of Orchidectomy alone.

REFERENCES

Byar D P (1980). Review of the Veterans' Administrative Studies of Cancer of the Prostate: The new results concerning treatment of Stage I and II tumours. In "Bladder Tumours and other Topics of Urological Oncology". Edited by Pavone Macaluso M, Smith P H and Edsmyr S. Page 471-492. Plenum Press, New York and London.

Bracci U (1977). Present Procedures in the Treatment of Prostatic Cancer. In "Hormonal Therapy of Prostatic Cancer". Editors Bracci U, Di Silverio F. Pages 177-192. Cofese, Palermo.

Fergusson J D and Phillips D E H (1962). Clin Eval of Radiation Pituitary Implantation /Carcinoma of Prostate. British Journal of Urology 34: 485to 492.

Huggins C, Hodges C V (1941). The Studies of Prostatic Cancer. Effect of Castration, Oestrogen and Androgen Injection on Serum Phosphatase in Metastatic Carcinoma of the Prostate. Cancer Research 1: 293-297.

Huggins C and Scott W W (1945). Bilateral Adrenalectomy in Prostatic Cancer. Annals of Surgery 122: 1031.

Labrie F, Dupont A and Bellanger A (1985). Complete Androgen Blockade for the Treatment of Prostatic Cancer. In "Important Advances in Oncology". Editors: De Vita V T, Helman S, Rosenberg S A, Lippincott Company Philidelphia.

Pavone Macaluso M, De Voogt H J, Vigginao G, Barasolo B, Lardenois B, De Pauw M, Sylvester R and the Members of the Urological EORTC Group. Comparison of Diethyl Stilboestrol and Cyproterone Acetate and Medroxyprogesterone Acetate in the Treatment of Advanced Prostatic Cancer: Final Analysis of a Phase III Trial of the EORTC Urological Group. To be published.

Smith P H, Sucio S, Robinson M R G, Richards B, Bastable J R G, Glashan R W, Buffioux C, Lardenois B, Williams R E, De Pauw M, Sylvester R. A Comparison of the Effect of Diethyl Stilboestrol and Low Dose Estramustine Phosphate in the Treatment of Advanced Prostatic Cancer: A Phase III Trial of the EORTC Urological Group. To be published.

Prostate Cancer, Part A: Research, Endocrine
Treatment, and Histopathology, pages 391–400
© 1987 Alan R. Liss, Inc.

TOTAL ANDROGEN BLOCKADE VS ORCHIECTOMY IN STAGE D2 PROSTATE
CANCER

G. Béland, M. Elhilali, Y. Fradet, B. Laroche,
E.W. Ramsey, P.M. Venner and H.D. Tewari
Universities of Montreal, (G.B.), McGill and
Sherbrooke, (M.E.), Laval, Quebec (Y.F. and B.L.),
Manitoba (E.W.R.), Alberta (P.M.V.) and St-John
Reg. Hospital (H.D.T.)

INTRODUCTION

The accepted treatment of metastatic prostate cancer
has been the suppression of testicular androgens. A small
amount of androgens remains from adrenal sources and it has
been suggested that complete androgen blockade might lead
to improved results. Excellent results have been obtained
in an open clinical trial using orchiectomy or LHRH agonists
and pure non steroidal antiandrogens and this combination
has been described as the only acceptable treatment for
advanced cancer of the prostate (Labrie et al., 1982, 1985).
To test this claim, a double-blind, randomized trial was
begun comparing total androgen blockade to simple testicular
androgen suppression. This can be obtained by the administration of estrogens, by LHRH agonists or by castration.
This latter approach, we feel, is the most reliable, safest
and simplest. It is independent of the patient's compliance,
has no side effects or serious complications and no possible
unknown influence on the evolution of the cancer that the
flare phenomenon described occasionnally with LHRH agonists
may have (Santen et al., 1984; Trachtenberg, 1983; Leuprolide
Study Group, 1984). Suppression of action of other androgens
is obtained by the use of antiandrogens (Raynaud et al.,
1979; Neumann and Schenck, 1976; Irwin and Prout, 1973).

MATERIAL AND METHODS

To be eligible for the study, the patients must have
proven carcinoma of the prostate with evaluable distant
metastases, no prior hormonal treatment and an anticipated

survival of 6 months.

When a patient is eligible and agrees to enter the study, he is castrated and randomly and double-blindly receives either a placebo or the antiandrogen. If the cancer progresses, the code is broken. If the patient had received a placebo, it is changed for the antiandrogen; if he had received the antiandrogen, appropriate therapy is given at the discretion of the investigator. If the patient refuses orchiectomy and requests the LHRH agonist, he is entered in a parallel non randomized group and given the antiandrogen automatically.

The drugs are provided by Roussel Canada. The LHRH agonist is Buserelin and is given by daily sub-cutaneous injections of 500 μg for the first 30 days followed by 250μg every day thereafter. The antiandrogen is Anandron and given by mouth at the dose of 100mg every 8 hours. This is the antiandrogen used by Dr Labrie in the early part of his study with which he obtained his excellent results.

In order to rapidly obtain a large number of patients, the study was conducted in all urology programs in the Province of Quebec and was later extended to other programs in Canada.

The patients are followed regularly (0.5, 1,2,3,4,6,9, 12,15,18 months) and submitted to a schedule of examinations including a record of symptoms, clinical examination, chest X-ray, bone scan and skeletal X-ray and intravenous urography. Blood samples are also obtained at each visit for the usual hematology and biochemistry tests, as well as for hormone assays. The patients are evaluated every 6 months and classified according to the N.P.C.P. criteria (Murphy and Slack, 1980).

RESULTS

211 patients have been entered in the study between February 1984 and April 1986. 22 were excluded and 189 are evaluable and are distributed as follows:

Castration and Placebo	75
Castration and Anandron	77
Buserelin and Anandron	37

The reasons for exclusion are given in Table 1, the totals being the same in the randomized groups and proportional in the parallel group. The characteristics of evaluable patients, e.g. number of patients with bone pain, impaired performance, abnormal serum acid phosphatase and mean age, were similar in the three groups. There was a delay between orchiectomy and the onset of drug treatment of 3.7 and 4.2 days for the placebo and Anandron groups respectively. Buserelin and Anandron were always begun at the same time in the parallel group.

Table 1. Reasons for exclusion

	Orchiectomy + Placebo	Orchiectomy +Anandron	Buserelin + Anandron
Incorrect staging :	1	2	-
Previous hormono-therapy :	2	4	1
Withdrawal for adverse events within the first 6 months:	1	1	1
Delay between orchiectomy and treatment:	2	1	-
Lost to follow-up within the first 6 months :	2	-	1
Treatment stopped by patient :	1	1	1
TOTAL	9	9	4

The drugs used were generally well tolerated. Impotence and hot flashes were very frequent and accepted as a normal consequence of therapy. Minor adverse reactions not necessitating a change in therapy were also frequent. They consisted of nausea and vomiting (24%), visual problems (43%) and alcohol intolerance (33%). Visual problems consisted mostly in "snow blindness" which is a slow adaptation to relative darkness after exposure to intense light. It is

interesting to note that half as many patients on placebo
as on Anandron presented nausea and vomiting and visual
problems. This demonstrates the difficulty of adequate evaluation of symptoms.

Table 2. Major adverse reactions

	Orchiectomy + Placebo	Orchiectomy +Anandron	Buserelin + Anandron
Nausea/vomiting	–	5 *	1
Visual problems	–	1	–
Rash	1	1	–
Interstitial pneumonitis	–	1	2
Hot flashes	–	3	–
Febrile reaction	–	–	1
TOTAL	1 (2%)	11 (18%)	4 (11%)

*Decrease of Anandron to 150 mg/day in 4 of 5 patients

Major adverse reactions leading to changes in medication also occurred (Table 2). Nausea and vomiting forced a
decrease in the dose of Anandron in 4 patients and complete
cessation in two. One patient refused his medication because of visual problems. 3 patients presented severe intolerance in the form of acute interstitial pneumonitis with
pulmonary insufficiency. This required cessation of medication and appropriate therapy. It completely regressed in
all instances. One febrile reaction was seen in a patient
receiving Buserelin and Anandron. A complete investigation
revealed no cause for the reaction which ceased when the
drugs were stopped. In the orchiectomy and placebo group,
there was only one discontinuation this being due to a rash.

The best objective response for those who have been in
the study for at least 6 months is shown in Table 3. A posi-

tive response can be either a complete response, a partial
response or no change as opposed to progressive disease. A
positive response was observed in 75% of orchiectomized
patients receiving placebo (36/48), 90% of orchiectomized
patients receiving Anandron (44/49) and 88% of patients
receiving Buserelin and Anandron (29/33). There is a slight
difference of response in favor of total androgen blockade.
However this difference is not statistically significant.

Table 3.   Best objective response according to NPCP criteria.

	Orchiectomy + Placebo N: 48		Orchiectomy +Anandron N: 49		Buserelin +Anandron N: 33	
Complete response	3(6%)		3(6%)		3(9%)	
Partial response	5(11%)	36(75%)	13(27%)	44(90%)	10(30%)	29(88%)
Stable disease	28(58%)		28(57%)		16(49%)	
Progressive Disease	12(25%)		5(10%)		4(12%)	

     As the disease has a tendency to progress after an
initial good response, the duration of response or progression rate was evaluated according to Kaplan and Meier's
method (Figure 1). The number and the percentage of patients
in whom the disease did not progress is seen for the two
randomized groups as well as for the non randomized group.
There is no significant difference in progression rate
between the three groups. However there is a not statistically significant difference in progression rate in favor
of total androgen blockade between 4 and 10 months which
disappears gradually thereafter.

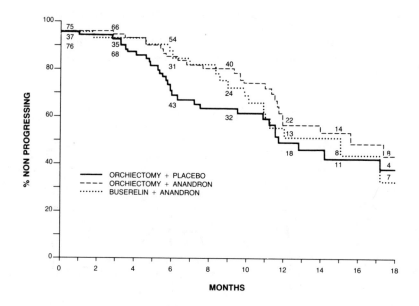

Figure 1. Time to first objective progression of disease
according to the Kaplan-Meier estimate.

Calculation of the actuarial survival rate, according
to the initial treatments, on the total number of patients
entered into the study (whether they had or had not been
treated for at least six months) did not show any statistically significant difference among the three groups
(Figure 2). However, the same small difference in favor of
total androgen blockade is again noted, the deaths occurring somewhat later in this group. The actuarial survival
at 18 months in all three groups is 60%.

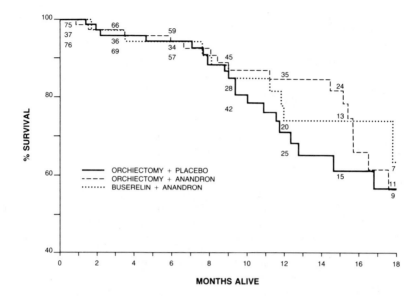

Figure 2. Time to death (survival analysis) according to the Kaplan-Meier estimate.

DISCUSSION

Standard treatment of advanced cancer of the prostate has been for many years the suppression of testicular androgens. Additional hormonal manipulation aiming at suppression of extratesticular androgens by different means has provided unpredictable results of short duration. These treatments were used mostly in relapsed cases when testicular androgen suppression had become ineffective with possible hormone resistance, rendering further improvement unlikely. A rationale for total androgen blockade as a primary therapy was introduced many years ago and recently reviewed (Geller, 1985; Schroeder, 1985). Excellent results were claimed for this approach (Labrie et al., 1985) and the present double-blind, randomized study was initiated to evaluate it more precisely.

The evaluation of any form of treatment in cancer of the prostate is very difficult and complex mostly because of its unpredictible course and the frequent intercurrent diseases occurring in these elderly patients. Multiple factors can individually influence the evolution of cancer of the prostate in a significant manner (Emrich et al., 1985). The precise evaluation of a new treatment, unless it is obviously better, is rendered difficult because it is compared with one which already provides a positive response in over 75% of patients. Therefore a large number of patients, followed for a long period, is necessary to arrive at a definitive and significant conclusion. We feel that our study has not as yet reached this stage.

Notwithstanding all these considerations, we can say that there is no significant difference in the number of best objective responses and the time to progression between total androgen blockade and simple testicular androgen suppression in the randomized groups. This is in contradiction to the claim for improved results reported with complete androgen blockade by others (Labrie et al., 1985). However, although not statistically significant, there is some difference in the percentage of responses and time to progression in favor of total androgen blockade which can not be ignored. Further follow-up may allow the identification of a group of patients who may benefit from this treatment. As far as the actuarial survival is concerned, the only other series available with LHRH agonists and antiandrogens reported a probability of survival at 2 years of 89.1% in stage D2 prostatic cancer (Labrie et al., 1986). Our study, using similar treatment, showed a probability of survival at 18 months of 60%. This is similar to the generally accepted figure for survival with simple testicular androgen suppression. Our results with Buserelin and Anandron started simultaneously do not differ from those with orchiectomy and Anandron despite a delay of 4.2 days after the orchiectomy before starting the antiandrogen. This does not support the opinion that cells lose their sensitivity to androgen ablation if it is not total from the beginning (Labrie et al., 1985).

The antiandrogen used caused many minor drug reactions and few serious ones. A small number of patients could not tolerate the medication because of nausea and vomiting at the regular dosage but did so when it was reduced by half. Other studies in this symposium reported equivalent results (Brisset et al., Navratil et al.) using a similarly reduced

dose. These patients were nevertheless dropped from the
study so as not to influence the statistics. A more dis-
tressing complication was seen in 3 patients who presented
a severe pulmonary insufficiency. This was completely reversible after cessation of the Buserelin and the antiandrogen and initiation of appropriate treatment.

CONCLUSION

Total androgen blockade has been compared to simple
testicular androgen suppression in a randomized and double-
blind study. Unfortunately, even with 189 evaluable patients, a definitive conclusion cannot be reached because of
the intrinsic difficulties and the short duration of this
study. Total androgen blockade can surely not be described
as the only acceptable treatment of advanced cancer of the
prostate based on the data available at present. A larger
number of patients with longer follow-up will be required
to determine if complete androgen blockade offers any advantage over testicular androgen ablation.

REFERENCES

Emrich LJ, Priore RL, Murphy GP, Brady MF, the investigators
   of the NPCP (1985). Prognostic factors in patients with
   advanced stage prostate cancer. Cancer Research 45:5173-
   5179.

Geller J (1985). Rationale for blockade of adrenal as well
   as testicular androgens in the treatment of advanced
   prostate cancer. Semin Oncol XII (suppl. 1): 28-35.

Irwin RJ, Prout GJ Jr (1973). A new antiprostatic agent
   for treatment of prostate carcinoma. Surg Forum 24:
   536-538.

Labrie F, Dupont A, Belanger A, Cusan L, Lacoursiere Y,
   Monfette G, Laberge JG, Emond JP, Fazekas ATA, Raynaud JP,
   Husson JM (1982). New hormonal therapy in prostatic
   carcinoma: Combined treatment with LHRH agonist and an
   antiandrogen. Clinic Invest Med 5: 267-275.

Labrie F, Dupont A, Belanger A (1985). Complete Androgen
  blockade for the treatment of prostate cancer.
  In De Vita VT, Hellman S, Rosenberg SA (eds): Important
  Advances in Oncology 1985, Philadelphia: J.B. Lippincott
  pp 193-217.

Labrie F, Dupont A, Belanger A, Poyet P, Giguere M,
  Lacoursiere Y, Emond J, Monfette G, Borsanyi JP (1986).
  Combined treatment with Flutamide and surgical or medical
  (LHRH agonist) castration in metastatic prostatic cancer.
  The Lancet, Jan 4: 48-49.

The Leuprolide Study Group (1984). Leuprolide versus
  diethylstilbestrol for metastatic prostate cancer.
  N Engl J Med 311: 1281-1286.

Murphy GP, Slack NH (1980). Response criteria for the
  prostate of the USA National Prostatic Cancer Project.
  Prostate 1:375-382

Neumann F, Schenck B (1976). New antiandrogens and their
  mode of action. J Reprod Fertil 24:129-145.

Raynaud JP, Bonne C, Bouton MM, Lagace L, Labrie F (1979).
  Action of a non-steroidal antiandrogen, RU 23908 in
  peripheral and central tissues. J Steroid Biochem 11:
  93-99.

SANTEN RJ, WARNER B, DEMERS LM, DUFAU M, SMITH J (1984).
  Use of GnRH hormone agonists analogs. In Vickery B,
  Nestor JJ Jr, Hafez ESE (eds): LHRH and its analogs. A
  new class of contraceptive and therapeutic agents.
  Boston: MTP Press.

Schroeder FH (1985). Total androgen suppression in the
  management of prostatic cancer. A critical review.
  In Schroder FH, Richards B (eds): Therapeutic Principles
  in Metastatic Prostatic Cancer. Prog Clin Biol Res 185A:
  307-317.

Trachtenberg J (1983). The treatment of metastatic prostatic cancer with a potent luteinizing hormone-releasing
  hormone analogue. J Urol 129:1149-1152.

Prostate Cancer, Part A: Research, Endocrine
Treatment, and Histopathology, pages 401–410
© 1987 Alan R. Liss, Inc.

DOUBLE-BLIND STUDY OF ANANDRON VERSUS PLACEBO
IN STAGE D$_2$ PROSTATE CANCER PATIENTS
RECEIVING BUSERELIN
Results on 49 cases from a multicentre study

H. Navratil
Faculty of Medicine, Montpellier-Nîmes.

Study centres : Centre Hospitalier Régional
Universitaire de Nîmes (H. Navratil, P. Costa,
J.F. Louis) ; Hôtel Dieu de Marseille (G. Serment,
J. Ducassou) ; Centre Hospitalo-Universitaire de
Reims (B. Lardennois) ; Hôpital de la Grave de
Toulouse (F. Pontonnier) ; Centre Hospitalo-
Universitaire de Rangueil, Toulouse (J.P.
Sarramon) ; Centre Hospitalo-Universitaire d'Alès
(G. Pugeat) ; Hôpital de la Durance, Avignon (M.
Levallois) ; Hôpital Goüin, Paris (B. Callet).

INTRODUCTION

    Complete androgen blockade with nonsteroid antiandro-
gens associated to medical castration is a modern therapeutic concept in the treatment of advanced prostate cancer
(Seguin et al., 1981 ; Labrie et al., 1983 ; Raynaud et
al., 1984). Its aim is to ensure a better control of
hormone-dependent cancers by suppressing hormonal stimulation by testicular androgens and opposing the action of
residual, in particular adrenal, androgens.

    We therefore decided to treat stage D$_2$ prostate cancer
patients entered into a controlled multicentre study by the
association : Buserelin + Anandron[R] versus Buserelin + placebo. A s.c. dose of 500 µg/day of the LH-RH analog buserelin suppresses testicular androgens (Borgmann et al.,
1982) ; the nonsteroid antiandrogen Anandron will oppose
the action of any residual androgens (Moguilewsky et al.,
1986).

Within 3 to 4 weeks of initiation of treatment, LH-RH analogs are known to inhibit the hypothalamo-pituitary axis leading to a decrease in FSH and LH levels and consequently to a fall in circulating testosterone similar to that observed after orchiectomy (Tolis et al., 1983). Efficacy is maintained throughout treatment and side-effects are minimal. However, a transient increase in circulating androgens can occur during the first ten days of treatment and can constitute a hazard to patients with metastases by inducing a flare-up of the disease (Donnelly, 1984 ; Smith et al., 1985 ; Waxman et al., 1985).

An appropriate dose of nonsteroid antiandrogen could also oppose the action of this increase in testosterone and consequently prevent the flare-up. The dose of 300 mg of Anandron per day represents a high dose that is well tolerated according to phase I studies. Its efficacy in potentiating the action of the LH-RH analog, buserelin, and in preventing a flare-up of the disease was investigated.

STUDY DESIGN

All patients had metastatic (stage D_2) prostate cancer and no patient had previously received hormone therapy. The study was double-blind. Patients were randomized into two groups : buserelin 500 µg s.c. + Anandron 300 mg orally per day, buserelin 500 µg s.c. + placebo. Administration of the two compounds was begun on the same day.

At the time of analysis, 26 patients had been enrolled into the buserelin + placebo group, 23 into the buserelin + Anandron group, and had started treatment 6 to 30 months previously. A total of 10 patients had to be excluded from the efficacy analysis since, for reasons of incorrect staging and previous hormone therapy, they should not have been admitted to the study. One patient receiving buserelin + placebo was excluded because of concomitant lung cancer. The efficacy analysis was thus performed on 22 patients receiving buserelin + placebo and 16 patients receiving buserelin + Anandron.

There was no significant difference in the main characteristics of the evaluable patients in the two groups at entry (Table 1).

TABLE 1. **Characteristics of evaluable patients**

	Buserelin		
	+ Placebo	+ Anandron	p
Patients included	26	23	
Patients evaluable for efficacy	22	16	
Median age (years)	75	72	n.s.
Patients with bone pain	10	12	n.s.
Patients with impaired performance status	14	10	n.s.
Patients with abnormal PAP	14	12	n.s.

n.s. : not significant (Fisher exact test)

Follow-up examinations were performed at 1, 3, 6, 12, and 18 months and included a physical examination, a record of symptoms, prostatic ultrasound (at each visit), intravenous pyelogram, bone scan, bone and chest X-rays (every 6 months), abdominal CT scan, lymphography (if necessary). An evaluation according to the National Prostatic Cancer Project (NPCP) criteria was performed every 6 months as from month 6.

We gave special attention to the bone scan for the detection of metastatic foci and to the study of prostate volume by ultrasound using a transrectal probe. This measured not only the diameter of the prostate but also its integrated volume, which was recorded by a video-recorder for a comparative follow-up.

Blood samples were obtained at each visit for the following assays :
- plasma prostatic acid phosphatase (PAP) by RIA
- plasma Anandron by RIA
- plasma hormones including testicular and adrenal androgens, LH, FSH, prolactin, cortisol
- blood parameters (RBC, WBC, haemoglobin, methaemoglobin, platelets, creatinine, uric acid, cholesterol, triglycerides, bilirubin, SGOT, SGPT, alkaline phosphatase, $Na+$, $K+$, $Cl-$).

PAP and plasma hormones were assayed by the same laboratory (J. Fiet, Hôpital Saint-Louis).

RESULTS

Several important observations were made before any
attempt to interpret the data :
- testosterone remained at castrate levels as from the
  first assay at the end of month 1,
- cortisol levels were within the normal expected range,
- Anandron levels were at the steady state (~ 7 mg/l),
- there was no significant difference in the biologic parameters between the two groups.

The analysis of the variations in PAP showed that the
return to normal levels was faster in the buserelin + Anandron group than in the buserelin + placebo group although
the difference was not statistically significant (Figure
1). A closer analysis of the patients whose abnormally high
PAP levels at entry were reduced by less than 50 % revealed
a lack of response of 14 % in the buserelin + placebo group
compared to 8 % in the buserelin + Anandron.

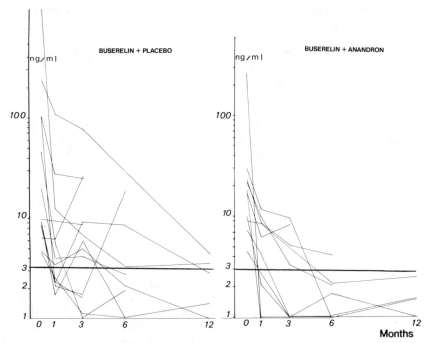

Figure 1. Individual variations in PAP in patients
          receiving buserelin + placebo (n = 13) or
          buserelin + Anandron (n = 10)

In patients complaining of bone pain from metastases, the visit at month 1 revealed an increase in bone pain in six patients receiving buserelin + placebo. No patient receiving buserelin + Anandron complained of such an increase (Table 2). This clinical observation suggests that Anandron may play an important role in controlling the LH-RH analog-induced flare up. The analysis of overall clinical response throughout the study showed that 36 % of patients receiving placebo did not respond to treatment compared to only 15 % receiving Anandron.

TABLE 2. **Evaluation of bone pain during the first month of treatment**

| | Buserelin | | p* |
	+ Placebo	+ Anandron	
Patients	22	14	
Increased pain	6	0	
No change	10	7	0.05
Decreased pain	6	7	

* Fisher exact test

A study of the performance status at months 1, 3 and 6 (Figure 2) revealed a significant difference at month 1 in favour of the buserelin + Anandron treatment. This difference between the two groups remained pronounced at month 3 but decreased slightly at month 6.

The best objective response recorded at any 6-monthly visit during treatment and evaluated according to the NPCP criteria is illustrated in Figure 3. (Progression at any moment **before** the first full-scale visit at month 6 was counted as a progression). The NPCP criteria take into account all the following parameters : PAP, bone pain, performance status, areas of increased uptake on bone scan, tumour mass volume, body weight, cancer-related anemia, cancer-related hepatomegaly, ureteral obstruction... When Anandron was combined to buserelin, the percentage of regressions was increased by 14 %.

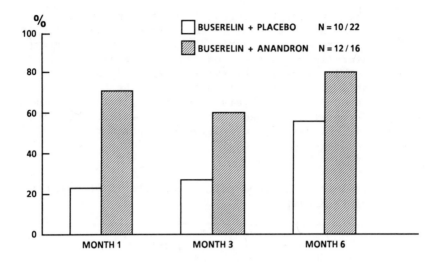

Figure 2. Performance status : percentage of patients improved

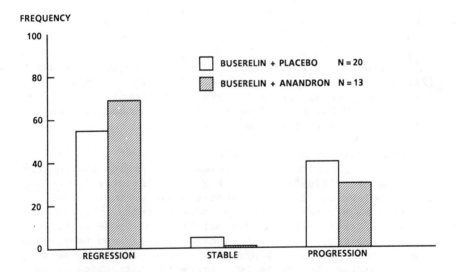

Figure 3. Best objective response to treatment

The time to progression is given in Table 3. Forty-five percent of patients progressed in the buserelin + placebo group compared to 37 % in the buserelin + Anandron group. At month 12, 63 % of patients in the Anandron group were improved or stable compared to 48 % in the placebo group. The median time to progression was 13 months on administration of Anandron compared to 10 months otherwise. However the number of patients evaluated for more than one year is still too small to make any judgement on longer follow-up periods.

TABLE 3. **Time to progression and time to death by cancer**

	Buserelin +		Buserelin +	
	Placebo	Anandron	Placebo	Anandron
N° patients	22	16	22	16
	Number of progressions		Number of deaths	
at 6 mths	7	4	3	2
6 - 12 mths	3	1	1	0
12 - 24 mths	0	1	3	1
Total	10	6	7	3
	(45 %)	(37 %)	(32 %)	(19 %)
	Progression free actuarial rate %		Actuarial survival rate %	
Month 6	68	73 (a)	86	87 (b)
Month 12	48	63	80	87
Month 18	48	47	45	70
Median (mths)	10	13	17	not reached

(a) Logrank test $p = 0.656$; (b) Logrank test $p = 0.579$

The number of deaths due to cancer is also given in Table 3. Although the difference between the two groups is not statistically significant, the death rate is markedly lower in the group receiving the combination buserelin + Anandron.

The adverse experiences which occurred during treatment are summarized in Table 4. There were no specific differences between the two groups except for three patients in the group receiving Anandron who complained of difficulties in visual adaptation when passing from light to dark.

TABLE 4. **Number of patients with adverse events**

	Placebo	Buserelin + Anandron	p*
Patients at risk	24	22	
Gastro-intestinal	5	4	0.60
Respiratory	3	3	0.62
Nervous system	1	4	0.15
Cardio-vascular	6	3	0.30
Renal	0	1	0.48
Skin	1	5	0.07
Bones & muscles	1	1	0.73
Endocrine (hot flushes)	2	4	0.29
Vision (adapt. to dark)	0	3	0.10
General (malaise, alcohol intolerance)	3	1	0.34
Patients with adverse events	13 (54%)	17 (77%)	0.09

* Fisher exact test

CONCLUSIONS

Analogs of gonadotropin-releasing hormone desensitize pituitary receptors and suppress testosterone but not adrenal androgen secretion in prostate cancer patients. A small proportion of patients do not respond fully to this treatment and, furthermore, about 10 % experience a flare-up of disease due to initial stimulation of LH and consequently of testosterone. This flare-up can have serious clinical consequences and should be avoided.

The nonsteroid anti-androgen Anandron has been shown to block the trophic action of adrenal androgens and to prevent the effect of the early increase in testosterone in castrated rats (Moguilewsky et al., 1986, this volume). In order to establish whether Anandron leads to an improvement in response in castrated patients with stage D_2 prostate cancer, we performed a double-blind clinical trial comparing the efficacy of a high dose (500 μg) of the LHRH-analog buserelin with or without concomitant administration of Anandron. Since, furthermore, animal studies have indicated that Anandron, unlike steroid anti-androgens, potentiates the inhibitory action of buserelin on the prostate (M. Moguilewsky et al., 1986, this volume), any improvement in response observed in this study could also be expected with lower buserelin doses.

Although the number of patients in this study is still insufficient to enable a statistically significant evaluation of all parameters, several conclusions can nevertheless be drawn on the basis of the observed trends.

The tolerance of the combination therapy buserelin + Anandron is acceptable for long term use.

The use of the antiandrogen Anandron, in association with buserelin, is particularly effective in preventing a flare-up of the disease as evidenced by the decreased incidence in bone pain during the first month of treatment.

The administration of Anandron also improves bone pain and performance status and consequently the quality of life, throughout treatment. It increases the regression rate and lengthens time to progression.

Complete androgen blockade with buserelin and Anandron seems to us at present to be a step forward in the hormone treatment of stage D_2 prostate cancer. However, it will be necessary to include a greater number of patients into the study to be able to establish statistically significant differences.

REFERENCES

Borgmann V, Hardt W, Schmidt-Gollwitzer M, Adenauer H,
    Nagel R (1982). Sustained suppression of testosterone
    production by the luteinizing-hormone releasing-hormone
    agonist Buserelin in patients with advanced prostate
    carcinoma. The Lancet, 1097-1099.
Donnelly RJ (1984). Continuous subcutaneous administration
    of "Zoladex" (ICI 118, 630 and LHRH-analogue) to patients
    with advanced prostatic cancer. J steroid Biochem
    20:137S.
Labrie F, Dupont A, Bélanger A, Lacoursière Y, Raynaud JP,
    Husson JM, Gareau J, Fazekas ATA, Sandow J, Monfette G,
    Girard JG, Emond J, Houle JG (1983). New approach in the
    treatment of prostate cancer : complete instead of part-
    ial withdrawal of androgens. The Prostate 4:579-594.
Moguilewsky M, Fiet J, Tournemine C, Raynaud JP (1986).
    Pharmacology of an antiandrogen, Anandron, used as an
    adjuvant therapy in the treatment of prostatic cancer. J
    steroid Biochem 24:139-146.
Raynaud JP, Bonne C, Moguilewsky M, Lefebvre FA, Bélanger
    A, Labrie F (1984). The pure antiandrogen RU 23908
    (Anandron^R), a candidate of choice for the combined
    antihormonal treatment of prostatic cancer : A review.
    The Prostate 5:299-311.
Seguin C, Cusan L, Bélanger A, Kelly PA, Labrie F, Raynaud
    JP (1981). Additive inhibitory effects of treatment with
    an LHRH agonist and an anti-androgen on androgen-
    dependent tissues in the rat. Mol Cell Endocr 21:37-41.
Smith JA, Glode LM, Wettlaufer JN, Stein BS, Glass AG, Max
    DT, Anbar D, Jagst CL, Murphy GP (1985). Clinical effects
    of gonadotropin-releasing hormone analogue in metastatic
    carcinoma of prostate. Urology XXV:106-114.
Tolis G, Faure N, Koutsilieris M, Lemay A, Klioze S,
    Yakabow A, Fazekas ATA (1983). Suppression of testicular
    steroidogenesis by the GnRH agonistic analogue buserelin
    (HOE-766) in patients with prostatic cancer : studies in
    relation to dose and route of administration. J steroid
    Biochem 19:995-998.
Waxman J, Man A, Hendry WF, Whitfield HN, Besser GM,
    Tiptaft RC, Paris AMI, Oliver RTD (1985). Importance of
    early tumour exacerbation in patients treated with long
    acting analogues of gonadotrophin releasing hormone for
    advanced prostatic cancer. Br Med J 291:1387-1388.

Prostate Cancer, Part A: Research, Endocrine
Treatment, and Histopathology, pages 411–422
© 1987 Alan R. Liss, Inc.

ANANDRON (RU 23908) ASSOCIATED TO SURGICAL CASTRATION IN
PREVIOUSLY UNTREATED STAGE D PROSTATE CANCER : A MULTICENTER
COMPARATIVE STUDY OF TWO DOSES OF THE DRUG AND OF A PLACEBO

J-M. Brisset, L. Boccon-Gibod, H. Botto, M. Camey,
G. Cariou, J-M. Duclos, F. Duval, D. Gontiès, R.
Jorest, L. Lamy, A. Le Duc, A. Mouton, M. Petit, A.
Prawerman, F. Richard, I. Savatovsky, G. Vallancien.

Centre Médico-Chirurgical de la Porte de Choisy,
Paris (J-M.B., G.V.), Hôpital Saint-Joseph, Paris
(J-M.B., J-M.D.) Hôpital Cochin, Paris (L.B-G), Centre
Medico-Chirurgical Foch, Suresnes (H.B., M.C., F.R.),
Hôpital Saint-Louis, Paris (G.C., A.L.D.), Clinique
Chirurgicale Mutualiste, Reims (F.D., M.P., A.P.),
Clinique Chantereine, Brou-sur-Chantereine (D.G.),
Centre Hospitalier Regional, Creil (R.J.), Hôpital de
Juvisy (L.L.), Clinique de l'Archette, Olivet (A.M.),
Hôpital R. Ballanger, Aulnay (I.S), France.

INTRODUCTION

Although testicular androgen suppression has not been
demonstrated to prolong survival of patients with metastatic
cancer of the prostate (Elder and Catalona, 1984), it has
been widely recognized to result in improvement of symptoms
in 70 to 80 % of patients when used as a first line therapy
(Klein, 1979; Resnick, 1984). Relapse usually occurs within
one to two years and could be due to growth of hormone-
insensitive tumor cells (Isaacs, 1985) or, alternatively,
could result from the continuing stimulation of androgen-
dependent cells by androgens of adrenal origin (Labrie, 1983;
Geller, 1985). Attempts to remove androgens of adrenal origin
by adrenalectomy or aminogluthetimide as a second line treatment have resulted in objective responses in 25 - 35 % of
cases and subjective responses in 25 - 80 % of patients but
most of these responses are of very short duration
(Schroeder, 1985). Rather than removing testosterone of testicular origin as a first step, and then suppressing adrenal

androgens upon relapse, it has been suggested that blocking
the effect of all androgens simultaneously would give better
results than orchiectomy alone. Excellent response rates have
indeed been reported with combinations of an LHRH agonist and
an antiandrogen (Labrie, 1983) or of a very small dose of DES
and an antiandrogen (Geller, 1985) in non-comparative
studies.

In order to definitively establish a beneficial effect
of administering an antiandrogen from the time of castration,
we designed a prospective randomized trial, in which orchiectomy was compared to the combination of orchiectomy and an
antiandrogen. Orchiectomy was used because it is a radical
means of eliminating testicular androgens and, once accepted
by the patient, does not raise any problem of compliance or
drug interaction. The antiandrogen chosen was Anandron, a non-
steroidal compound devoid of any hormonal or antihormonal
activity other than its antiandrogenic activity (Raynaud,
1979). Two daily doses were compared: the higher dose of 300
mg per day was selected after a tolerance study had shown it
to be appropriate for long-term use; its safety, tolerance
and probable efficacy had been confirmed by a non-comparative
study (Labrie, 1983). The lower dose was 150 mg per day.

PATIENTS AND METHODS

In this prospective multicenter double-blind trial, 195
patients with stage D biopsy-proven prostatic carcinoma, who
had received no previous surgical, hormonal or radiation
treatment for their cancer and with a life expectancy of at
least 3 months were randomized into one of three treatment
groups: orchiectomy and placebo; orchiectomy and Anandron 150
mg per day; orchiectomy and Anandron 300 mg per day. The test
drug was taken orally and provided by Roussel- UCLAF,
Romainville, France.

Before study and every 6 months, the work-up included
clinical examination, measurement of prostate volume (through
transrectal ultrasonography in several centers), chest X-ray,
bone scan, bone X-rays, and intravenous pyelogram. Abdominal
CT scan and lymphography were performed when necessary to
evaluate lymph node involvement. After 1 and 3 months of
treatment, a shorter work-up included clinical examination
and measurement of prostate volume. At each visit a blood

sample was obtained for usual hematology and biochemistry
parameters, as well as for radioimmunoassay (RIA) of prostatic acid phosphatases (PAP) and of several hormones : LH,
FSH, testosterone, dihydrotestosterone (DHT), dehydroepiandrosterone (DHA), dehydroepiandrosterone sulfate (DHA-s)
Δ 4-androstenedione, estradiol, cortisol and prolactin. All
radioimmunoassays were performed in a central laboratory
(J. Fiet, Hôpital Saint-Louis, Paris, France). Plasma concentrations of Anandron were assayed, also by RIA, in order
to document compliance to treatment (Centre de Recherches
Roussel-UCLAF, Romainville, France).

The National Prostatic Cancer Project (NPCP) criteria
(Schmidt, 1976) were used to evaluate objective response at
each of the 6-monthly follow-ups. The best objective response (at any of the 6-monthly follow-ups), with the time-to-
progression and the survival time, were the main efficacy
criteria.

Individual subjective and objective criteria (bone
pain, performance status, PAP, primary tumor volume, number
of areas of increased uptake on bone scan) were analyzed as
well. In each center, successive bone scans were read and
compared by independent assessors who did not know to which
group the patient belonged.

The patients continued taking the test medication
(Anandron or placebo) as long as they tolerated it well and
their disease did not progress. When progression occurred,
the code was broken and the investigator could then give the
patient the treatment he thought most appropriate, including
Anandron when the patient had been on placebo.

The statistical methods were the following : For qualitative variables, comparisons between groups were made using
a chi-square test. For laboratory data, treatment groups
were compared using a Kruskall-Wallis test performed on
differences with baseline values. For time-to-progression
and time-to-death, actuarial rates were computed using
Kaplan-Meier estimate and compared using the Logrank test.
The significance level was $p < 0.05$.

RESULTS

One hundred and sixty patients had been included
between 6 and 33 months before the analysis (median : 20

months) and were therefore evaluable for tolerance and safety variables. Among them, 33 patients were not evaluable for efficacy, most often because, in retrospect, it was not absolutely certain that they had metastases at entry or because they had received previous hormonal treatment. Two patients were lost to follow-up before the 6 month-evaluation, three started treatment more than 3 months after orchiectomy. Thus 127 patients could be evaluated for efficacy:
- . 43 in the orchiectomy plus placebo group
- . 46 in the orchiectomy plus Anandron 150 mg group
- . 38 in the orchiectomy plus Anandron 300 mg group.

The three groups were similar with regard to their main characteristics: age; number of patients with stage D1 and stage D2 disease; frequency of bone pain and of abnormal PAP levels. The number of patients with impaired performance status was higher in the 150 mg group than in the two other groups (Table 1). Median time between orchiectomy and onset of test treatment was 3 days and the same in the three groups.

TABLE 1. Characteristics of evaluable patients

| | Orchiectomy | | | |
	Placebo	Anandron 150 mg	Anandron 300 mg	p*
Number of patients	43	46	38	
Median age (years)	72.0	72.5	70.0	NS
Stage D1	5	4	1	
D2	38	42	37	NS
Number of patients with bone pain	18	28	17	NS
Number of patients with impaired performance status	12	24	12	<0.05
Number of patients with abnormal PAP (>3 ng/ml)	26	30	28	NS

* Chi-Square test - NS = not significant

Among patients who complained of bone pain on entry, a greater percentage was improved in the Anandron 300 mg group after 1, 3 and 6 months of treatment and in the Anandron 150 mg group after 3 and 6 months of treatment than in the placebo group (Table 2).

TABLE 2. Percentage of patients improved among patients with bone pain on entry.

		Placebo	Orchiectomy Anandron 150 mg	Anandron 300 mg	p*
Number of patients with bone pain on entry		18	28	17	
Percentage improved	Month 1	61 %	67 %	93 %	<0.10
	Month 3	67 %	81 %	94 %	NS
	Month 6	44 %	71 %	94 %	<0.01

* Chi-square test – NS = not significant

Similarly, among patients with impaired performance status on inclusion, all were improved in the Anandron 300 mg group on months 1, 3 and 6 of treatment, compared to 50 to 67 % in the placebo group (Table 3).

TABLE 3. Percentage of patients improved among patients with impaired performance status on entry.

		Placebo	Orchiectomy Anandron 150 mg	Anandron 300 mg	p*
Number of patients with impaired performance status on entry		12	24	12	
Percentage improved	Month 1	67 %	57 %	100 %	<0.01
	Month 3	60 %	78 %	100 %	<0.05
	Month 6	50 %	80 %	100 %	<0.01

* Chi-square test

Although the differences were not statistically significant, there was a tendency for abnormally high PAP
values to return to normal levels in a greater percentage
of cases in the two Anandron groups than in the placebo
group (Table 4).

TABLE 4. Percentage of patients whose PAP became normal
among patients with abnormal PAP on entry.

| | | Orchiectomy | | | |
		Placebo	Anandron 150 mg	Anandron 300 mg	p*
Number of patients with abnormal PAP on entry		26	30	28	
Percentage normalized	Month 1	37 %	56 %	58 %	NS
	Month 3	52 %	70 %	78 %	NS
	Month 6	59 %	65 %	72 %	NS

* Chi-square test – NS = not significant

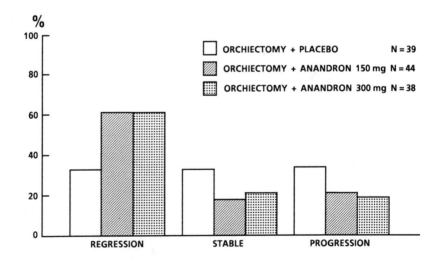

Figure 1. Best objective response according to NPCP
criteria (6 patients were not evaluable on this basis due to
a missing parameter, usually bone scan, at month 6).

Using NPCP criteria the best objective response to treatment was regression in 61 % of patients in the two Anandron-treated groups compared to 33% in the "orchiectomy and placebo" group and the difference was statistically significant. The percentage of patients who did not respond or who had already progressed at the 6-month visit were 20% and 19% in the two Anandron groups and 34 % in the placebo group. The remaining patients had stable disease as their best response (Figure 1).

The progression-free actuarial rate was higher at 6 months in the two Anandron groups (83 % and 84 %) than with orchiectomy alone (70 %). However, at 12 and 18 months the rates were similar in the 3 groups and there was no overall difference (Table 5). Likewise, the survival rate was similar in the three groups with medians of the distribution of 24, 22 and 22 months (Table 5).

TABLE 5. Progression and survival data *

| | | | Orchiectomy | |
		Placebo	Anandron 150 mg	Anandron 300 mg
Number of patients		43	46	38
Progression free actuarial rate	Month 6	70 %	83 %	84 %
	Month 12	58 %	57 %	49 %
	Month 18	40 %	42 %	35 %
Median time to progression (months)		13	13	12
Survival Actuarial rate	Month 6	98 %	98 %	97 %
	Month 12	83 %	82 %	79 %
	Month 18	70 %	59 %	61 %
Median time to death (months)		24	22	22

* The Logrank test revealed no significant differences among the three groups.

Analysis of hormone assay results demonstrated increases in LH and FSH and decreases in testosterone, DHT and estradiol to levels which were similar in the three groups. Prolactin and cortisol did not change in any of the groups while $\Delta 4$ - androstenedione, DHA and DHA-s decreased in a dose dependent manner in the groups treated with Anandron compared to the groups treated by orchiectomy alone. Plasma mean concentrations of Anandron were 7.3 mg/l (s.d. = 3.9, n = 31) in the 300 mg group and 3.5 mg/l (s.d. = 1.2, n = 32) in the 150 mg group. They were stable after 1, 3, 6 and 12 months of treatment.

For 8 patients in the higher dose group, 3 in the lower dose group, and none of the placebo group, treatment was stopped because of adverse experiences which were considered drug-related in four instances : two cases of interstitial lung disease, one case of visual disturbances and one of nausea, all of which disappeared upon discontinuation of the drug.

There was an overall dose-dependence of the number of intercurrent events in the three groups. The most frequently reported adverse events were hot flushes, the frequency of which was about 50 % in each of the three treatment groups. Two symptoms more specific to Anandron were an impairment in visual adaptation to darkness and alcohol intolerance. The former occurred in 19 % of patients in the 150 mg group and 28 % of patients in the 300 mg group and the latter in 17 % of patients of the higher dose group.

With regard to hematology and biochemistry parameters, there was no clinically relevant difference between the three groups.

DISCUSSION

This double-blind study which compared the combination of the antiandrogen Anandron and orchiectomy to treatment with orchiectomy alone gives good evidence that the former treatment results 1) subjectively in more frequent improvement in bone pain and performance status and 2) objectively in a greater decrease in tumor masses and a more frequent normalisation of prostatic acid phosphatase.

As in many trials in D2 prostate cancer performed in the last few years, the NPCP criteria were used to evaluate the objective response to treatment, and the categories regression (partial or complete), stable disease and progression were computed separately.

The percentage of patients whose best objective response was regression was 33 % in the group treated with orchiectomy alone : this percentage is similar to those reported in the literature for patients with Stage D2 prostate cancer treated with orchiectomy or DES : Smith et al. (1984) reported partial or complete regression in 23 % of 32 patients and 32 % of 44 patients included in two separate EORTC studies and treated with DES, 3 mg per day. Murphy et al. (1984) found objective regression in 41 % of 83 patients treated with DES or orchiectomy.

In our study both Anandron-treated groups demonstrated the same percentages of objective regressions (61 %) which were significantly higher than what was observed in the group treated with orchiectomy. A difference between the orchiectomy alone group and the two Anandron-treated groups was also found in the progression-free actuarial rate : at 6 months, it was 70 % in the former and 83 and 84 % in the latter two groups. The difference, however, was not maintained after 12 and 18 months of treatment : median time-to-progression was 12 or 13 months in the three groups, similar to the 60 and 61 weeks reported with DES or Leuprolide by the Leuprolide Study Group (1984). Nor was there any difference in survival time. Thus, this comparative study confirms the better symptomatic response and the improved objective response rate reported by Labrie et al. (1983) but not the dramatic improvement in survival which they later claimed (Labrie, 1984).

However, it may not be that surprising to find no difference in survival time between a group treated with orchiectomy alone and groups treated with orchiectomy and Anandron since it is not certain that endocrine therapy will increase survival in stage D2 patients. Although it will improve symptoms and prevent growth of hormone-sensitive tumor cells, it will have no impact on hormone-independent tumor cells which probably continue growing and eventually cause relapse of the disease.

Which of the two doses was the more effective? A greater improvement in pain and performance status was demonstrated after one month of treatment with the higher dose. However, the objective regression rate was the same in both Anandron-treated groups. This, together with the relatively long time needed to attain the steady-state in plasma Anandron concentration, leads us to propose a treatment regimen of 300 mg per day during the first month and 150 mg per day afterwards.

An interesting finding of this study, already reported by Bélanger et al. (1984) in their non-comparative study, was the decrease in plasma adrenal androgens observed in the Anandron-treated groups. Although the mechanism of this decrease has not yet been elucidated (decreased synthesis, enhanced catabolism or increased elimination), it could also contribute to the antiandrogenic activity of Anandron. However, since both doses have the same efficacy on tumor regression rate despite the lesser effect of the lower dose on adrenal androgen concentrations, it is probable that the prime mechanism of the antiandrogenic activity of Anandron is through competitive inhibition on the androgen receptor as suggested in experimental animal models (Moguilewsky et al. 1986).

CONCLUSION

Conventional endocrine treatment is unanimously recognized to improve symptoms of advanced prostate cancer but statistical studies have never demonstrated that it increases survival. In this prospective randomized study the combination of orchiectomy and Anandron was effective in improving the quality of life and objective tumor regression rate. Adding this antiandrogen to orchiectomy therefore enhances the known beneficial effects of castration.

REFERENCES

Bélanger A, Dupont A, and Labrie F (1984). Inhibition of basal and adrenocorticotropin-stimulated plasma levels of adrenal androgens after treatment with an antiandrogen in castrated patients with prostatic cancer. J Clin Endocrinol Metab 59: 422-426.

Elder JS, Catalona WJ (1984). Management of newly diagnosed metastatic carcinoma of the prostate. Urologic Clinics of North America 11: 283-295.

Geller J, Albert JD, (1983). Comparison of various hormonal therapies for prostatic carcinoma. Seminars in Oncology, Suppl. 4, 10: 34-41.

Geller J (1985). Rationale for blockade of adrenal as well as testicular androgens in the treatment of advanced prostate cancer. Seminars in Oncology, Suppl 1, 12: 28-35

Isaacs JT (1985). New principles in the management of metastatic prostatic cancer. In Schroeder FH, Richards B (eds) : "EORTC Genitourinary Group Monograph 2, Part A: Therapeutic Principles in Metastatic Prostatic Cancer". New-York: Alan R. Liss, p. 383-405.

Klein LA (1979). Prostatic carcinoma. N Engl J Med 300: 824-833.

Labrie F, Dupont A, Bélanger A, Lacourcière Y, Raynaud JP, Husson JM, Gareau J, Fazekas ATA, Sandow J, Monfette G, Girard JG, Emond J, Houle JG (1983). New approach in the treatment of prostate cancer : complete instead of partial withdrawal of androgens. The Prostate 4: 579-594.

Labrie F, Bélanger A, Dupont A, Emond J, Lacourcière Y, Monfette G (1984). Combined treatment with LHRH agonist and pure antiandrogen in advanced carcinoma of prostate. Lancet 8411: 1090

Moguilewsky M, Fiet J, Tournemine C, Raynaud JP (1986). Pharmacology of an antiandrogen, Anandron, used as an adjuvant therapy in the treatment of prostate cancer. J Steroid Biochem 24: 139-146.

Murphy GP, Slack NH and participants in the National Prostatic Cancer Project (1984). Current status of the National Prostatic Cancer Project Treatment Protocols. In Denis L, Murphy GP, Prout GR, Schroeder F (eds): "Controlled Clinical Trials in Urologic Oncology". Raven Press: New-York p. 119-133.

Raynaud JP, Bonne C, Bouton MM, Lagacé L, Labrie F, (1979). Action of a non steroid androgen, RU 23908, in peripheral and central tissues. J. Steroid Biochem 11 : 93-99.

Schroeder FH (1985). Total androgen suppression in the management of prostatic cancer. A critical review. In Schroeder FH, Richards B (eds): "EORTC Genitourinary Group Monograph 2, Part A: Therapeutic Principles in Metastatic Prostatic Cancer". New-York: Alan R. Liss, p. 307-317.

Schmidt JD, Johnson DE, Scott WW, Gibbons RP, Prout GR, Murphy GP (1976). Chemotherapy of advanced cancer. Evaluation of response parameters. Urology 7: 602–610

Smith PH, Pavone-Macaluso M, Viggiano G, de Voogt H, Lardennois B, Robinson MRG, Richards B, Glashan RW, de Pauw M, Sylvester R and the EORTC Urological group (1984). In Denis L, Murphy GP, Prout GR, Schroeder F (eds): "Controlled Clinical Trials in Urologic Oncology". Raven Press: New-York p. 107–117.

The Leuprolide Study Group (1984). Leuprolide versus diethylstilbestrol for metastatic prostate cancer. N Engl J Med 311: 1281–1286.

Prostate Cancer, Part A: Research, Endocrine
Treatment, and Histopathology, page 423
© 1987 Alan R. Liss, Inc.

HORMONAL PROFILE DURING TREATMENT OF PROSTATIC CANCER WITH LH-RH DEPOT (ICI 118630) OR FLUTAMIDE ALONE AND UNDER COMBINED THERAPY

Krüger H., Möhring K., Dörsam J., Haack D., Vecsei P., Röhl L.
Dept of Urology, Surgical Center and Dept. of Pharmacology, University of Heidelberg, R.F.A.

The influence of LH-RH agonists or pure antiandrogens and their combination on the gonadotrophins, testicular and adrenal androgens is of clinical importance in the antihormonal treatment of prostatic cancer. Since 1985, a complete endocrine profile was examined in 22 patients under therapy with LH-DH Depot (3.6mg/28d; n = 9), flutamide (3x 250mg/d; n = 10) and combined therapy (n = 3). Plasma testosterone (T), free T (fr.T), dehydrotestosterone (DHT), LH, prolactine (P), 17 β−estradiol (E), androstenedione (A), dehydroepiandrostenedione (DHEA), and DHEA-sulphate (DHEAS) were estimated at 4-week intervals. Median treatment time was 20 months (10-23) for the flutamide group, 9.5 months (1-16.5) for the LH-RH group, and 3 to 14 months under combined therapy.

A significant decrease (p < 0.05) in plasma concentrations was found for T, fr. T, DHT, E and LH after 4 weeks under LH-RH. After therapy with flutamide for 6 months, however, a significant increase in T, fr.T, E and LH was found. For DHEA, A and P no significant change has been demonstrated to date though DHEAS showed a tendency to drop with treatment time. This drop was pronounced and included DHEA under combined therapy or if LH-RH was added to initial flutamide monotherapy in case of progression.

These findings suggest that LH-RH agonists and pure antiandrogens may have an additive effect on adrenal or testicular androgen metabolism.

Prostate Cancer, Part A: Research, Endocrine
Treatment, and Histopathology, page 425
© 1987 Alan R. Liss, Inc.

TREATMENT OF PROSTATIC CANCER WITH D Trp 6 LH-RH, AN LH-RH AGONIST. LONG TERM RESULTS IN FORTY ONE CASES.

Chiche R., Steg R., Boccon-Gibod L., Debré B.
Clinique Urologique - Hôpital Cochin, PARIS

Forty-one patients with advanced prostate carcinoma were treated from 28 to 36 months with D Trp 6 LH-RH, a luteinizing hormone releasing hormone agonist. Thirty-eight of them had advanced cancer with either metastases or major local spread. Sixteen patients (39%) have been treated previously by other hormonal therapy, but treatment was interrupted because of cardio-vascular trouble, or escape of the disease, or by the patient himself. The twenty five others (61%) had not undergone hormonal manipulation.

In all the cases in which the testosterone levels were normal before treatment, the treatment led to a decline to the levels observed after castration (0.5 ng/ml). Similarly, LH decreased to a mean of 1.4 ± 1 mUI/ml. In nine patients out of the thirty three who had hormonal determination on the first days, a rise of testosterone was observed in the very first days of the treatment.

After three months, thirty patients (73%) reacted favorably to the "medical castration" resulting from LH-RH agonists (16 improved and 14 remained stable). All but one of the sixteen patients who improved were in the previously untreated group. After twenty-eight to thirty-six months, results dramatically deteriorated : only twelve patients remained improved or stable. Twenty-one deaths were registred, the majority cancer related. In two patients with bone and lung metastases pain dramatically increased early after the first injections, requiring major narcotic analgesia, a very similar and rapidly progressive delirious statement occurred, and in one of these cases a sudden paraplegia due to spinal cord compression by epidural metastases. These patients died within two weeks. The role of the agonists in such a sudden deterioration of the tumor after the first injection cannot be ruled out.

LH-RH agonists is an efficient treatment of the prostatic cancer allowing a good medical castration but after a few months, escape of the disease appears as in conventional hormonotherapy.

Prostate Cancer, Part A: Research, Endocrine
Treatment, and Histopathology, page 427
© 1987 Alan R. Liss, Inc.

RANDOMISED STUDY OF LONG ACTING D-TRP-6-LHRH vs ORCHIDECTOMY IN ADVANCED PROSTATIC CARCINOMA

H. Parmar, L. Allen, R.H. Phillips
Edgware General Hospital and Westminster Hospital, London, G.B.

104 patients were randomised for the study. 55 patients were entered into the D-Trp-6-LHRH group and 49 patients into the orchidectomy group. All pre-treatment patient characteristics were similar and no significant difference was found between the groups. Mean duration of treatment was 18 months.

20 patients (36%) in the D-Trp-6-LHRH group and 16 patients (33%) in the orchidectomy group had a partial remission at 3 months or later. 26 patients (47%) in the D-Trp-6-LHRH group and 24 patients (49%) in the orchidectomy group had stable disease. 9 patients in each group (16% and 19% respectively) had evidence of progressive disease.

8 patients in the D-Trp-6-LHRH group and 7 patients in the orchidectomy group have died. The mean survival of the dead patients was 16 months in the D-Trp-6-LHRH group and 13 months in the orchidectomy group. There was no significant difference between the groups for response or survival.

3 patients in the D-Trp-6-LHRH group had a disease "flare" in the first 10 days of treatment. The flare symptoms resolved by the end of 4-6 weeks.

39 patients (76%) in the D-Trp-6-LHRH group and 32 patients (73%) in the orchidectomy group had symptoms of facial flushing. Decreased libido was reported in 59% of the D-Trp-6-LHRH group and 68% of the orchidectomy group. 82% of the patients in the D-Trp-6-LHRH group and 89% of the orchidectomy group were reported to be impotent. Psychological tests showed that there was a trend showing decreased morbidity in the D-Trp-6-LHRH offers a safe and highly effective alternative to orchidectomy and can be recommended as first line treatment of advanced prostatic carcinoma.

Prostate Cancer, Part A: Research, Endocrine
Treatment, and Histopathology, pages 429–434
© 1987 Alan R. Liss, Inc.

THE TREATMENT OF PROSTATIC CANCER BY LH-RH AGONIST

Kyoichi Imai, Hidetoshi Yamanaka, Hisako Yuasa,
Masaru Yoshida, Masaharu Asano and Isao Kaetsu
Department of Urology, School of Medicine,Gunma,
University, Maebashi, Japan, 371, (K.I.,H.Y.,
H.Y.) and Takasaki Radiation Chemistry Research
Establishment, Japan Atomic Energy Research,
Takasaki, Japan, 370, (M.Y.,M.A,I.K.).

INTRODUCTION

The chronic administration of pharmacological doses
of LH-RH agonist results in initial stimulation but subsequent inhibition of the release of LH and FSH (Sandow, 1983).
The resultant decrease in testicular steroidgenesis has proved the therapeutic efficacy in the patients with prostatic
cancer (Wenderoth and Jacobi, 1983; Yamanaka et al, 1985).
However this treatment has the disadvantage of requiring
the administration of daily injections for the optimal clinical efficacy. Therefore we have studied controlled slow
release of the drug.

MATERIALS AND METHODS

Preparation of VPC and PLAC: VPC (vinyl polymer composite) is made by radiation-induced polymerization of glass
-forming co-monomers at low temperature (Imai et al., 1986)
and the appearance of leuprolide-VPC is shown in Fig. 1. Two
kinds of low molecular weight ($\overline{M}n=1850$ and 2200) poly-(DL-
lactic acid) (PLA) were prepared by polycodensation of DL-
lactic acid in the abscence of a catalyst. A mixture of powdered PLA and leuprolide was molted at 70°C in order to dis-
tribute the drug in PLA homogeneously. The molten mixture
was charged into a teflon tube of 2 mm inside diameter and
then cooled to 20°C. A piston rod inserted into the above
tube under a pressure of 100kg/cm^2 at 40°C (Asano et al.,
1985). It was named PLA composite (PLAC). From four kinds
of PLAC (Fig. 2), leuprolide releasing profile was studied
in the patients with porstatic cancer.

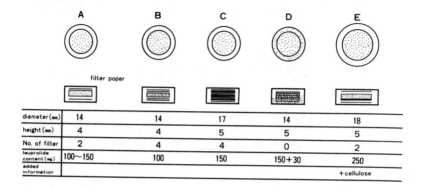

Figure 1. Schematic appearance of VPC.

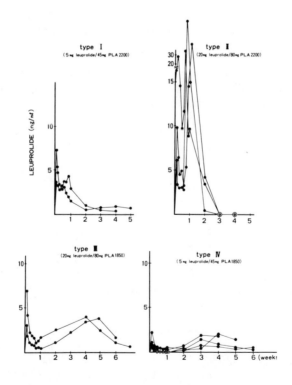

Figure 2. Leuprolide releasing profile from PLAC.

Animal experiments: Male Wister rats (3 rats/group) weighted about 300 to 360 gr were used. VPC which contains 5 mg of leuprolide was implanted subcutaneously in the back of rats. For an injection-administration of leuprolide, the drug was given to the rats at a dose of 20 μg subcutaneously once a day.

Clinical studies: Subcutaneous injection (SC) group; 1 or 20 mg of leuprolide was injected subcutaneously once a day. VPC group; One of five types of VPC was implanted subcutaneously for more than three months. And then to some patients, same and/or different types of VPC were implanted. PLAC group; Leuprolide releasing profile from four types of PLAC was studied by subcutsneous every five week injection and the clinical effects of type-1, -3 and -4 of PLAC were evaluated. IN group; Buserelin was administrated with intranasal spray application (600 or 900 μg/day).

Fifty nine patients with prostatic cancer were treated by LH-RH agonist. Five patients previously treated were included in them. The clinical effects of LH-RH agonist therapy were evaluated according to NPCP criteria (Murphy and Slack, 1980).

Hormone assay: Blood samples were assayed for leuprolide, testosterone, LH and FSH by radioimmunoassay. The radioimmunoassay sensitivity of leuprolide was 50 pg /assay tube.

RESULTS AND DISCUSSION

Animal experiments clearly demonstrated that the weight of ventral prostate, dorsolateral prostate, seminal vesicle and testis were decreased by continuous LH-RH agonist administartion (VPC) more effectively than that by intermittent administration (SC). However the weight of adrenal gland was not affected by LH-RH agonist administration (Fig. 3).

By each of those LH-RH agonist administration methods, serum testosterone was decreased below 1 ng/ml in all patients, except one patient treated by IN. It was estimated that the failure of serum testosterone suppression was not caused by his sensitivity to LH-RH agonist, but the administration method, because serum testosterone in this patient was decreased by VPC. Fifty two patients who were treated by LH-RH agonist for up to three months (excluded two patients; one patient treated by IN described above and the other died of cardiac attack at the 2nd month.) and not previously treated by any other therapy were evaluated. Thirty one patients had PR (59.6%), eighteen had stable (34.6%) and three had progression (5.8%).

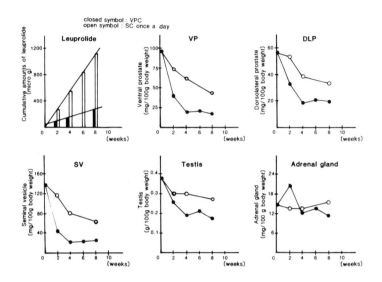

Figure 3. LH-RH agonist effect on organ weight in male Wister rats.

Neither significant clinical nor hormonal difference between 20 mg/day of SC and 1 mg/day of SC was observed. However serum leuprolide concentration was obviousely different between both doses, namely 24 hrs serum leuprolide concentration was 75 ng/ml in the case of 20 mg of SC but undetectable in the case of 1 mg of SC. Therefore it was estimated that 1 mg/day was the lowest dose to obtain the therapeutic efficacy by daily SC.

Five patients in VPC group were treated by one or several types of VPC for more than one year. One patient (case #8 in Fig. 4) among them was treated for 615 days by one VPC which contains 180 mg of leuprolide. Serum testosterone was suppressed below 1 ng/ml during this period and leuprolide still detectable on the 615th day. In this patient, average daily leuprolide releasing dose was below 0.29 mg/day.

Leuprolide releasing speed from PLAC-2 (20 mg of leuprolide in 80 mg of PLA Mn2200) was too rapid to obtain the optimal injection interval. Therefore the clinical effect was evaluated in the patients treated by PLAC-1, -3 and -4. Average daily leuprolide releasing dose was below 0.14 mg/ml.

These results clearly demonstrate that LH-RH agonist therapy by continuous administration (VPC and PLAC) was more

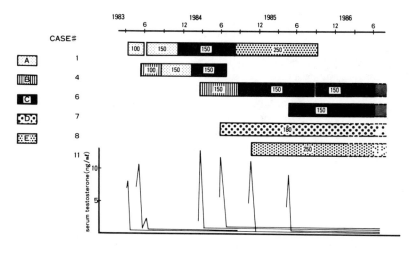

Figure 4. LH-RH agonist therapy by several types of VPC.

efficient than that by intermittent administration (SC), in regard to the cost effectiveness. And this conclusion was also supported by the animal experimental results described above.

Methods	Patients #	CR	PR	S	PD	Others
SC	30 (3)	0	16	10 (1)	3 (2)	1
VPC	11 (1)	0	7	2 (1)	2	0
PLAC	7 (1)	0	4	3 (1)	0	0
IN	11	0	4	6	0	1
total	59 (5)	0	31	21 (3)	5 (2)	2

Table 1. LH-RH agonist effect on Prostatic cancer. Numbers in parentheses are patients number treated previously.

In one case treated by VPC for more than one year, serum leuprolide was not detectable, but serum testosterone was below 1 ng/ml. This promoted us to investigate the testicular morphological change. The testicular biopsy samples after prolonged (for more than one year) tretment by LH-RH agonist demonstrated marked spermatogenic suppression, thickening of the tubular wall and decreased number of the Leidig cells. These results agree approximately with those reported by others (Joseph et al., 1985). We estimate that the number of Leidig cells may not be reversible.

REFFERENCES

Asano M, Yoshida M, Kaetsu I, Imai K, Mashimo T, Yuasa H, Yamanaka H, Suzuki K (1985). Biodegradability of a hot-pressed poly (lactic acid) formulation with controlled release of LH-RH agonist and its pharmacological influence on rat prostate. Makromol Chem Rapid Commun 6:509

Imai K, Yamanaka H, Yuasa H, Yoshida M, Asano M, Kaetsu I, Yamazaki I, Suzuki K (1986). The sustained release of LH-RH agonist from LH-RH agonist-polymer composite in patients with prostatic cancer. The Prostate 8:

Murphy GP, Slack NH (1980). Response criteria for the prostate of the USA National Prostatic Cancer Project. The Prostate 1:375

Sandow J (1983). Clinical application of LHRH and its analogues. Clin Endocrinology 18:571.

Smith J, Urry R (1985). Testicular histology after prolonged treatment with a gonadotropin-releasing hormone analogue. J Urol 133:612.

Wenderoth UK, Jacobi GH (1983). Gonadotropin-releasing hormone analogues for palliation of carcinoma of the prostate, A new approach to the classical concept. World J Urol 1: 40.

Yamanaka H, Makino T, Yajima H, Saruki K, Shida K (1985). Efficacy of (D-LEU^6-DES GLY-NH$_2$^{10}-LHRH ethylamide against prostatic cancer. The Prostate 6:27.

Prostate Cancer, Part A: Research, Endocrine
Treatment, and Histopathology, pages 435–437
© 1987 Alan R. Liss, Inc.

PHARMACOKINETICS OF D-Trp6 LHRH IN MAN: SUSTAINED RELEASE POLYMER MICROSPHERE STUDY (I.M. ROUTE)

K. Drieu*, J.P. Devissaguet, R. Duboistesselin, F. Dray, E. Ezan
*Institut Henri Beaufour, Le Plessis-Robinson, France

A specific and sensitive (70 pg/ml) radio-immuno-assay of DTRP6-LHRH* in biological fluids has been previously developed and applied to animal pharmacokinetic studies. A study was subsequently performed in man and is reported here :

METHODOLOGY

- a reference study was conducted in 6 healthy volunteers with a single S.C. administration of an aqueous solution of 0.1 mg of DTRP6-LHRH,

- another study was conducted in 6 patients with prostatic cancer, who successively received : 0.1 mg of DTRP6-LHRH solution by S.C. injection for 7 days, then an I.M. injection of 3 mg (bioavailable) of DTRP6-LHRH in the form of an aqueous suspension of microspheres designed to ensure therapeutic cover for one month with a single injection.

These microspheres, with a mean diameter of 30-40 µm, constitute a porous biocompatible and biodegradable matrix (poly d, 1 lactide-coglycolide) in which DTRP6-LHRH is dispersed. A

---

* decapeptyl (IPSEN Biotech)

histological study in the rat demonstrated the progressive biodegradation of the microspheres in the muscle tissue and confirmed the normal appearance of the injection site after resorption of the polymer vector.

RESULTS

In healthy subjects (S.C. route, single dose), the chronological variation in the plasma concentrations was very similar in each of the 6 subjects : peak concentrations : 1.85 ± 0.23 ng/ml were reached within 0.63 ± 0.26 hr and, after a distribution phase lasting 3 to 4 hours, the plasma concentration decreased with a half-life of 7.6 ± 1.6 hr to reach 0.11 ± 0.04 ng/ml after 24 hours. The total plasma clearance of DTRP6-LHRH was 161.7 ± 28.6 ml/min, associated with a volume of distribution of 104.1 ± 11.7 litres.

An earlier study in the dog demonstrated that the bioavailability of DTRP6-LHRH was total after S.C. injection and the calculation of the volume and the clearance in man was based on this hypothesis.

In patients (S.C. route, repeated doses), the peak concentrations were 1.28 ± 0.24 ng/ml and remained similar for the 7 days of repeated administration, indicating the absence of accumulation. The total plasma clearance was 118.1 ± 32.0 ml/min, lower than in healthy subjects, due to delayed elimination, confirmed by the biological half-life of 11.7 ± 3.4 hours. The volume of distribution did not appear to be modified : 113.4 ± 21.6 litres.
These results can be explained by the age and state of health of the patients.

After I.M. administration of a suspension of microspheres, an initial peak was noted, probably corresponding to the release of the superficial DTRP6-LHRH. The concentrations stabilised after 24 hours and remained at a plateau for 4 weeks. The level of this plateau was 0.22 to 0.48 ng/ml, depending on the subject and was inversely proportional to the total plasma clearance of DTRP6-LHRH. The stability of the individual concentrations is due to the constant rate of release of DTRP6- LHRH from the polymer support, estimated to be 50 µg/day and homogeneous from one subject to another.

CONCLUSION

Despite a lower total clearance than in healthy subjects, which can be explained by the age and general state of the patients, DTRP6-LHRH was not accumulated.

The pharmacological (chemical castration) and therapeutic activity observed after repeated S.C. administration was maintained for more than 4 weeks after a single I.M. injection of the sustained release form. The aptitude of the polymer vector to deliver DTRP6-LHRH at a constant rate is demonstrated by the stability of the plasma concentrations.

Prostate Cancer, Part A: Research, Endocrine
Treatment, and Histopathology, pages 439–443
© 1987 Alan R. Liss, Inc.

EFFECT OF SURGICAL AND BIOCHEMICAL CASTRATION AND AN
ANTIANDROGEN ON PATIENTS WITH STAGE D2 PROSTATIC CANCER:
PRELIMINARY RESULTS

Morris L. Givner and Oliver H. Millard

Departments of Pathology (MLG) and Urology (OHM)
Dalhousie University, Halifax, N. S., Canada

The purpose of this study was to determine the effects
of orchiectomy, orchiectomy plus Flutamine and (D-trp)
LHRHEA plus Flutamide on 30 patients with stage D2 prostatic
cancer.

The treatment groups were as follows:

Group 1: Orchiectomy (5)[a]
Group 2: Orchiectomy + Flutamide (16)[b]
Group 3: D-trp LHRHEA[c,d] + Flutamide (9)[b]

[a] No. of Patients
[b] 250 mg p.o.t.i.d.
[c] L-pyroglutamyl-L-histidyl-L-tryptophyl-
L-seryl-L-tyrosyl-D-tryptophyl-L-leucyl-
L-arginyl-L-prolyl-ethylamide
[d] 600 µg s.c. O.D. x 30, 300 µg s.c. O.D. thereafter

The biochemical changes are shown in Figs. 1-15.
Patients treated with LHRH analogue plus Flutamide, had
significant decreases in serum LH, FSH, prolactin,
testosterone, DHEAS, progesterone, 17 α-hydroxyprogesterone
estradiol-17 β, prostatic acid phosphatase, alkaline
phosphatase and uric acid. Calcium levels were increased
by this treatment.

Patients treated by orchiectomy plus Flutamide had
significant decreases in testosterone, DHEAS, progesterone,
prostatic acid phosphatase and uric acid.

Effect of Orchiectomy, Orchiectomy plus Flutamide, [D-Trp]₆ LHRHEA plus Flutamide on Serum Luteinizing Hormone Levels in Patients with Advanced Prostatic Cancer

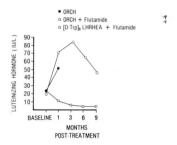

Figure 1.

Effect of Orchiectomy, Orchiectomy plus Flutamide, [D-Trp]₆ LHRHEA plus Flutamide on Serum FSH Levels in Patients with Advanced Prostatic Cancer

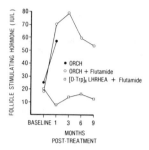

Figure 2.

Effect of Orchiectomy, Orchiectomy plus Flutamide, [D-Trp]₆ LHRHEA plus Flutamide on Serum Prolactin Levels in Patients with Advanced Prostatic Cancer

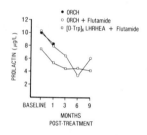

Figure 3.

Effect of Orchiectomy, Orchiectomy plus Flutamide, [D-Trp]₆ LHRHEA plus Flutamide on Serum Testosterone Levels in Patients with Advanced Prostatic Cancer

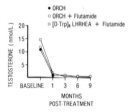

Figure 4.

Effect of Orchiectomy, Orchiectomy plus Flutamide, [D-Trp]₆ LHRHEA plus Flutamide on Serum DHEA-Sulphate Levels in Patients with Advanced Prostatic Cancer

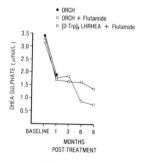

Figure 5.

Effect of Orchiectomy, Orchiectomy plus Flutamide, [D-Trp]₆ LHRHEA plus Flutamide on Serum Progesterone Levels in Patients with Advanced Prostatic Cancer

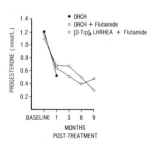

Figure 6.

Effect of Orchiectomy, Orchiectomy plus Flutamide, [D-Trp]₆ LHRHEA plus Flutamide on Serum 17αOH Progesterone Levels in Patients with Advanced Prostatic Cancer

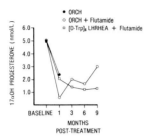

Figure 7.

Effect of Orchiectomy, Orchiectomy plus Flutamide, [D-Trp]₆ LHRHEA plus Flutamide on Serum Estradiol-17 β Levels in Patients with Advanced Prostatic Cancer

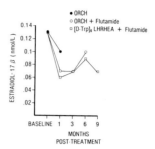

Figure 8.

Effect of Orchiectomy, Orchiectomy plus Flutamide, [D-Trp]₆ LHRHEA plus Flutamide on Serum Prostatic Acid Phosphatase Levels in Patients with Advanced Prostatic Cancer

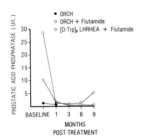

Figure 9.

Effect of Orchiectomy, Orchiectomy plus Flutamine, [D-Trp]₆ LHRHEA plus Flutamide on Serum Alkaline Phosphatase Levels in Patients with Advanced Prostatic Cancer

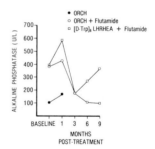

Figure 10.

Effect of Orchiectomy, Orchiectomy plus Flutamide, [D-Trp]₆ LHRHEA plus Flutamide on Serum Uric Acid Levels in Patients with Advanced Prostatic Cancer

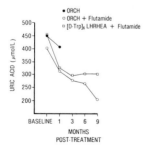

Figure 11.

Effect of Orchiectomy, Orchiectomy plus Flutamide, [D-Trp]₆ LHRHEA plus Flutamide on Serum Calcium Levels in Patients with Advanced Prostatic Cancer

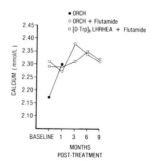

Figure 12.

Effect of Orchiectomy, Orchiectomy plus Flutamide, [D-Trp]₆ LHRHEA plus Flutamide on Serum Cortisol Levels in Patients with Advanced Prostatic Cancer

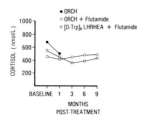

Figure 13.

Effect of Orchiectomy, Orchiectomy plus Flutamide, [D-Trp]₆ LHRHEA plus Flutamide on Serum Albumin Levels in Patients with Advanced Prostatic Cancer

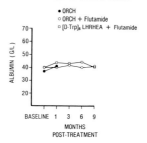

Figure 14.

Effect of Orchiectomy, Orchiectomy plus Flutamide, [D-Trp]₆ LHRHEA plus Flutamide on Serum Total Protein Levels in Patients with Advanced Prostatic Cancer

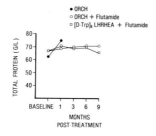

Figure 15.

Patients treated by orchiectomy alone had elevated levels of LH, FSH and calcium. Decreased levels of testosterone, DHEAS, progesterone, 17 α-hydroxyprogesterone, prostatic acid phosphatase and uric acid were effected by this treatment.

All 30 patients in the 3 treatment groups had decreases in serum testosterone levels to castrate values during the first 3 months of treatment.

The preliminary responses to the three different treatments are shown in Table 1 and no definite conclusions can be drawn, at this stage of the study.

Table 1

Effect of Three Different Treatments on Patients with
Stage D Prostatic Cancer: Preliminary Results

| Clinical Response | Treatment | | |
(3 months)	Group 1 (5)[a]	Group 2 (16)	Group 3 (9)
Complete	0	0	1
Partial	4	13	8
Stable	1	3	0
Progression	0	0	0

a   No. of Patients

Acknowledgements

        We wish to thank Mr. Edward C. Kavalec of Schering
Canada (Montreal) for supplying Flutamide and D-TrpLHRHEA
and for their support and encouragement.

        The authors also wish to express their appreciation to
Ms. Carole Kennedy, our study coordinator and Ms. Marcelle
Comeau, who supervised the hormone assays in the
Endocrinology Laboratory, The Victoria General Hospital,
Halifax, Nova Scotia, Canada. Our sincere thanks to
Ms. Joanne McGinis for assistance in the preparation of
the manuscript.

Prostate Cancer, Part A: Research, Endocrine
Treatment, and Histopathology, pages 445–475
© 1987 Alan R. Liss, Inc.

PROGRESS IN PATHOLOGY OF CARCINOMA OF PROSTATE

F. K. Mostofi, I. A. Sesterhenn & C. J. Davis

Armed Forces Institute of Pathology

Washington, D. C. 20306

INTRODUCTION

The role of the pathologist is to assist the clinical
colleagues in the management of a patient with a malignant
tumor. This involves confirming or ruling out the diagnosis of malignancy, providing an estimate of the degree of
malignancy, predicting the response of the tumor to the
therapy, and contributing to better understanding of the
biology and natural history of the tumor.

This presentation will deal with progress in these
areas.
1. Progress in pathologic diagnosis

As a preliminary to the discussion, we must consider
criteria for diagnosis of prostatic cancer.

Pathological criteria for diagnosis of any tumor are
anaplasia, invasion and metastasis. In many tumors the
pathologist usually has no information about the existence
of metastasis so he must depend entirely on anaplasia and
invasion.

Three features of nuclei are generally considered diagnostic of prostatic carcinoma: (PCa) variations in size and
shape, vacuolization, and the presence of a large prominent
but ill defined nucleolus. Unfortunately, many PCas do not
show these features even after the tumor has demonstrated
its invasive and metastatic potential. (Figs. 1 & 2) Sometimes the nuclei are homogeneously dark staining without

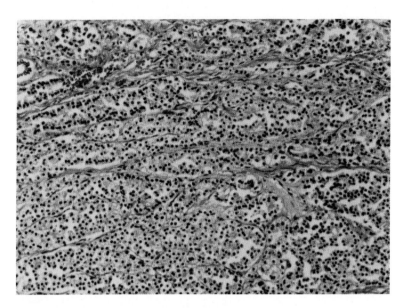

Fig. 1. Carcinoma. Nuclear Grade 1. The
nuclear are uniform. AFIP Neg. 86-9490 X 160.

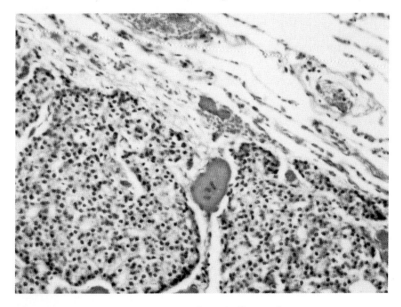

Fig. 2. Carcinoma metastatic to lung from
the tumor shown in Fig. 1. AFIP Neg. 86-9494
X 160.

any discernible structure, sometimes they have a pale staining delicate chromatin distribution with a small usually
centrally placed nucleolus and sometimes they are vacuolated and have a large ill-defined nucleolus.
Perhaps the problem is that the criteria for anaplasia in
PCas have not been clearly defined.

Brawer et al (1985) in a study of 19 benign and 32 malignant prostates stained with antikeratin antibody 902 and
antikeratin antibody 903 demonstrated that the former labeled all columnar secretory cells of normal and hyperplastic
prostatic epithelium as well as neoplastic cells. On the
other hand antikeratin antibody 903 labeled only the basal
cells and not the secretory cells or any of the malignant
glands even the well differentiated PCa and intraductal
dysplasias. They thought this could be used to help in
diagnosing PCa ·   The proposal has not been confirmed.

Invasion is another criterion that pathologists use
for diagnosis of malignancy. In the prostate, although the
acini are surrounded by a delicate basement membrane, detection of breakthrough the basement membrane with currently available staining technics is not reliable. However,if
the acini are seen in intimate relationship to smooth muscle bundles (Fig. 3) stromal invasion can be diagnosed, but
again, unfortunately, this is not seen very often.

Bostwick et al (1986) have proposed that disruption of
basal cell layer as demonstrated by the absence of antikeratin monoclonal (basal cell specific) antibody reaction :sug -
gested invasive potential. Unfortunately, most PCas do not
have a basal cell layer.

Perineural invasion (Fig. 4) has generally been recognized as sine qua non evidence of PCa. We have demonstrated that given adequate tissue, perineural invasion is demonstrable in over 90% of PCas, but, unfortunately, many
needle biopsies or transurethrally removed tissues do not
show perineural invasion. Invasion of the seminal vesicles,
bladder neck, pericapsular tissue, lymphatics and vascular
channels, if present, and detected, can readily establish
the diagnosis of malignancy but many of the biopsies or
surgically removed tissues do not demonstrate any of these
features.

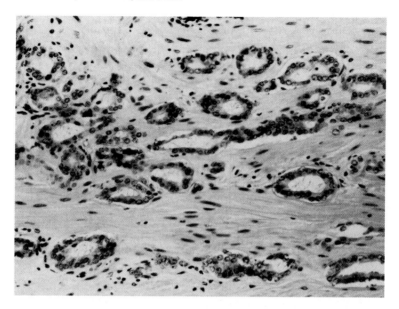

Fig. 3. Carcinoma with stromal invasion.
AFIP Neg. 86-9491 X 100.

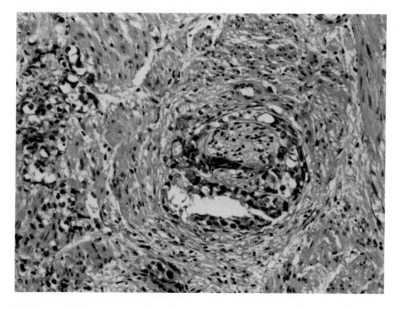

Fig. 4. Carcinoma with perineural invasion.
AFIP Neg. 86-9492 X 100.

In the absence of anaplasia and invasion pathologists have come to depend on disturbances of architecture to diagnose PCa. These consist of small glands (Fig. 5), large glands without convolutions (Fig. 6), glands closely packed together (Fig. 7), fused glands (Fig. 8), glands in glands (Fig. 9), large and small glands side by side, and haphazardly distributed glands (Fig. 10).

Looking at the glands themselves, the double layer of nuclei of secretory and basal cells commonly observed in normal and in hyperplastic glands is replaced by a single layer of cells (Fig. 11).

While the presence of one or more such disturbances in the architecture has been recognized as indicative of carcinoma, two features create problems:
a) The criteria are subjective. What may look like small glands to one pathologist, may be normal to another.
b) A number of benign prostatic lesions simulate carcinoma.

Elsewhere Mostofi (1952 & 1973) and more recently Dhom (1985) discussed lesions that simulate PCa. On the clinical side, prostatic calculi and chronic granulomatous prostatitis are lesions that, by virtue of their hardness and/or induration, may simulate carcinoma. Fortunately, urologists have been alerted to this phenomenon and total prostatectomy is rarely done in the United States solely on the basis of rectal findings.

Four benign lesions of the prostate are most frequently confused with carcinoma: chronic prostatitis, prostatic atrophy, intra-acinar, (cribriform) hyperplasia, and involutional changes in the seminal vesicles.

Chronic prostatitis may be manifested in one or more of several reaction patterns. A typical granulomatous prostatitis showing multinucleated giant cells, epithelioid cells and chronic inflammatory cells is easily diagnosed but in cases where there are sheets of cells with pale pink staining or clear cytoplasm surrounding small dark staining nuclei, the appearance may simulate PCa. It is principally the cells with clear cytoplasm (Fig. 12) that may be misdiagnosed as carcinoma. Careful examination will demonstrate that these cells are, in fact, balooned lymphocytes. The distinguishing features are the small

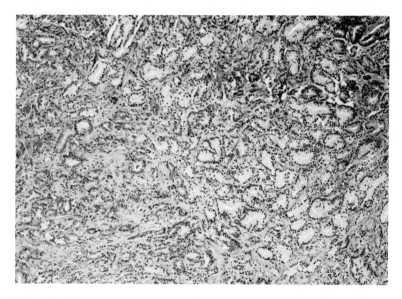

Fig. 5. Carcinoma consisting of small glands.
AFIP Neg. 86-9493 X 100.

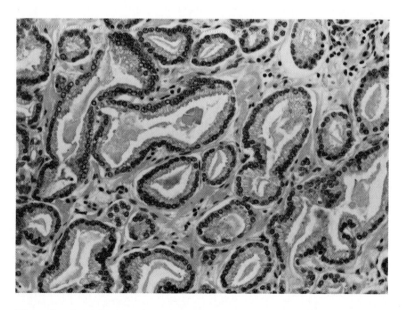

Fig. 6. Carcinoma consisting of large glands.
AFIP Neg. 86-9494 X 100.

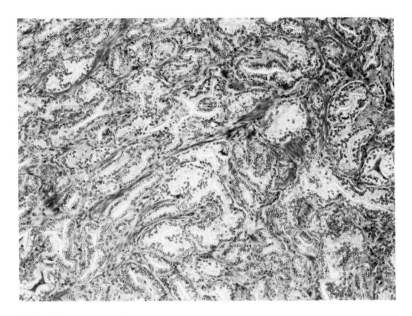

Fig. 7. Carcinoma. The glands are closely
packed. AFIP Neg. 86-9495 X 100.

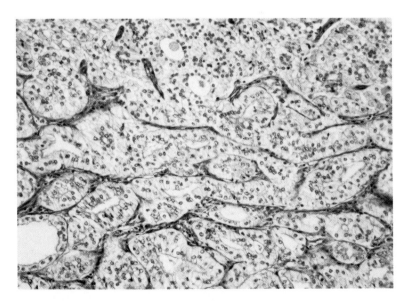

Fig. 8. Carcinoma consisting of fused
glands. AFIP Neg. 86-9496 X 160.

dark nuclei, absence of any acinar or tubular structural
arrangement (although there may be an occasional preexist-
acinus) and the invariable association of the infiltrate
with a duct, sometimes with a loss of the epithelial lining
and presence of exudate in the lumen. (Fig. 12)

Another benign lesion that is often confused with PCa
is the so-called atrophy. The term quiescent is perhaps a
better designation but atrophy is commonly used in the
literature. In this condition the acini may be collapsed,
but they are small, closely packed and lined by a single
layer of cuboidal cells with small dark staining nuclei.
(Fig. 13) The supporting stroma consists of fibrous sometimes hyalinized connective tissue. The entire structure
has an organoid pattern with the acini arranged around a
duct.

Intra-acinar (cribriform) hyperplasia is another
benign lesion that is often misdiagnosed PCa. As the name
indicates, there is gland in gland growth but certain features indicate the benign nature of the lesion. In cribriform hyperplasia the glands have a delicate fibrovascular
stroma. They show a distinct basal layer of cells with
vesicular nuclei (Fig. 14). The cell population is fairly
uniform with nuclei that are identical throughout. Intra-
acinar hyperplasia is frequently associated with acini that
show basal cell hyperplasia. There is always some stromal
hyperplasia. In contrast, cribriform carcinoma usually
lacks a basal cell layer, there is no delicate fibrovascular stroma supporting the glands, the nuclei are invariably
pyknotic at the center, there is usually small acinar or
large acinar carcinoma nearby and the stroma is not hyperplastic.

Perhaps the most frequent source of confusion is the
seminal vesicle that is the seat of involution. In older
patients biopsy may consist of tissue that has several
acinar (ductal) structures that are closely packed together
and lined either by a single layer or 2 - 3 layers of cells.
The luminal cells are often bizarre. The nuclei are large,
sometimes giant sized, and intensely dark staining (Fig.15).
Viewed by themselves the nuclei are quite bothersome.
Several features, however, lead to proper recognition of the
lesion. The large and bizarre nuclei have no visible architecture. They are densely staining, have no vacuoles or
nucleoli. The nuclear cytoplasmic ratio is normal. Many

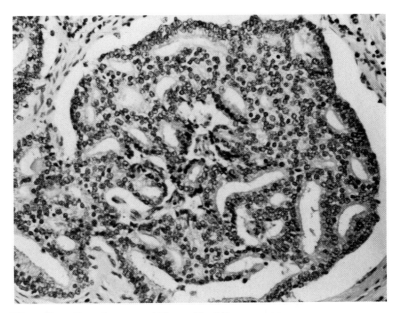

Fig. 9. Carcinoma with cribriform pattern.
AFIP Neg. 86-9497 X 100.

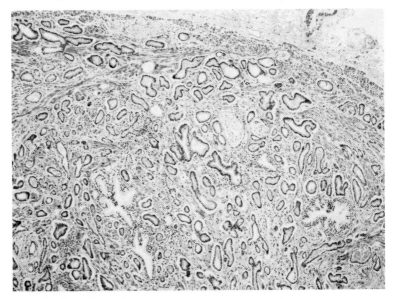

Fig. 10. Carcinoma showing haphazard distribution of glands & large & small glands side
by side. AFIP Neg. 86-9498 X 60.

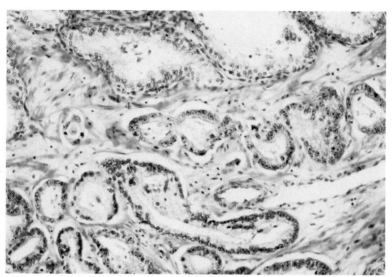

Fig. 11. Hyperplasia & carcinoma double layer
of nuclei of hyperplastic glands versus single
layer of nuclei in the carcinoma. AFIP Neg.
86-9499 X 250.

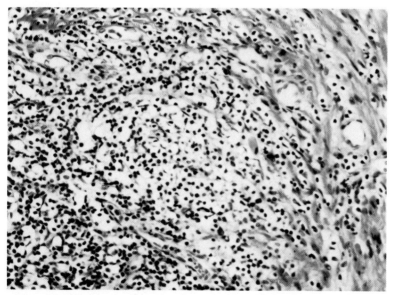

Fig. 12. Chronic prostatitis with balooned
lymphocytes simulating carcinoma. AFIP Neg.
86-9500 X 250.

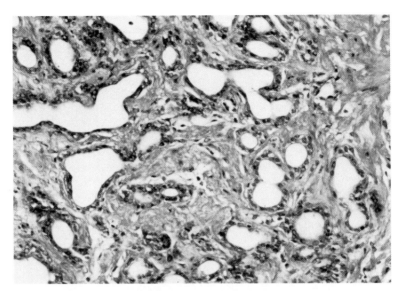

Fig.13. Atrophy. The acini are lined by a
single layer of small cells simulating
carcinoma. AFIP Neg. 86-9501 X 160.

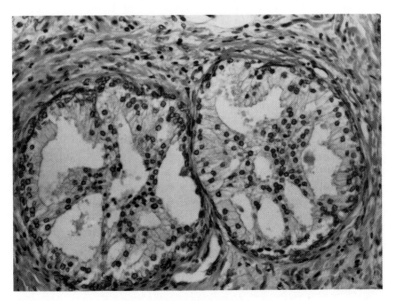

Fig. 14. Intra acinar cribriform hyperplasia
simulating carcinoma. Compare to Fig. 9.
AFIP Neg. 86-9502 X 100.

of the cells contain brownish pigment, the abnormal cells
are either luminal or desquamated, the acini have an organoid pattern arranged around a central duct.

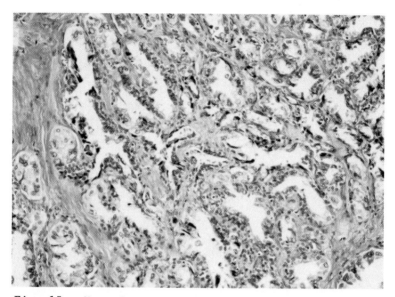

Fig. 15. Normal seminal vesicle. Closely
packed ducts simulate carcinoma. AFIP Neg.
86-9503 X 60.

Misdiagnosis includes not only over diagnosis but under
diagnosis as well. Not infrequently well differentiated
carcinomas are dismissed as atypia. The acini are small,
closely packed. The nuclei are more or less the same size
and shape. At other times the neoplastic cells permeate the
tissue and are interpreted as macrophages.(Figs 16-17)Care-
ful examination will reveal variation in the shape of nuclei,
nuclear vacuolization and a large, prominent ill defined
nucleolus.

The continued misdiagnosis of carcinoma of prostate is
very disturbing. In 1986 in our material which is highly
selected, over 10% of prostatic biopsies that are sent in
for consultation continue to be misdiagnosed. It can reliably be said that progress in diagnosis of PCa has been
limited. There is need for research to improve the criter-

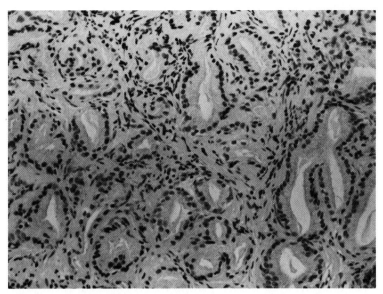

Fig. 16. Missed well differentiated carcinoma.
Small & large acini lined by a single layer of
cells. AFIP Neg. 86-9504 X 100.

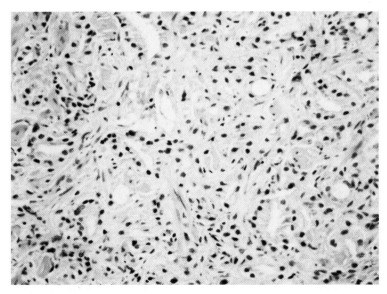

Fig. 17. Missed carcinoma of prostate. Infil-
trating cells misinterpreted as reactive cells.
AFIP Neg. 86-9505 X 250.

ia for diagnosis of anaplasia and invasion, and detection of metastatic potential of PCa. Secondly, there is need for education of the pathologist.

2. Progress in pathologic prognostication

The situation relative to prognosis is more complicated. There are 2 important factors in prognosis: The host and the tumor.* We know very little about the host. Many tumors remain dormant during the life of the patient and are discovered only by the pathologist if he happens to examine the prostate carefully at post mortem examination. Some patients live for many years with their prostatic cancer even with metastasis, with or without treatment. In contrast in others the disease takes a rapid downhill course.

As far as the tumor is concerned, Broders (1926) introduced grading as a method of prognostication. The system was based on differentiation. There has been much controversy about reliability of grading of any tumor and the problem is magnified in PCa. From 1926, when Broders introduced his grading system, to 1976, over 30 grading systems had been proposed for PCa. Mostofi (1976) has discussed the situation in detail. Suffice it to say that in addition to confusion about anaplasia and differentiation that PCa has along with other tumors, in PCa we have some other problems. Many PCas are slow growing tumors. Many have an unpredictable behavior and with treatment or even without treatment the patient may live for many years. PCas have a wide range of histologic patterns.

In 1966 Gleason, of the Veterans Administration observing that the majority of PCas had more than one growth pattern, proposed that a primary and a secondary pattern be recognized. In both categories he identified 5 different patterns. These have been described in detail (Gleason 1966, 1977; Mellinger et al 1967, 1977). If only one pattern was seen the value was doubled. If several patterns were seen, the 2 most prominent were taken. The primary and the secondary patterns both were equally important, regardless of their relative proportions.

---

*We have excluded the urologist's role in altering the prognosis of PCa because there is some evidence that the urologist probably does not change the course of PCa.

Mellinger et al (1977) claimed that by adding the tumor stage (calculated from 1 to 4) to the primary and secondary patterns they obtained better prognostic results. Gleason (1977) has correlated his own system to other grading systems. His 2-4 are grouped as Grade 1, his 5-7 are grouped as grade II, his 8, 9, 10 as grade III.

Although in several publications Gleason (1966,1977) and Mellinger et al (1967, 1977) claimed good correlation of Gleason system with clinical behavior the system was not accepted by pathologists as evidenced by lack of any reports.

In 1979 the NPCP called a meeting in Buffalo, N. Y. to evaluate four of the many existing grading systems for PCa. The details of the 4 systems have been reported elsewhere. (Murphy & Whitmore 1979, Mostofi 1986).

The NPCP recommended that PCas be graded and the Gleason system be used tentatively at least in conjunction with any other system; that nuclear and cytologic characteristics be considered in prospective studies to further the discriminative capabilities of the Gleason system and that data be accumulated on the correlation between grade of the tumor, the natural history of the disease and the response to various forms of therapy. At the time of the recommendation it was claimed that the system was readily learned, reproducible and reliable. In this claim the NPCP relied heavily on Gleason (1966 & 1977), Gleason & Mellinger (1974),Mellinger et al (1967) and Mellinger (1977). The only other report on the system was by Harada et al (1977) but these authors had had 2 tutorials from Gleason and reported a reproducibility of 70%. They also recorded reproducibility by the same individual on two different occasions to be 64% for primary patterns and 44% for secondary and only 38% for the sum of the two. Gleason's personal reproducibility has been reported to be 80%. (Murphy & Whitmore, 1979).

Many pathologists, including the authors, have found it necessary to have personal tutorial from Gleason, to obtain reasonable competence in using the system.

Is the Gleason system reliable?

In 2 surveys of the literature (Grayhack & Assimos,1982 and Mostofi, 1986)it has been surmised that about one-third of the reports found the Gleason system reliable, the other two-thirds, that it was unreliable. But the number of cases studied in all these reports was small.

Dissatisfaction with the Gleason system has led to several other grading systems (Dhom (1977, 1985), Gaeta et al (1980), Brawn et al, 1981, and Mostofi et al, 1980, and Bocking et al, 1982. These systems are based on differentiation and/or anaplasia as recommended by WHO Panel of Experts on PCa. (Mostofi et al, 1980). The Panel had endeavored to clarify anaplasia and differentiation. Anaplasia was defined as variation in size, shape and staining of nuclei, and divided into slight, moderate and marked.(Figs. 18-20) Differentiation was defined as formation of glands. Tumors that formed glands were differentiated. Glands were further subclassified into large glands, small glands, fused glands or glands in glands. (Figs. 8-10) Tumors that did not form glands occurred as columns, cords or solid sheets. (Fig.21-22)

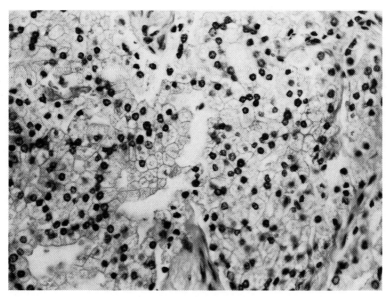

Fig. 18. Carcinoma nuclear grade I. AFIP Neg.86-9506 X 160.

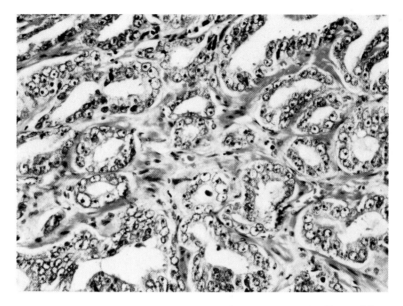

Fig. 19. Carcinoma nuclear grade II. AFIP Neg. 86-9507 X 160.

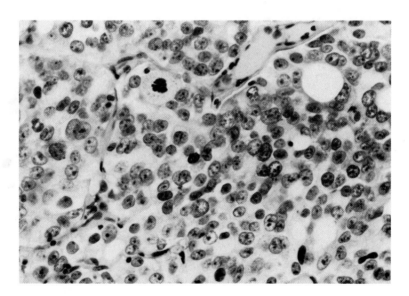

Fig. 20. Carcinoma - nuclear grade III. AFIP Neg. 86-9508 X 160.

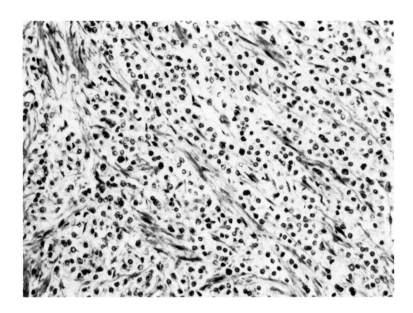

Fig. 21. Carcinoma forming columns and cords.
AFIP Neg. 86-9509 X 100.

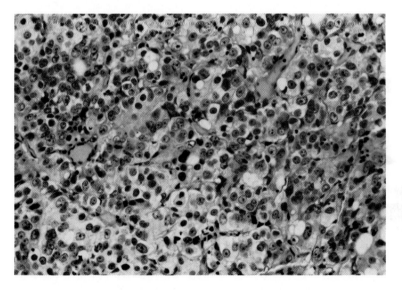

Fig. 22. Carcinoma forming solid sheets.
AFIP Neg. 86-9509 X 100.

In a study of about 1,000 PCa, Harada et al (1977) demonstrated that slight nuclear anaplasia was associated with
no cancer deaths (0 out of 107), whereas, tumors with marked
nuclear anaplasia showed 14.88 deaths (63 in 127) and those
with moderate nuclear anaplasia had an intermediate death
rate (144 in 564). Adding nuclear grade (1 to 3) to stage
(1 to 4) gave the following results: For 97 patients
with sum of 7 the rates were 25.92: for 357 with sum of 6,
the rates were 8.53; for 342 with sum of 5, the rates were
2.75, and for 191 patients with stage and grade sum of 2 to
4 death rates were 0.46.

In 758 patients Bocking et al (1982) combined histologic grading with nuclear grading. Four histologic grades
were recognized based on glandular differentiation and 3
cytologic grades based on nuclear anaplasia.

The sum of 2 - 3 was classed as grade 1, 4 - 5 as
grade ll and 6 - 7 as grade III. Thirty-five percent of
patients with grade III PCa had metastases at the time of
admission, whereas, none of grade I PCa had metastases.
The histologic and cytologic grading system utilized by
Bocking et al were essentially those of WHO (Mostofi et al
1980).

All of the grading systems, including those for PCa,
have several deficiencies: They all recognize good tumors
and bad tumors to varying degrees of accuracy but most of
the patients fall in the intermediate category; no grading
system is applicable to the individual patient; none of the
systems can reliably predict the lethal potential of a tumor
in an individual patient, nor the responsiveness of the
tumor to various forms of therapy.

In summarizing the situation relative to pathologic
prognostication in PCa, one must conclude that progress in
pathological grading and prognostication has been limited
and disappointing - it has not given the urologist reliable
information on the management of the patient with PCa.

Before leaving the subject 2 other attempts at pathologic prognostication may be mentioned. Tannenbaum et al
(1982) measured nucleolar surface area by stereoscopically
analyzing pictures obtained by the back-scattered electron
imaging attachment to a scanning electron microscope. The
details are given elsewhere (Tannenbaum et al 1982). They

reported that progressive disease was always accompanied by nucleolar surface area measurement larger than 2.40 um ^{2}. The number of cases was small and, unfortunately, the method is not practical for every day use.

A second approach has been reported by Diamond et al (1982). Briefly stated, the shape and morphology of the nuclei were determined by computer assisted image analysis using fixed sections studied by light microscopy. The mean nuclear roundness factor for all PCa nuclei was 1.059, for benign nuclei it was 1.034. The mean nuclear roundness factor for those who were alive and well 14 years or more post-operatively was 1.047, for those which had metastasized it was 10.69. Epstein et al (1984) have confirmed the observations. This study has focused attention on the nuclei of PCa and introduced quantitative morphometry and the computer - the former valuable for accuracy and reproducibility and the latter for easy storage and recall. But the number of cases reported are small.

The introduction of fine needle aspiration for diagnosis of PCa - a technic that has been extensively utilized in Europe, especially Scandinavia, and is coming into the USA, will, in fact, require diagnosis and grading of PCa primarily in the individual tumor cells and not on pattern of growth.

3. Progress in predicting response of the tumor to therapy.

Treatment of PCa has increasingly become dependent on the stage of the tumor. In each stage, however, one or more of several therapeutic regimens are available, and to some degree the decision has been based on histology. Should a patient with Stage A disease be followed? Should he have total prostatectomy or radiation therapy? In some centers the number of fragments involved, the grade and the presence of residual carcinoma on second TUR are used to separate those to be followed from those to be treated. For stage B patients radical prostatectomy is favored in many centers but radiation therapy has many advocates. For C and D patients the problem is more complicated: radiotherapy (which type) anti androgen therapy (which type) or chemotherapy (which agent).

Understandably, the urologist would like the pathologist to reliably predict the response of the tumor to the
specific therapy.

Kastendieck & Altenahr (1975) in a study of 28 histologically proven PCas, could not relate the various histological or cytological elements to response to therapy.
Sinha et al (1977) reported the ultrastructural
features of 22 PCa, of whom 8 had been treated with 1-5 mg
of DES and 30 mg provera daily for varying periods and 14
untreated patients. They recognized 2 distinct basal cells:
Type I (light) and type II dark cells. The detail of the
cell types is discussed elsewhere. (Sinha et al 1977).
Suffice it to say that PCas which were or subsequently became
refractory to estrogen therapy showed more abundant type II
basal cells than responsive patients. They postulated that
type II basal cells as well as some type I basal cells are
endocrine unresponsive from the onset.

Dhom & Degro(1982) noted that low differentiated PCas
often show lymph node metastases and skeletal metastasis and
are frequently resistant against hormone therapy. These
observations have not been confirmed.

Evaluation of the response to specific form of therapy
has received some attention. Elsewhere we have discussed
in detail the changes induced by estrogen therapy in PCa
cells. (Mostofi & Price, 1973).

Responsive neoplastic cells show the following changes:
A decrease or loss of secretions, and of acid phosphatase
and other enzyme activity,reduction of 50% in size of the
nuclei, condensation of chromatin and pyknosis, loss of
nucleoli, vacuolization of cytoplasm beginning in the basal
layer, coalescence of vacuoles, rupture of cell membrane,
fragmentation of pyknotic nuclei and cessation of mitotic
activity.

A less well known phenomenon is the development of
squamous carcinoma in patients who have been given estrogen
therapy. Some of these may originate from prostatic ductal
epithelial cells, others may come from the tumor cells themselves. We have seen the changes both in the primary and in
metastases.

Pertschuk, L. P., et al (1985) have discussed the positive value of androgen and estrogen receptors in tumor cells
as determined biochemically and histochemically. These may
be valuable in predicting which tumors will respond to
hormone therapy.

The changes brought about by radiation therapy have been
subject of controversy. Radiotherapists have insisted that
the tumor cells in post-radiation biopsy that appear viable
are, in fact, incapable of growth and multiplication.

Kastendieck et al (1975), Dhom & Degro (1982) and Dhom
(1985) have clarified the nature of the radiation induced
changes. Although the regressive changes in tumor cells
after radiation therapy are identical to those of estrogen
therapy, there are some differences: The cytoplasm shows a
considerable dilatation and vacuolization. The cells may be
flattened into tubules leading to cystically dilated spaces.
The nuclei are pyknotic; nucleoli are not detectable. The
nuclei are often bizarre. In other areas shrunken tumor cells
or small complexes of tumor can be found which can hardly be
recognized as complexes of tumors. Prostatic acid phosphatase and prostatic specific antigen are positive in many of
these cells. The stroma may show edema and polymorphonuclear
infiltration in early stages; in later stages there is fibro-
sis and radiation vasculopathy.

Dhom & Degro (1982), Dhom (1985) have offered a grading
system for regression. The unaffected tumor is given a score
of ten (10), those showing marked regression are given a
score of zero (0).

10-8 No or only slight regression.
6-4   Moderate to marked regression.
2-0   Marked regression or - no detectable tumor.

The significance of these observations is that if the
biopsy does not manifest these changes the cells must be considered viable. In evaluating post therapy changes, it is
obviously necessary to have pre-treatment tissue for comparison.

In summary there has been progress in evaluating response to therapy and hope that we may be able to predict
which tumors will respond to hormone therapy.

4. <u>Progress in understanding the biology and natural history of PCa cell</u>.

A. Heterogeneity of PCa Cell

By light microscopy as many as 5 different cells may be found:

Clear cells, dark cells, eosinophilic cells, vacuolated cells and cells with amphophilic cytoplasm. Most of PCa contain at least 2 cell types but the clinical significance of the variations in cell types has not been investigated.

Kastendieck and Altenahr (1975) studied 28 PCas ultra-structurally. They found 5 different cells: Immature cells, highly differentiated cells, functionally deranged cells and degenerative tumor cells. The authors did not relate the cell type to behavior or response to therapy.

Mention has already been of the observations of Sinha et al (1977) that 2 distinct basal cells were present in their PCas and that PCas which were or became refractory to therapy showed more abundant type II basal cells.

Application of immunopathology has demonstrated the heterogeneity of the cytoplasm of cells which, by H&E stains seem identical. Sesterhenn et al (1985) have reported that in studies of several hundred PCas for prostatic acid phos-phatase (PAP) and prostatic specific antigen (PA), all grades of PCA have some cells that are negative for one or the other or both, others that are strongly positive for one or the other or both, and some that are weakly positive. Of special interest is their observation that in histologically undifferentiated tumors (tumors that do not form glands but consist of sheets of cells)cells that are identical with H&E stains may give strongly positive, slightly positive or entirely negative reaction with either PAP or PA. These ob-servations indicate that despite apparent homogeneity of tumor cells as seen in H&E stained sections, PCa cells have heterogeneity of immune reactive population. The authors did not relate the observations to response to therapy or survival and mortality.

Epstein & Eggleston (1984) studied 19 patients with PCa. Of 12 PCa with areas of either weak or negative PAP reaction 9 progressed. Two of the seven PCas that did not have these foci also progressed. Of 12 patients with only moderate or

intense staining the tumor did not progress in 8. This correlation was said to be statistically significant. They
reported the superiority of PA over PAP, and concluded that
the presence of cells that lack sufficient differentiation
to express normally present immunologically recognizable
antigens is an indication of potentially more aggressive
behavior.

More interesting and exacting is the report of Benson & Walsh
(1980). By the use of flow cytometry they proposed a grading index related to pathologic stage. In one patient confined tumor had a mean grade of 1.5; 4 patients with capsular penetration only had a mean grade of 2.5 and 2 patients
with capsular penetration and seminal vesicle invasion had
a mean grade of 3.5. These authors used fresh tissue but
flow cytometry can now be applied to fixed tissues and it
is hoped that these observations will be confirmed by a
larger number of cases.

Sesterhenn et al (1985) observed some interesting reaction with peanut lectin staining. Generally speaking, it
was the basal cell that seemed to react; however, some secretory cells also reacted raising the question of heterogeneity of cell population in normal and hyperplastic
prostates.

Summarizing the situation we can state that diversion
of long overdue attention to the PCa cell has revealed that
we are dealing with a heterogeneous cell population observed
not only by light and electron microscopy but functionally
as well as evidenced by the reaction to PAP and PA.

B. Precancerous States

Mostofi & Price (1973) were the first to call attention
to certain alterations in atrophic and hyperplastic glands
which they interpreted as malignant transformation of the
epithelium. In atrophic glands this consisted of nuclear
enlargement,vacuolization,and the presence of a distinct
nucleolus. They demonstrated that while the cells lining
glands retained their small size resembling atrophic acini
the nuclei were distinctly anaplastic and the glands in-
vaded the stroma and the perineural spaces.

In hyperplastic glands while the acini maintained the
hyperplastic pattern, the benign secretory epithelium was

replaced by anaplastic cells with vacuolated nuclei and large irregularly outlined nucleoli. The epithelium was sometimes piled up.

The authors reported that they had observed these changes in prostates removed for carcinoma. Although they believed that these constituted early malignant transformation of the epithelium, they had not observed progression of the lesion to distinct PCa.

Kastendieck & Altenahr (1976), Kastendieck et al (1976), Kastendieck (1980) proposed the term "dysplasia" to denote unusual or atypical proliferation in glands, cytological atypia of proliferating epithelium and disorganization of morphologic unity between glandular epithelium and fibromuscular stroma. In 1980, Kastendieck substituted atypical primary hyperplasia for dysplasia, which he defined as irregular architecture of glands lined by atypical cells together with focal indistinct demarcation of glandular epithelium and stroma.

Kastendieck (1980) found atypical hyperplasia in 106 of 180 patients with PCa. Early stages of PCa were associated with atypical primary hyperplasia in 83.3%. For other details the reader is referred to Kastendieck (1980a)

Helpap (1980) compared typical hyperplasia with atypical hyperplasia and PCa by the use of tritiated (3H) thymidine autoradiography. Briefly summarized Helpap reported the average labeling index in 65 cases of simple glandular hyperplasia to be 0.49 $\pm$ 0.4%. In 11 cases of prostatic hyperplasia with cellular atypia but without carcinoma labeling index averaged 1.60$\pm$ 0.8%. In atypical hyperplasia with pronounced cellular and structural atypia adjacent to adenocarcinoma the labeling index was 1.50 $\pm$ 0.84 percent. Single values, however, ranged from 0.2 to 4.1%. This range of labeling indices was comparable to that of poorly differentiated adenocarcinoma (0.2 - 2.4 percent) and cribriform carcinoma (0.4-5.7 percent).

McNeal & Bostwick have reported a study of 100 serially blocked prostates with carcinoma and 100 benign prostates obtained at autopsy. Referring to the atypia as intraductal dysplasia and grading it 1 to 3, they found 82% of the former and 43% of the latter contained such foci. Grade 3 dysplasia was found in 33% of the prostates with cancer but in only 4%

of benign prostates. They reported that the frequency of multiple independent invasive carcinomas was high among prostates with multiple foci of dysplasia and concluded that dysplasia is probably a direct biologic precursor of PCa and may be the antecedent lesion in the majority of PCas.

We find some problems with this report. While their figures 3, 4 and 9 may represent ducts, figs. 1, 2, 5,6,8&10 are obviously not ducts. The introduction of dysplasia into prostatic malignancy after the problems it has created in the cervix and the bladder is most regrettable. If the lesion fulfills the criteria of PCas as their figures 8 and 10 do, it should be called carcinoma. If it does not fulfill the criteria (e.g.,their figures 1, 2,3 & 4) atypia would seem to be a more desirable term.

Bostwick & Brawer (1986) have added to the confusion by introduction of the term intraepithelial neoplasia (PIN) as substitute for McNeal & Bostwick's dysplasia. PIN is by far preferable to the term "dysplasia".

Earlier in this manuscript reference was made to the claim of these authors that the negative reaction to the antikeratin monoclonal antibody indicated disruption of basal cell layer and evidence of invasion. The authors reported close correlation between such disruption of basal cell layer and PIN grades. It was present in 0.7% of PIN 1, 15% of PIN 2 and 56% of PIN 3. The amount of disruption also increased with increasing grades of PIN, with loss of more than one-third of basal layer in 52% of foci of PIN 3 compared with less than 2% in lower grades of PIN. If invasion occurs commonly in association with high grade intraepithelial neoplasia as the authors claim, how can these be distinguished from PCas that do not show invasion and why should it be called PIN?

Oyasu et al (1986) reported the frequency and distribution of atypical hyperplasia in 51 total prostatectomy specimens for cancer. They had 13 major findings. Atypical hyperplasia was more frequent in prostatectomy (48 of 51) than in autopsy specimens (14 of 37) noncancerous patients. The distribution of atypical hyperplasia and carcinoma in prostatectomy specimens was similar; in majority of prostatectomy specimens atypical hyperplasia, when found, was located at sites separate from carcinoma as well as in contiguous areas.

In a detailed review of precancerous states of the prostate, Mostofi (1984) discussed the relationship of hyperplasia and its variants (atypia, atypical hyperplasia, atypical adenomatous hyperplasia), to carcinoma. To this list may be added dysplasia and PIN. As already noted, there is considerable confusion as to what is meant by these terms and the published descriptions and illustrations from different reports record a bewildering variety of changes - a group of closely packed acini, intra-acinar hyperplasia with papillary or cribriform growth, secondary, post-atrophic hyperplasia, basal cell hyperplasia, transitional cell metaplasia, anaplastic epithelium lining hyperplastic acini and even well differentiated carcinoma. We believe that if a lesion can be identified as some form of hyperplasia, it should be so designated.

The term "atypia" should be reserved for 2 categories of change: When the growth pattern is disturbing but not typical of carcinoma and when nuclear changes are abnormal but do not fulfill the criteria for diagnosis of carcinoma. When hyperplastic or atrophic acinar epithelium displays changes that resemble carcinoma we prefer to designate the area as malignant change.

Our objection to dysplasia is that it has been found confusing when applied to cervix and bladder, and the same is applicable to the prostate. For 2 reasons we have refrained from using carcinoma in situ (CIS): CIS has been used for several different lesions in the prostate, and secondly, it has not been demonstrated that left alone such lesions will progress to carcinoma. This also applies to PIN.

When such areas are found in specimens from transurethral resection for benign hyperplasia the urological surgeon should be alerted to the possible presence of a carcinoma elsewhere in the gland, and this should be ruled out.

In summary, it may be said that attention has been focused on certain changes in the epithelium but, unfortunately, the multiplicity of the terms used for these changes has resulted in considerable confusion. It is hoped that if the changes can be recognized as some type of hyperplasia or metaplasia they would be so labeled, if they resemble carcinoma they should be so designated, if the histology or cytology is disturbing but not pathognomonic of carcinoma, they should be designated as atypia.

C. Relationship of Metastases to the Primary

Information relative to the relationship between the
structure of the primary and that of the metastases has been
meager. In preliminary studies in our laboratory we have
found that in over 90% of cases, the structure of the
metastases is identical to that of the primary.

The majority of metastatic tumors showed more than one
pattern and more than one grade of anaplasia. Taking differentiation alone, in 95% all patterns seen in the primary
were found in the metastases. Looking at anaplasia alone,
in 70% all grades seen in the primary were present in the
metastases. In addition one or more grades seen in the
primary were present in the metastases. Thus in 97% the
grades of the tumors in the metastases reflected those seen
in the primary. These observations, if confirmed, would
suggest that true dedifferentiation is very rare and whatever is seen in the metastases was probably present but
perhaps missed in the primary.

(The opinions or assertions contained in this paper are
the personal views of the authors and are not to be con-
strued as official or as reflecting the views of the
Department of the Army or the Department of Defense.)

REFERENCES

1. Benson, MC, Walsh PC (1986). The application of
flow cytometry and the assessment of tumor cell heterogeneity and the grading of human prostatic cancer; a preliminary
report. J. Urol. 135:1194-1198.
2. Bocking, A., Kiehn, J., Heinzel-Wach, M.: (1982)
Combined histologic grading prostatic carcinoma. Cancer 288-
294.
3. Bostwick, DG, Brawer, MK (1986) Prostatic intraepi-
theliel neoplasia (PIN) and early neoplasia in prostatic
cancer. Lab Investigation 54:7A (Abstract)
4. Brawer, MK, Peeble, DM, Stamey, TA, Bostwick, DG
(1985) Keratin immunoreactivity in the benign and neoplastic
human prostate. Cancer Research 45:3663-3667.
5. Brawn, PN, Ayala AA, von Eschenbach AC, Hussey DH,
Johnson DE(1981) Histologic grading study of prostatic adenocarcinoma. The development of a new system and comparison with other methods. Cancer 49:113-120.

6. Broders AC (1925) The grading of carcinoma. Minn. Med. 8:726-730, 1925.

7. Dhom G (1985) Histopathology of prostatic carcinoma. Diagnosis and differential diagnosis. Path. Res. Pract. 179: 277-3-3.

8.Dhom, G. (1977) Classification and grading of prostatic carcinoma. Rec Results. Cancer Research 60:14-26.

9. Dhom, G., Degro, S. (1982) Therapy of prostatic cancer and histopathologic follow up. Prostate 3:531-542.

10. Diamond, DA, Berry, SJ, Umbricht, C, Jewett, HJ, Coffey, DC (1982). Computerized image analysis of nuclear shape as a prognostic factor for prostatic cancer. The Prostate 3:321-332.

12. Epstein, J.I., Eggleston JC (1984). Immunohistochemical localization of prostatic specific acid phosphatase and prostatic-specific antigen in stage A2 adenocarcinoma of the prostate. Human Path. 15:853-859.

13. Gaeta JF, Asirwatham JE, Miller G, Murphy GP: Histologic grading primary prostatic cancer: A new approach to an old problem (1980). J Urol 123:689-693.

13.Gleason, DF (1966) Classification of prostatic carcinomas. Cancer Chemother Rep:125-128.

14. Gleason DF (1977) Histologic grading and clinical staging of prostatic carcinoma. In Tannenbaum, M. (Ed) Urologic Pathology: The Prostate. Phila., Lea & Febiger,171-198.

15. Gleason DF, Mellinger GT, The Veterans' Administration Cooperative Urological Research Group.(1974)Prediction of prognosis for prostatic adenocarcinoma and combined histological grading and clinical staging. J Urol 111:58-64.

16. Grayhack, JT, Assimos, DG (1983) Prognostic significance of tumor grade and stage in patients with carcinoma of the prostate. (1983) The Prostate 4:13-31.

17. Harada, M., Mostofi, FK, Corle,DK, Byar, DP, Trump, BF (1977) Preliminary studies of histological prognosis in cancer of the prostate. Cancer Treat. Rep. 61:223-225.

18. Helpap, B.(1980) The biologic significance of atypical hyperplasia of the prostate. Virchows Arch. A Path Anat. 387:307-317.

19. Kastendieck, H. (1980) Morphologie des Prostatakarzinoms in Stanzbiopsien und totalen Prostatektomien. Pathologe 2:31-43.

20. Kastendieck, H. (1980) Prostatic carcinoma. Aspects of pathology prognosis and therapy.J. Cancer Res clin Oncol 96:131-156.

21. Kastendieck, H. (1980) Correlation between atypical primary hyperplasia and carcinoma of the prostate. (1980 a) Path Res Pract 169:366-387.

22. Kastendieck, H. Altenahr, E.(1976) Cyto - and Histomorphogenesis of the prostatic carcinoma. A comparative light and electron microscopic study. Virchows Arch. Path Anat. 370:207-224.

23. Kastendieck, H., Altenahr, E., Husselman, H. and Bressel, M. (1976) Carcinoma and dysplastic lesions of the prostate. A histomorphological analysis of 50 total prostatectomies by step section technique. Z. Krebsforsch (1976) 88:33-54.

24. McNeal, J.E. & Bostwick, D.G.(1986)Intraductal dysplasia:A premalignant lesion of the prostate. Human Pathol. 17:64-71.

25. Mellinger, GT, Gleason, DF and Bailar, J. III. (1967) The histology and prognosis of prostatic cancer. J. Urol. 97:331-337.

26. Mellinger, GT (1977) Prognosis of prostatic carcinoma. In:Grundmann,E., Vahlsieck, W.Eds. Tumors of the Male Genital System: Recent Results in Cancer Research. Vol. 60,Berlin, Springer-Verlag,61-72.

27. Mostofi, FK (1952) Criteria for pathologic diagnosis of carcinoma of the prostate. In Proceedings of the Second National Cancer Conference. Phila. Amer. Cancer Soc., Inc.

28. Mostofi, FK. Problems of grading carcinoma of prostate. (1976) In Jarbo,JW (Ed)Seminars in Oncology, Vol. 3, Washington, Grune & Stratton.

29. Mostofi, FK, Sesterhenn, I.,Sobin,LH (1980) International Histological Classification of Prostatic Tumors. Geneva, WHO.

30. Mostofi, FK (1984)Precancerous lesions of the prostate. In Precancerous States. (Ed) Carter, RL, London, N.Y., Toronto, Oxford University Press.

31. Mostofi, FK, Price,EB Jr:(1973) Tumors of the Male Genital System (Fasc.8) Atlas of Tumor Pathology, 2nd Series, Armed Forces Inst. of Pathology, Wash. DC.

32. Murphy, GP, Whitmore, WF (1979) A report of the workshops on the current status of the histologic grading of prostate cancer. Cancer 44:1490-1494.

33. Oyasu, M., Balinson, RR, Nowels, K.,Garnet,JE. (1986) Cytological atypia in the prostate gland: frequency, distribution and possible relevance to carcinoma. J Urol 135:959-962.

34. Pertschuk LP, Eisenberg, KB, Macchia, RJ, Feldman JG (1985) Heterogeneity of steroid binding sites in prostatic carcinoma:morphological demonstration and clinical implications. The Prostate 6: 35-47.

35. Sesterhenn,I., Mostofi, FK, Davis, CJ Jr.: (1985) Immunopathology in prostate and bladder tumors in Immunocytochemistry. In Tumor Diagnosis. Ed:J. Russo. Boston, Dordrecht & Lancaster. Martinius Nijhoff Publ.

36. Sinha, A.A., Blackard, C.E., Seal, U.S.(1977) A critical analysis of tumor morphology and hormone treatments in the untreated and estrogen treated response and refractory human prostatic carcinoma. Cancer 40:2836-2850.

37. Tannenbaum, M., Tannenbaum, S., DeSandis, P.N, and Olson, C.A. (L982)Prognostic significance of nucleolar surface area in prostatic cancer. Urology 19:546-551.

Prostate Cancer, Part A: Research, Endocrine
Treatment, and Histopathology, pages 477–483
© 1987 Alan R. Liss, Inc.

IMMUNOHISTOCHEMISTRY IN THE DIAGNOSIS OF DIFFICULT CASES OF PROSTATIC CANCER

J.M. Caillaud, M.C. Mathieu, C. Carlu
Histo-pathologie, Institut Gustave Roussy,
Villejuif, France

Immunohistochemistry (IMH) of prostatic lesions is essentially based on the study of prostatic acid phosphatase (PSAP) and prostatic specific antigen (PSA). The technical modalities of IMH and the distribution of the labelling of PSAP and PSA in the normal prostate and in prostatic cancer have been described previously.

IMH may be an aid to the diagnosis of prostatic adenocarcinoma (PC) in several situations : 1) identification of a metastatic site in a patients with no known primary ; 2) identification of a new tumour site, metastatic or otherwise in a patients with known PC ; 3) identification of the primary prostatic tumour : undifferentiated prostatic carcinoma, differential diagnosis between bladder and prostatic cancer, unusual appearance of PC, differential diagnosis between PC and basal cell hyperplasia or atypical hyperplasia.

I - IDENTIFICATION OF A METASTATIC LESION IN A PATIENT WITH NO KNOWN PRIMARY TUMOUR

In the majority of cases this consists of a bone or lymph node metastasis.

The prostatic tumour is confirmed by clinical examination in most cases. In the 9 cases which we have studied (4 bone biopsies and 5 lymph node biopsies), PC was detected in 8 cases. In the other case, the clinical context (bone metastases, raised serum PSAP, IMH results) was judged to be sufficient to commence treatment for PC.

CONCLUSION

IMH of prostatic lesions is valuable from several points of view. It can be performed on classical fixed, paraffin-imbedded material enabling retrospective studies. It has the advantage of a system with two different inputs, PSAP and PSA with good specificity. However, the conjoined study of these two proteins is necessary. In fact, they are different substances which can demonstrate non-identical results on IMH. Moreover, the specificity of PSAP is not strictly limited to the prostate.

IMH of the prostate is a definite aid to diagnosis.

In the study of metastases of adenocarcinoma of unknown origin, the prostatic origin can be easily determined ; this has been demonstrated by a large number of studies. IMH of metastases of adenocarcinoma of unknown origin should not be limited to the study of PSAP and PSA, it should also include thyroglobulin, NSE (neuron specific enolase and CEA to increase the accuracy of the diagnosis of the primary tumour. The same approach should be applied when identifying a new tumour site (metastasis or second tumour ?) in a patient with known PC. Comparison of the reactivities of PC and the new tumour with the different antibodies studied will provide the most accurate conclusion possible.

In undifferentiated carcinomas of the prostate, the positivity to PSAP and/or PSA is preserved in a large number of cases. Some cases remain negative in which case other antibodies should be studied. The detection of NSE appears to be of particular interest, as it allows the identification of neuroendocrine tumours of the prostate.

Cases of PC with unusual morphology may raise the problem of extension of an adjacent gastrointestinal or vesical adeno- carcinoma. In our experience, bladder adenocarcinomas and bladder carcinomas with glandular metaplasia are negative for PSAP and PSA. Gastrointestinal adenocarcinomas are also negative. In contrast, the majority of PC are positive for PSAP : 92 to 100 % and for PSA : 82 to 100 %.

In the prostate itself, IMH can help to distinguish between well differentiated PC and atypical hyperplasia However, although this approach appears to be possible, it must be interpreted very cautiously. The diagnostic criteria in this case are qualitative and are defined by comparison with the reactivity of normal prostatic tissue. In order to confirm the diagnosis of PC of a well differentiated lesion by IMH, the following three features must be associated : decreased intensity of the positivity, variation of the positivity from cell to cell and reinforcement of the positivity in the apical pole of the cell. These features have been demonstrated on electron microscopy for PSAP. The interpretation of the results should be based on well preserved areas away from peripheral zones of the sample and away from areas of prostatitis and degenerative features of the prostate. This type of interpretation also requires good IMH technique and good quality reagents. The constancy of monoclonal antibodies appears to be particularly valuable. The comparison with normal tissues presupposes the persistence of such tissue in the samples examined. In problem cases, which do not present all three of the above criteria, it is impossible to be more precise and the final interpretation will be based on classical histopathological criteria. As in any IMH study, a negative result is difficult to interpret and a positive result should always be interpreted in association with histological findings and the clinical context in order to ensure coherency.

In addition to PSAP and PSA, anti leu-7 (HNK-1) monoclonal antibodies also react with normal and cancerous prostatic tissue. The nature of the corresponding antigen is unknown. This antibody also reacts with certain lymphocytes and, most importantly, with various tissues of neuro-ectodermal origin, which make its diagnostic use delicate.

Cytokeratins are expressed on normal and cancer cells of the prostate. Brawer et al. have described an anti-keratin monoclonal antibody which allows the identification of basal cells of the prostate. The use of this antibody allows the demonstration of the disappearance of the basal cells during malignant transformation of the glandular structures of the prostate.

GENERAL BIBLIOGRAPHY

Allhoff E P, Proppe K H, Chapman C M, Lin C W, Prout G R
(1983). Evaluation of prostate specific acid phosphatase
and prostate specific antigen in identification of prostatic cancer. J. Urol. 129:315-318.

Banerjee D, Thibert R F (1983). Natural killer-like cells
found in B-cell compartments of human lymphoid tissues.
Nature. 304:270-272.

Bates R J, Chapman C M, Prout G R, Lin C W (1982). Immunohistochemical identification of prostatic acid phosphatase:
correlation of tumor grade with acid phosphatase distribution. J. Urol. 127:574-580.

Bentz M S, Cohen C, Demers L M, Budgeon L R (1982). Immuno-
chemical acid phosphatase level and tumor grade in prostatic carcinoma. Arch. Pathol. Lab. Med. 106:476-480.

Bentz M S, Cohen C, Budgeon L R, Demers L M (1984). Evaluation of commercial immunoperoxidase facts in diagnosis of
prostate carcinoma. Urology 23:75-78.

Brawer M K, Peehl D M, Stamey T A, Bostwick D G (1985).
Keratin immunoreactivity in the benign and neoplastic
human prostate. Cancer Res. 45:3663-3667.

Caillaud J.M., Benjelloun S, Bosq J, Braham K, Lipinski M
(1984). HNK-1-defined antigen detected in paraffin-embedded
neurectoderm tumors and those derived from cells of the
amine precursor uptake and decarboxylase system. Cancer
Res. 44:4432-4439.

Dauge M C, Grossin M, Doumecq-Lacoste J M, Vinceneux P,
Delmas V, Bocquet L (1985). Tumeur "carcinoide" de la
prostate. Une nouvelle observation anatomoclinique avec
revue de la litterature. Arch Anat. Cytol. Pathol. 33:73-
79.

Ellis, D W, Leffers S, Davies J S, Alan B P (1984). Multiple
immunoperoxidase markers in benign hyperplasia and adenocarcinoma of the prostate. Am. J. Clin. Path. 81:279-284.

Gleason, D P (1985). Atypical hyperplasia, benign hyperplasia
and well-differentiated adenocarcinoma of the prostate.
Am.J. Surg. Pathol. 9:53-67.

Jobsis A C, De Vries G P, Anholt P R H, Sanders G T B (1978).
Demonstration of the prostatic origin of metastases.
Cancer 41:1788-1793.

Lam K W, Li O, Li C Y, Yam L T (1973). Biochemical properties of human prostatic acid phosphatases. Clin. Chem.
19:483-487.

Li C Y, Lam W K W, Yam L T (1980). Immunohistochemical diagnosis of prostatic cancer with metastasis. Cancer 46:706-712.

Mathieu M C, Caillaud J M (1985). Carcinomes prostatiques: etude en immunoperoxydase avec des antiserums diriges contre la phosphatase acide prostatique (PAP) et contre l'antigene specifique de la prostate (PSA). Bull. Cancer 72:405-413.

Molino A A, Meiss R P, Leo P, Sens A I (1985). Demonstration of cytokeratins by immunoperoxidase staining in prostatic tissue. J. Urol. 134:1037-1040.

Mori K, Wakasugi C (1985). Immunocytochemical demonstration of prostatic acid phosphatase: different secretion kinetics between normal, hyperplastic and neoplastic prostates. J. Virol. 133:877-883.

Nadji M, Tabei S Z, Castro A, Chu T M, Morales A R (1980). Prostatic origin of tumors. An immunohistochemical study. Am. J. Clin. Pathol. 73:735-739.

Nadji M, Tabei S Z, Castro A, Chu T M, Murphy G P, Whang M C, Morales A R (1981). Prostatic specific antigen: an immuno-histological marker for prostatic neoplasms. Cancer 48: 1229-1232.

Stein B S, Peterson R O, Vangore S, Kendall A R (1982). Immuno-peroxidase localization of prostate-specific anti-gen. Am. J. Surg. Pathol. 6:553-557.

Wahab Z A, Wright G L (1985). Monoclonal antibody (anti-Leu 7) directed against natural killer cells reacts with normal, benign and malignant prostate tissues. Int. J. Cancer 36:677-683.

Wang M C, Valenzuella L A, Murphy G P, Chu T M (1979). Puri-fication of a human prostate specific antigen. Invest. Urol. 17:159-163.

Prostate Cancer, Part A: Research, Endocrine
Treatment, and Histopathology, pages 485–487
© 1987 Alan R. Liss, Inc.

ANTI-HUMAN PROSTATIC ACID PHOSPHATASE (P.A.P.) MONOCLONAL ANTIBODIES: CHARACTERISATION AND PRACTICAL APPLICATION

P. Teillac*, M. Leroy**, B. Rabaud*, A. Le Duc*, Y. Najean **

Service d'Urologie (*) et Service de Médecine Nucléaire (**) Hôpital Saint Louis - Paris

INTRODUCTION

When diagnosed sufficiently early in a subject in good general condition, prostatic cancer may be suitable for radical treatment.

Before considering such treatment, staging must be performed including, in particular : bone scintigraphy and lymphography. Areas of increased uptake detected on bone scans do not always correspond to bone metastases and may reflect old trauma or arthrosis.

Bipedal lymphography is only reliable in about 60 % and does not visualise the first set of nodes. Some authors therefore propose pelvic lymphadenectomy in the staging of prostatic cancer.

Monoclonal antibodies could constitute a useful tool in the diagnosis of the tumour, its lymph node extensions and its metastases as a result of their specific localisation. If such antibodies are labelled by a radioactive isotope, they can then be detected by immunoscintigraphy. We selected a specific marker for prostatic tissue : prostatic acid phosphatase (PAP) in order to produce monoclonal anti-PAP antibodies. We then selected 5 of these labelled monoclonal anti-PAP antibodies to perform immunoscintigraphy in the Nude mouse with a transplanted tumour.

The monoclonal antibodies were produced according to the classical fusion protocol established by KOHLER and MILSTEIN, using splenocytes from mice immunised with purified human PAP, form 2A and murine myeloma Sp20 Ag14 cells.

Forty two microcultures gave positive results, indicating the synthesis of anti-PAP antibodies. Five cultures were selected for their proliferative and secretory properties : clones 146, 227, 243, 468 and 802.

Analysis of the properties of these monoclonal antibodies involved the study of isotypy by OUCHTERLONY's method and the affinity by SCATCHARD's analysis.

The epitopic recognition was studied by solid phase binding inhibition and the tissue localisation was studied by immuno- histochemistry on frozen sections of prostatic biopsies. The affinity coefficients ranged from 1.5×10^9 l/mole for 243 to 2×10^9 l/mole for 227 and 802.

Epitopic cartography was used to identify 4 partially overlapping epitopic groups. Antibodies 227 and 243 were able to recognise sufficiently distant epitopes to allow their simultaneous binding to PAP. This property could be used to develop a one-stage immunoradiometric assay for PAP.

The antibodies tested on frozen sections of prostatic biopsy were all found to be positive for prostatic epithelial cells. None of the antibodies bound to the connective tissue.

Overall, the principal characteristics of the 5 antibodies demonstrated that, in each case, they were immunoglobulin G1 specific for PAP.

Antibody 227 was selected for the study of the biodistribution in the Nude mouse. The Nude mouse received 10^7 cells of either mammary adenocarcinoma 466 B cell line or prostatic carcinoma DU 145 cell line. The tumours developed within 3 to 5 weeks. The results were compared with a tumour-free control mouse. Antibody 227 labelled with Iodine 125 by the iodogenic method was injected subcutaneously. The mice were sacrificed 4 days after the injection of antibody ; the organs were removed, weighed and the radioactivity was counted.

The results obtained in the mouse with tumour 466 B were identical to those obtained in the control mouse. However, in the mouse with the DU 145 prostatic tumour, intense accumulation of the antibody was detected in the tumour.

Finally, immunoscintigraphy was performed in the mouse ; it revealed the localisation of the tumour with a ratio of activity in the tumour region to the non-tumour region of about 3.

In conclusion, we can consider the practical application of anti-human PAP monoclonal antibodies :

- for immunoradiometric assay of PAP,
- for histolocalisation of PAP allowing identification of the origin of a metastasis or a doubtful tumour
- for the scintigraphic immunodetection of metastases and lymph node extension of prostatic cancer.

Prostate Cancer, Part A: Research, Endocrine
Treatment, and Histopathology, pages 489–502
© 1987 Alan R. Liss, Inc.

PEPTIDE HORMONES, SEROTONIN, AND OTHER CELL DIFFERENTIATION
MARKERS IN BENIGN HYPERPLASIA AND IN CARCINOMA OF THE
PROSTATE

Per-Anders Abrahamsson, Jan Alumets, Lars B.
Wadström, Sture Falkmer and Lars Grimelius

Departments of Urology, University of Lund, Malmö
General Hospital, Malmö, Tumour Pathology,
Karolinska Hospital, Stockholm, and Pathology,
University of Uppsala, Uppsala, Sweden.

INTRODUCTION

In a recent report (Abrahamsson et al., 1986 a,b) we
could demonstrate a cell population of endocrine type in
the epithelium of the ducts and acini in normal and hyperplastic prostate glands, as well as in the urothelium of
the prostatic urethra. Ultrastructurally, these cells are
equipped with secretion granules of endocrine appearance,
and the cells may be of either open or closed type (di
Sant´Agnese and de Mesy Jensen, 1985). The fine structure
of the secretion granules can differ so much that it has
been concluded that several types of such endocrine cells
exist. These cells have also been described, occasionally,
in adenocarcinomas of the prostate (Azzopardi and Evans,
1971; Kazzaz, 1974; Capella et al., 1981; Fetissof et al.,
1983). However, no comprehensive studies of the existence
of several types of endocrine cells, under normal and
pathological conditions, with regard to their content of
the biogenic amines and peptide hormone immunoreactivities
have been made so far.

In order to identify, localize and characterize the
presence of endocrine cells in normal, hyperplastic and
neoplastic prostate glands, three silver-staining procedures and three kinds of immunohistochemical methods with
a broad battery of antisera against neurohormonal peptides
were used, as well as antisera raised against serotonin,
neuron-specific enolase and chromogranin A (O´Connor and
Deftos, 1986).

MATERIAL AND METHODS

Two kinds of specimens were investigated. One was fresh material, obtained from patients with urinary obstruction who had undergone transurethral resection (groups 2 A & 3 A). From every case at least five specimens were taken. They were fixed within 10 min by immersion in Bouin's fluid for 18-24 h. After rinsing in tap-water and 70% ethanol, the specimens were dehydrated, cleared and embedded in paraffin. Sections about 4-5 µm thick were stained with hematoxylin and eosin (H&E) or with van Gieson's stain. In addition, the Grimelius' silver-nitrate procedure (Grimelius, 1968) and the Churukian-Schenk technique (Churukian and Schenk, 1979) for detecting argyrophil cells were applied, as well as the Masson-Fontana argentaffin reaction (Masson, 1956). The histopathological diagnosis of benign hyperplasia and prostatic carcinoma was checked by at least two experienced pathologists on the H&E- and van Gieson-stained sections in every case. The tumours were classified according to the WHO grading system (Mostofi, 1976).

The second kind of specimen consisted of archival paraffin blocks. All the specimens had been formalin-fixed. New sections were cut from the paraffin blocks and stained as described above.

Group	No. of cases	Histopathological diagnosis
Group 1	2 (age 28 & 31)	Normal (autopsy)
Group 2 A	24 (mean age 69; range 52-79 yr)	Benign nodular hyperplasia
Group 2 B	40 (mean age 71; range 49-83 yr)	Benign nodular hyperplasia
Group 3 A	40 (mean age 72; range 55-86 yr)	Adenocarcinoma
Group 3 B	80 (mean age 74; (range 53-87 yr)	Adenocarcinoma

Immunohistochemical Techniques

On paraffin sections, the following three immunohistochemical procedures were applied, viz., the indirect
immunofluorescence technique (Coons, 1958), the per-
oxidase-antiperoxidase (PAP) method (Sternberger, 1979),
and the avidin-biotin variant of the latter (Hsu et al.,
1981).

In order to relate the results of the silver-staining
procedures to those of the immunohistochemical investigations, a re-staining technique was developed according to
Kishimoto et al. (1981). The more conventional technique
with two consecutive 2-3 µm thick sections was also used,
to identify the cell or group of cells "stained" with different antisera.

RESULTS

Normal and Hyperplastic Prostate Gland

The endocrine cells could easily be visualized by
means of silver-staining techniques, even using conven-
tionally formalin-fixed, paraffin-embedded specimens.
However, the immunoperoxidase techniques showed greater
sensitivity than the Masson-Fontana procedure and greater
specificity than the Grimelius or Churukian-Schenk technique in the visualization of endocrine cells in the normal
prostatic gland and in the nodules of benign prostatic
hyperplasia of man. The avidin-biotin variant of the
immunoperoxidase technique, with monoclonal antibodies
raised against chromogranin A, proved to be the most
sensitive and specific test for endocrine cells, both in
Bouin-fixed and in formalin-fixed specimens. These cells
were also found to be immunoreactive with antisera raised
against neuron-specific enolase, but with a somewhat lower
specificity and sensitivity.

The endocrine cells were located in the epithelium of
the acini and the ducts of all the different parts of the
gland, as well as in the urothelium of the prostatic part
of the mucosa of the urethra. They were either of open or
of closed type and usually occurred widely scattered as
single cells. Three kinds of endocrine cells were observed

Fig. 1 A & B. Photomicrographs of two consecutive sections of a few glands in a hyperplastic prostate gland incubated with antisera against TSH (Fig. 1 A) and serotonin (Fig. 1 B). One and the same cell shows a distinct immunoreactivity (black) against both antisera, indicating co-existence of this neurohormonal peptide with the biogenic amine. In addition, a paracrine process of the immunoreactive cell along the basal membrane can be seen, particularly in Fig. 1 B.

PAP procedure; x 594.

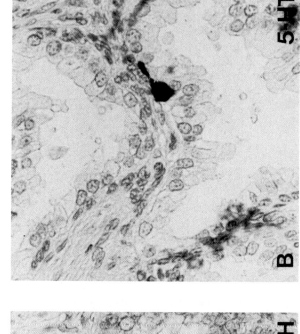

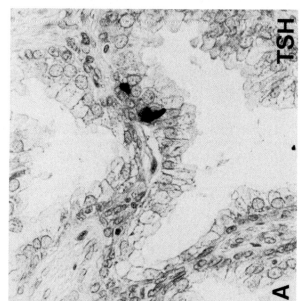

both in the normal gland and in the hyperplastic parenchyma. In the by far most prevalent type, serotonin was
found to co-exist with a peptide immunohistochemically
related to the thyroid stimulating hormone (TSH) (Fig. 1 A
& 1 B). In a more rare type serotonin co-existed immunohistochemically with calcitonin (Fig. 2). A third kind of
endocrine cells was somatostatin-immunoreactive cells; they
were also rare. The only difference observed between the
normal and hyperplastic parenchyma was an increase in the
number of all the three kinds of endocrine cells in certain
areas of diffuse hyperplasia, especially in the periurethral ducts/acini, where an epithelial cell proliferation is common.

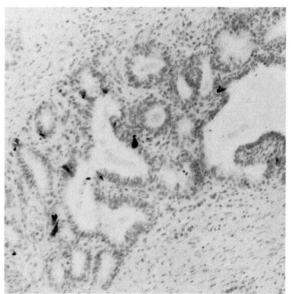

Fig. 2. Calcitonin-immunoreactive endocrine cells (black)
in a few prostatic acini in a benign prostatic hyperplasia.
PAP procedure; x 211.

Neoplastic Prostate Gland

The incidence of the endocrine cells was higher in the
fresh Bouin-fixed biopsy specimens than in the formalin-
fixed specimens from archival paraffin blocks. All carcinomas were found to have endocrine cells as an integral
element of the tumour. In highly differentiated carcinomas

TABLE 1

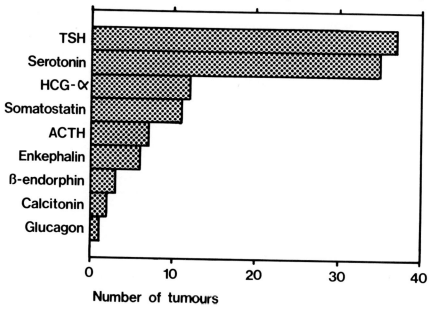

Immunohistochemical features of prostatic cancers

(grade I) these cells were scattered focally, intermingled with non-endocrine cells in typical adenocarcinomas; their incidence was estimated to be about the same as in benign prostatic hyperplasia. Most of them were immunoreactive with antisera raised against serotonin and thyroid stimulating hormone (TSH) (see Table 1). In moderately and poorly differentiated (grades II–III) carcinomas, however, the endocrine cells were more numerous (Fig. 3) and showed greater variation in growth pattern (Fig. 4); only occasionally they displayed a typical carcinoid-like structure (Fig. 5). Moderately and poorly differentiated carcinomas also showed a greater variation in the number and kinds of peptide immunoreactivities than the highly differentiated carcinomas. In addition to serotonin- and TSH-immunoreactive cells as the most prevalent type, now also human chorionic gonadotrophin (HCG-α), adrenocortico-

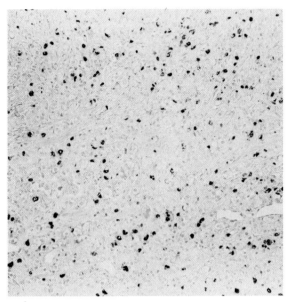

Fig. 3. Chromogranin A immunoreactive tumour cells (black) in a poorly differentiated prostatic carcinoma.
ABC (avidin-biotin complex) procedure; x 166.

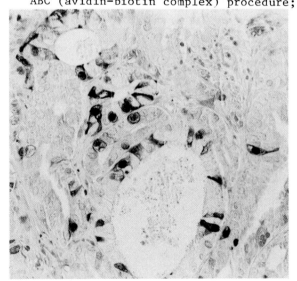

Fig. 4. Neuron-specific enolase immunoreactive tumour cells (black) in a highly and moderately differentiated prostatic carcinoma.   ABC procedure; x 330.

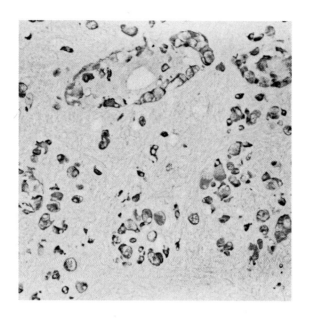

Fig. 5. Numerous tumour cells (black) in a poorly differentiated prostatic carcinoma showing positivity with
Grimelius´ silver-staining procedure; notice the organoid
(carcinoid-like) pattern.

Grimelius; x 224.

----

tropic hormone (ACTH), leu-enkephalin, β -endorphin,
somatostatin, glucagon and calcitonin-immunoreactive cells
could be found within certain tumour areas (see Table 1)
and often with a distinctly patchy distribution. In two
cases, the tumour cells in the metastases were found to be
immunoreactive with the same antisera as those of the
primary tumour (Fig. 6).

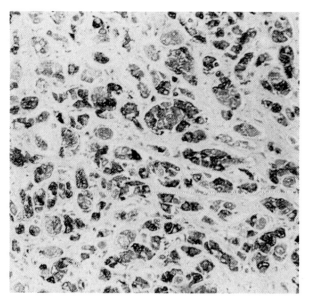

Fig. 6. Thyroid stimulating hormone (TSH) immunoreactive, metastatic tumour cells (black) in a pelvic lymph node in a poorly differentiated prostatic carcinoma.

ABC procedure; x 211.

DISCUSSION

The presence of serotonin-storing cells and soma-tostatin-immunoreactive cells in the human prostate gland has previously been described (Fetissof et al., 1983; di Sant'Agnese and de Mesy Jensen, 1984). Likewise, earlier ultrastructural and histochemical works confirm the pre-sence of cells storing biogenic amines in the epithelium of the ducts and acini, as well as in the prostatic urothelium (Casanova et al., 1974; Lendon et al., 1976; Capella et al., 1981).

A new observation made in our study is the immuno-histochemical fact that serotonin co-exists with a TSH-like peptide in the most prevalent type of endocrine cells in the human prostate parenchyma. In the second type of endocrine cells serotonin co-exists with a calcitonin-like immunoreactive peptide. The functional significance of this observation has to await further biochemical analyses of these hormonal peptides. Nevertheless, a high concentration of immunoreactive calcitonin of prostatic origin has earlier been demonstrated in human semen (Sjöberg et al., 1980).

In endocrine glands of classical type, it is known that biogenic amines often co-exist with cells producing biologically important peptide hormones. The fact that the third type of endocrine cells in the normal and hyperplastic prostate gland, viz., the somatostatin-immunoreactive cells, lacks the co-existence with serotonin, indicates a fundamental difference between the TSH-like and calcitonin-like immunoreactive cells on one hand and the somatostatin cells on the other. It has been anticipated that the biogenic amine plays a role in the release mechanism of the peptide hormone. Such a mechanism does not seem to exist for the somatostatin cells. As a matter of fact, the major role for the somatostatin cells seems rather to be a local paracrine inhibitor of hormone release. Thus, somatostatin is apparently antagonistic to the biogenic amines in the neuroendocrine system (Larsson et al., 1979; Reichlin, 1983).

Another interesting result of our study, from a biomedical point of view, is the fact that a benign, nodular, fibro-myo-glandular hyperplasia of a prostatic gland implies only an increase in the number of endocrine cells in the epithelium of the ducts and acini, as well as in the urothelium of the prostatic part of the urethra but no appearance of any new cell types. Thus, there are only the same three kinds of endocrine cells as in the normal prostatic parenchyma as described above. Consequently, the hyperplasia does not seem to induce any fundamental changes at the genome level with expression of new products in the hyperplastic cells. This finding is the basic difference between a benign hyperplasia and a malignant neoplasm.

Our observations confirm and underline the previous report by di Sant´Agnese et al. (1985) that endocrine cells are more frequent in certain areas of diffuse hyperplasia, especially in the periurethral ducts and acini. In the periurethral ducts, where epithelial cell proliferation is common, the most pronounced discrepancy in number of endocrine cells between the normal and hyperplastic gland could be demonstrated.

As described in the results, our findings do not only confirm previously made, rather sporadic demonstrations of endocrine cells in adenocarcinomas of the prostate gland, but also make the important extension of this observation that serotonin and peptide hormone immunoreactive cells can be found as an integral element of virtually all prostatic adenocarcinomas. This statement could be made by using fresh biopsy specimens and more sensitive and specific immunohistochemical procedures. It should be emphasized, however, that these endocrine cells were mostly focally localized and formed only a minority of the total number of carcinomatous cells. Nevertheless, our findings emphasize the possibility that prostatic carcinomas may be more complex and heterogenous than previously thought.

Our observations also estimate that endocrine cells increase in number and variability with decreasing degrees of differentiation of the prostatic adenocarcinoma. Thus, in addition to the three kinds of immunoreactive cells observed in normal and hyperplastic prostate glands no less than five other kinds of endocrine cells could be found in the prostatic carcinomas (see Table 1). The multitude of immunoreactive cells was particularly obvious in the poorly differentiated neoplasm. This fact indicates that with decreasing maturity of the tumour cells, the number of active genes increases with increased expression of the genomic products. A spectrum of endocrine differentiation in a traditionally non-endocrine neoplasm may simply represent divergent differentiation of tumour cells along a line different from the normal or non-neoplastic state. The complex tumours sometimes found in mammary, pancreatic and prostatic carcinomas, simply imply a de-differentiation from the usual histopathologic and functional form towards a mutually multipotent epithelial stem cell. This stem cell could be both exo- and endocrine (DeLellis et al., 1984; Chejfec et al., 1985) in its nature, i.e., the same tumour cell could be capable of divergent functional modalities as demonstrated by immunostaining against prostate-specific acid phosphatase, prostate-specific antigen, serotonin, neuron-specific enolase, chromogranin A, and neurohormonal peptides, even ultrastructurally.

The clinical significance of the presence of endocrine cells in prostatic carcinomas still essentially remains unknown. There are, however, some prostatic carcinomas that have been associated with clinical signs of ectopic hormone production. Thus, nine cases have been reported of prostatic carcinomas associated with Cushing's syndrome (Dauge et al., 1985); one of them also had inappropriately high serum levels of an antidiuretic hormone. Most of these tumours were histopathologically classified as moderately and poorly differentiated adenocarcinomas.

It is, however, quite clear that carcinomas of the prostate only rarely give rise to clinical symptoms of endocrine type. Thus, we could not observe any well-defined, so-called paramalignant endocrine syndromes in any of our patients. This seemingly paradoxical situation could be explained by the fact that the hormonal substances produced do not attain any high serum levels. Another plausible explanation could be that these immunohisto-chemically detected hormonal peptides are not exactly identical with the peptides against which the antisera used have been raised. Nevertheless, the presence of these peptides may contribute to the knowledge of the patho-physiology in prostatic carcinoma and indicate, in association with other endocrine markers such as NSE and chromogranin A, new possible tumour markers. Endocrine prostatic cells most likely have both paracrine and endocrine activity and may directly and/or indirectly regulate prostatic secretion and cell growth, and have a trophic effect on prostatic carcinoma.

REFERENCES

Abrahamsson PA, Wadström LB, Alumets J, Falkmer S, Grimelius L (1986 a). Peptide-hormone- and serotonin-immunoreactive cells in normal and hyperplastic prostate glands. Pathol Res Pract. In press.
Abrahamsson PA, Wadström, LB, Alumets J, Falkmer S, Grimelius L (1986 b). Peptide-hormone- and serotonin-immunoreactive tumour cells in carcinoma of the prostate. In manuscript.
Azzopardi JG, Evans DJ (1971). Argentaffin cells in prostatic carcinoma: Differentiation from lipofuscin and melanin in prostatic epithelium. J Pathol 104:247-251.

Capella C, Usellini L, Buffa R, Frigerio B, Solcia E
(1981). The endocrine component of prostatic carcinomas,
mixed adenocarcinoma-carcinoid tumours and non-tumour
prostate. Histochemical and ultrastructural identification of the endocrine cells. Histopathology 5:175-192.

Casanova S, Corrado F, Vignoli G (1974). Endocrine-like
cells in the epithelium of the human male urethra. J
Submicr Cytol 6:435-438.

Chejfec G, Capella C, Solcia E, Jao W, Gould VE (1985).
Amphicrine cells, dysplasias, and neoplasias. Cancer
56:2683-2690.

Churukian CJ, Schenk EA (1979). A modification of Pascual's
argyrophil method. J Histotech 2:102-103.

Coons AH (1958). Fluorescent antibody methods. In Danielli
JD (ed): "General Cytochemical Methods," New York:
Academic Press, p 399.

Dauge MC, Grossin M, Doumecq-Lacoste JM, Vinceneux Ph,
Delmas V, Bocquet L (1985). "Carcinoid" tumor of the
prostate. A new clinically and pathologically documented
case with a review of the literature. Arch Anat Cytol
Pathol 33:73-79.

DeLellis RA, Tischler AS, Wolfe HJ (1984). Multidirectional
differentiation in neuroendocrine neoplasms. J Histochem
Cytochem 32:899-904.

Fetissof F, Dubois MP, Arbeille-Brassart B, Lanson Y,
Boivin F, Jobard P (1983). Endocrine cells in the
prostate gland, urothelium and Brenner tumors. Immuno-
histological and ultrastructural studies. Virchows Arch
(Cell Pathol) 42:53-64.

Grimelius L (1968). A silver nitrate stain for α_2 cells
in human pancreatic islets. Acta Soc Med Ups 73:243-
270.

Hsu SM, Raine L, Fanger H (1981). Use of avidin-biotin-per
oxidase complex (ABC) in immunoperoxidase techniques: A
comparison between ABC and unlabeled antibody (PAP)
procedures. J Histochem Cytochem 29:577-580.

Kazzaz BA (1974). Argentaffin and argyrophil cells in the
prostate. J Pathol 112:189-193.

Kishimoto S, Polak JM, Buchan AMJ, Verhofstad AAJ,
Steinbusch HWM, Yanaihara N, Bloom SR, Pearse AGE
(1981). Motilin cells investigated by the use of
region-specific antisera. Virchows Arch (Cell Pathol)
36:207-218.

Larsson LI, Goltermann N, de Magistris L, Rehfeld JF, Schwartz TW (1979). Somatostatin cell processes as pathways for paracrine secretion. Science 205:1393-1395.

Lendon RG, Dixon JS, Gosling JA (1976). The distribution of endocrine-like cells in the human male and female urethral epithelium. Experientia 32:377-378.

Masson P (1956). "Tumeurs humaines. Histologie, Diagnostics et Techniques." (2nd Ed), Paris: Maloine, p 1131.

Mostofi FK (1976). Problems of grading carcinoma of prostate. Semin Oncol 3:161-169.

O'Connor DT, Deftos LJ (1986). Secretion of chromogranin A by peptide-producing endocrine neoplasms. N Engl J Med 314: 1145-1151.

Reichlin S (1983). Somatostatin. N Engl J Med 309:1556-1563.

di Sant'Agnese PA, de Mesy Jensen, KL (1984). Somatostatin and/or somatostatinlike immunoreactive endocrine-paracrine cells in the human prostate gland. Arch Pathol Lab Med 108:693-696.

di Sant'Agnese PA, de Mesy Jensen KL (1985). Endocrine-paracrine cells of the prostate and prostatic urethra: An ultrastructural study. Hum Pathol 15: 1034-1041.

di Sant'Agnese PA, de Mesy Jensen KL, Churukian CJ, Agarwal MM (1985). Human prostatic endocrine-paracrine (APUD) cells. Arch Pathol Lab Med 109:607-612.

Sjöberg HE, Arver S, Bucht E (1980). High concentration of immunoreactive calcitonin of prostatic origin in human semen. Acta Physiol Scand 110:101-102.

Sternberger LA (1979). "Immunocytochemistry." (2nd Ed), New York: John Wiley & Sons.

Prostate Cancer, Part A: Research, Endocrine
Treatment, and Histopathology, page 503
© 1987 Alan R. Liss, Inc.

VALUE OF P.A. (prostate-specific-antigen) IN THE STAGING AND FOLLOW-UP OF PROSTATIC CANCER. PRELIMINARY RESULTS OF A COMPARATIVE STUDY WITH P.A.P. AND BONE SCAN.

Caty A., Gosselin P, Dehaut J.P., Blin B.,
Adenis L.
Centre de Lutte contre le Cancer Oscar Lambret, rue
Frédéric Combemale. 59000-LILLE

Prostatic tissue specific Prostate Antigen (P.A.) is a glycoprotein (molecular weight 33 000 daltons). The quantitation of serum P.A. was performed using the standard double body R.I.A. method (Lab Yang). The sensitivity is 0.2 ng/ml. The normal level is lower than 2.5 ng/ml. 115 serum sample analyses and P.A.P. analyses were carried out at the same time on 82 patients. 17 controls, 22 with apparently benign prostatic hyperplasia (P.B.H.) and 43 prostatic cancers. The controls showed normal P.A. and P.A.P. levels. Out of the 22 P.B.H., 4 P.A.were positive with normal P.A.P. levels.

The staging of the 43 cancers after bone scan and CT scan was : 6 localised disease (2 AL - 2 BL - 2 B2) and 37 metastatic disease (2 DL - 35 D2). Of the 6 localised disease, only 2 BL were P.A. positive (P.A.P. normal). 1 patient DL, never treated was P.A. positive (P.A.P. normal). The other DL, in remission, was P.A. and P.A.P. negative. 68 serum samples were collected from 35 D2 patients. In 52 sera there was a correlation between both markers (13 normal determinations for patients in remission). In 10 patients with active disease P.A. was positive while P.A.P. was normal. The preliminary results show a better sensitivity for P.A. compared with P.A.P. in the diagnosis and follow-up of prostatic cancer. Its positivity in apparently P.B.H. is either false positive or the expression of a misdiagnosed cancer.

Prostate Cancer, Part A: Research, Endocrine
Treatment, and Histopathology, page 505
© 1987 Alan R. Liss, Inc.

PROSTATIC SPECIFIC ANTIGEN AND PROSTATIC ACID PHOSPHATASE
IN CARCINOMA OF THE PROSTATE.

E.H. Cooper, J.K. Siddall and J.W. Hetherington.

The Unit for Cancer Research.

The University of Leeds, Leeds LS2 9NL.

Serum prostatic specific antigen (PSA) and prostatic acid
phosphatase (PAP) were measured using double monoclonal
radioimmunoassays (Hybritech, Calif.). Normal limits are:
PSA 0.1-2.7, mean 1.01 ng/ml, PAP 0.2-2.8 mean 1.09 ng/ml.
In 91 untreated patients with non-metastatic disease 42.8%
had a PSA >10 ng/ml and 18.6% had a PAP >2 ng/ml. In 90
patients with untreated metastatic disease the PSA was
>10 ng/ml in 91.1% and the PAP >2 ng/ml in 68.9%. In
prolonged remission the PSA was generally <5 ng/ml and the
PAP <2 ng/ml. Longitudinal studies of 2-4 years showed
the independence of these markers and a higher correlation
of changes in the PSA level and clinical status than given
by parallel PAP measurements.

The incidence of metastases developing within 3 years of
presentation was compared to the levels of PSA and PAP.
Nine out of seventy patients with PAP levels <2 ng/ml
progressed, whereas in the group with PSA <10 ng/ml, only
1/51 patients progressed. In the group with PAP >2 ng/ml
7/16 progressed, all of whom had levels of PSA >10 ng/ml.
The group with PSA >10 ng/ml, 15/35 progressed within 3
years, 8 of these however, had levels of PAP within the
normal range. It appears that the level of PSA carries
greater prognostic significance than the level of serum
PAP.

Prostate Cancer, Part A: Research, Endocrine
Treatment, and Histopathology, pages 507–510
© 1987 Alan R. Liss, Inc.

VALUE OF DIFFERENT MARKERS IN PROSTATIC CARCINOMAS. AN IMMUNOHISTOLOGICAL STUDY

Daher N., Bove N., Bara J., Abourachid H.
ER 277 CNRS, IRSC - Villejuif - France
C.H.U. 80000 Amiens -

We studied 52 specimens of prostatic tissue fixed in 95% ethanol and embedded in paraffin wax according to the technic of Sainte Marie because when we compared different fixatives, we found that formalin altered or masked the antigenic sites in contrast with ethanol and we found that formalin specimens only presented good staining for prostatic specific antigen. The specimens included 8 normal prostates of young males, 18 benign hypertrophies and 26 carcinomas.
We used either an immunoperoxidase or IP technic on 3u serial sections. We studied different antigenic systems that we report briefly here.

KERATIN RELATED ANTIGENS
Keratins are one of the five types of proteins that constitute the intermediate-sized filaments. Recent results have indicated that keratins can be divided into an acidic and a basic subfamily and that each acidic keratin formed a pair with a specific basic keratin, and all epithelia contained at least one keratin each of the two subfamilies.
4 monoclonal antibodies and 2 antisera against various types of keratins (T.T. Sun, L.B. Chen, R. Mouaad) were used in this study :
AE1 (Acidic Specificity : 40, 48, 50, 50', 56.5 KD)
AE3 (Basic Specificity : 52, 54, 56, 58, 59, 64, 65-67 KD)
AE2 (Epidermal pair keratin 56.5/65-67 KD)
B16 (40 KD)
D66 (52 KD) antiserum
An antiserum against the total keratins was also used.
The keratin acidic pattern of staining in normal prostate was either cytoplasmic or more frequently located at the plasma membrane and either in basal or in basal and luminal cells of ductal and acinar structures.

The same pattern was observed in benign hypertrophy but in a lesser intensity, while in carcinomas the staining was observed focally and predominantly in the plasma membrane of acinar cells. Moreover, the staining was more occasional or absent in differentiated structures.

The keratin basic pattern of staining was much more frequently and constantly observed than the acidic pattern, in normal or benign or even malignant tissues. The epidermal keratin pair was absent in acinar structures or either normal or malignant tissues but it was expressed in ductal structures in a supranuclear location. (AE2) The 40 KD keratin was more scarcely observed as compared to the acidic pattern of staining as well as for the 52 KD keratin when compared to the basic pattern, while the antiserum against the total keratins stained most of the prostatic structures either normal or tumoral and in the latter mainly when tissues still have some differentiation.

These preliminary results suggest that keratins may be an important tool for understanding the cellular origin and the differentiation program in prostatic carcinomas.

ABH AND LEWIS RELATED ANTIGENS
During recent years, the expression of blood group antigens has been studied in various tumors and correlated to the behaviour of these tumors. We tried to study the status of ABH antigens and Lewis (Le^a, Le^b, Sialyted Le^a, Le Y) antigens by twelve monoclonal antibodies in normal, benign or malignant prostatic tissue.

Normal tissue expressed the ABH antigens corresponding to the patient blood group and for A and B patients an occasional H expression was observed. The staining was mainly cytoplasmic and concerned frequently more than the half up to the whole prostatic normal areas while in malignant tissue only occasional and focal staining was observed.

For the Lewis antigens, the staining concerned the ductal rather than the acinar structures. It was mainly cytoplasmic and in occasional foci. There was no evident difference between normal and malignant tissue staining of Lewis related antigens and these latter antigens seemed to be conserved in malignant as well as in normal prostatic tissue. However, these results are still questionable because the Lewis status of patients in unknown and further investigations are needed.

SOME ONCOFETAL ANTIGENS
Because the only available monoclonal antibodies in our laboratory were against oncofetal antigens of the gastro-intestinal tract, we undertook this study in order to see if there is any relation between digestive and prostatic carcinomas.

Carcinoembryonic and related antigens were studied by four monoclonal antibodies and the results showed us that only occasional cells in either benign or malignant scare specimens were stained. Monoclonal antibodies against a feta-acinar pancreatic protein did not show any staining.

Five monoclonal antibodies against fucomucin associated antigens were tried and we were surprised to find that these antibodies always stained (in normal specimens) an area in the "veru montanum" with cylindrical cells corresponding probably to the prostatic utriculus because none of the four pathologists questioned could affirm the nature of these positive cells and if they are truly cells of the prostatic utriculus.

This fact is very important because it could help to understand the rare endometrioid differentiation in some prostatic carcinomas; however this remains open to debate because the origin and type of the cells stained by these antibodies have not yet been identified.

BASEMENT MEMBRANE ANTIGENS
Our group and others recently demonstrated the important role that basement membrane antigens can play in invasion and prognosis of various carcinomas.

In this preliminary study of some prostatic specimens, we only looked for type IV collagen in normal benign and malignant basement membranes. Normal tissue and benign hypertrophy have their basement membrane stained for type IV collagen while in prostatic carcinomas the staining sometimes was conserved as in well-differentiated structures or altered and even absent in less differentiated structures. This study is preliminary and we have not yet investigated wether there is any correlation between alteration of basement membrane antigens and prognosis.

PROSTATIC SPECIFIC ANTIGEN
Only for this study, tissues fixed in formalin were used because no difference could be found between ethanol or formalin fixatives. More than one hundred specimens were studied : seventy five of them concerned either normal, benign or malignant prostatic tissues and the remainder included carcinomas of other urologic or colorectal tissues.

The antisera used in this study stained nearly all structures of the normal and benign tissues while in prostatic carcinomas the staining was a little heterogeneous and not all glands were stained and this mainly in less differentiated carcinomas, but we never observed a negative specimen. The most important fact was the study of fifteen specimens in patients presenting unusual features (rectal mass with rectitis, trigonal mass with hematuria, papillary tumors of urethra, testis metastasis). As in these latter cases, the prostate specific antigen could be helpful for pathologists in recognizing the origin of some carcinomas.

Prostate Cancer, Part A: Research, Endocrine
Treatment, and Histopathology, page 511
© 1987 Alan R. Liss, Inc.

PROSTATIC CANCER: HISTOLOGICAL GRADE AND INDICATION FOR CHEMOTHERAPY

G. Arvis, G. Tobelem
Service d'Urologie,
Hôpital St. Antoine, Paris, France

A large number of studies together with everyday clinical experience demonstrate that when prostatic cancer fails to respond to hormone therapy, it is useless to increase the doses of hormones or to change the type of hormone used. Only chemotherapy, administered alone or in combination, can induce stabilisation or even regression of the lesions.

Now that active chemotherapy is available and in view of the fact that prostatic cancer is frequently either initially hormone-resistant or rapidly becomes so, especially in stage D tumours, one wonders in which cases it would be wiser, taking into account the histological type of the cancer, to start treatment with chemotherapy.

High grade prostatic cancers (undifferentiated cancer) have a particularly unfavourable prognosis, especially in young patients. They are virtually insensitive to hormone therapy. We consider these tumours to be a good indication for initial chemotherapy.
Conversely, it is logical to consider well differentiated tumours to be hormone sensitive and this is confirmed by experience.

The most doubtful cases are the intermediate tumours, where it is difficult to determine the exact degree of differentiation (or undifferentiation). Are these tumours hormone sensitive ? Do they have a homogeneous histological structure ? These questions remain unanswered at the present time.

We personally consider that as soon as the loss of differentiation becomes "important", it is preferable to commence treatment with chemotherapy.

Prostate Cancer, Part A: Research, Endocrine
Treatment, and Histopathology, pages 513–516
© 1987 Alan R. Liss, Inc.

EFFECTS OF OESTROGEN ON GROWTH AND MORPHOLOGY OF THE DUNNING R3327H PROSTATIC CARCINOMA

J.-E. Damber, L. Daehlin, A. Bergh, M. Landström
and R. Tomic.
Departments of Physiology, Urology and Andrology,
Pathology, University of Umeå, S-901 87 Umeå,
Sweden.

INTRODUCTION

The use of oestrogen in the management of prostatic carcinoma patients is widespread. The main effect of oestrogen
in such patients is considered to be due to arrest of testicular testosterone production. However, inhibitory effects
of oestrogen per se on the prostatic tumour have also been
reported (1). The H-subline of the transplantable Dunning
rat adenocarcinoma (R3327H) is androgendependent for its
growth, histologically well-differentiated, contains 5α-reduc-
tase and androgen and oestrogen receptors. (2). The R3327H
tumour is therefore considered to be a useful model for studies of prostatic carcinoma. The aim of the present investigation was to study whether oestradiol-17β has any additive
inhibitory effect on tumour growth when compared to castration alone. The morphological studies were done to elucidate
the effects of oestrogen on the different tissue components
of the Dunning R3327H carcinoma.

MATERIAL AND METHODS

Thirty male Copenhagen X Fisher F_1 rats bearing R3327H
tumours in their flanks were castrated, randomly allocated
to one of four groups and treated by daily subcutaneous injections for four weeks: I; controls = C, II; testosterone
proprionate 0.1 mg (T) = C + T, III; oestradiol benzoate 0.05
mg (E2) = C + E2, IV; the combined treatment of testosterone
(T) and oestradiol (E2) = C + T + E2. Tumour diameters were
measured weekly by microcalipers and volume was calculated
by using the formula of an ellipsoidal mass. Morphometric

measurements were performed at 250 x magnification using a square lattice mounted in the eyepiece of a light microscope and by counting the number of testpoints over each of the tissue compartments (3).

RESULTS

Tumour volumes in % of value at start of treatment are given in Fig. 1. When compared to testosterone supplementation the growth of tumours after castration alone or with additional oestradiol was significantly (p < 0.01) decreased after 2, 3 and 4 weeks of treatment, while oestradiol in combination with testosterone inhibited tumour growth significantly (p < 0.05) after 4 weeks of injection. Oestradiol injection in castrated rats resulted in significantly (p < 0.01) smaller tumour volumes than after castration alone at 4 weeks of treatment.

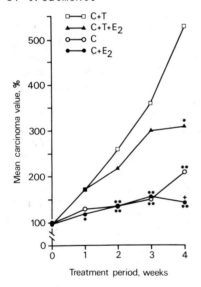

Fig 1. Growth plots of the R3327H prostatic carcinoma after different hormonal treatments. For abbreviations, see text.
* = p < 0.01 when compared to testosterone-supplemented rats (C+T).
+ = p < 0.05 when compared to castration alone (C).

The morphometric analyses of the tumours are summerized in table 1. Treatment of castrated rats with testosterone induced a decrease (p < 0.01) of stroma volume density and a increase (p < 0.01) of epithelium volume density. Oestradiol-treatment of castrated rats induced a decrease (p < 0.01) of epithelium volume density and an increase (p < 0.01) of the volume density of glandular lumina. The addition of oestradiol to testosterone induced a significant (p < 0.05) increase of stroma volumed density, whereas the volume density of glandular epithelium decreased significantly ($p < 0.05$). The volume density of glandular lumina was significantly ($p < 0.05$) increased. Testosterone stimulated the glandular epithelium as demonstrated by the significant ($p < 0.05$) increase of volume density of glandular epithelium after addition of testosterone to oestradiol treatment.

Table 1. Volume densities of tumour stroma, glandular epithelium and glandular lumina after different hormonal treatments of Dunning R3327H – implanted rats.

Group	n	Volume density (%)		
		Stroma	Epithelium	Lumen
C	10	50.9 ± 7.5	32.2 ± 4.6	10.4 ± 2.1
C+T	10	$32.9 \pm 2.7^{a)}$	$57.4 \pm 3.2^{a)}$	9.7 ± 2.6
C+E$_2$	10	49.8 ± 5.7	$25.4 \pm 3.1^{a)}$	$24.6 \pm 3.2^{a)}$
C+T+E$_2$	10	$47.1 \pm 7.8^{b)}$	$34.2 \pm 3.9^{b)c)}$	$18.9 \pm 5.0^{b)}$

For abbreviations, see text. Mean values $\pm$ SD are given. a = $p < 0.01$ when compared to castrated rats (C); b = $p < 0.05$ when compared to testosterone substituted rats (C+T); c = $p < 0.05$ when compared to oestradiol treatment alone (C+E$_2$). n = number of tumours studied.

The total volume of different parts of tumours after different treatments are shown in Fig. 2. Testosterone treatment of castrated rats induced an increase ($p < 0.01$) of the volumes of both the stroma and epithelium while oestradiol-treatment of castrates induced an increase ($p < 0.05$) of the stroma.

In rats given the combined treatment of testosterone and oestradiol, the total volume of tumour stroma was significantly ($p < 0.05$) larger than in animals injected with testosterone alone. Concomitantly, the total volume of glandular epithelium tended to decrease on addition of oestradiol to testosterone supplementation. The total volumes of tumour stroma and glandular epithelium were significantly ($p < 0.05$ and $p < 0.01$, respectively) larger after the combined treatment with testosterone and oestradiol when compared to oestradiol injection alone.

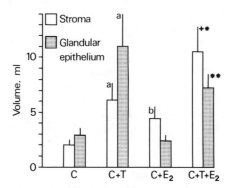

Fig. 2. Total volume (ml) of stroma and glandular epithelium in R3327H prostatic tumours after different hormonal treatment. For abbreviations, see text. Mean values ± SEM are given. a = p < 0.01 and b = p < 0.05 when compared to castrated rats (C). + = p < 0.05 and ** = p < 0.01 when compared to oestradiol treatment alone (C+E$_2$).

CONCLUSIONS

Oestradiol-17β has a direct inhibitory effect on the overall growth of prostatic carcinoma after castration or testosterone supplementation. This observation support the view that oestrogens are superior to surgical castration in the primary treatment of prostatic carcinoma, at least in this model. The inhibitory effect of oestrogen on the overall tumour growth is compounded by increase of tumour stroma volume, while the epithelium volume decreased. Further studies of stromal-epithelial interaction in prostatic carcinoma should be undertaken.

REFERENSES

1. Shessel F S et al. 1980. Inves Urol 17: 529.

2. Smolev J K et al. 1977. Cancer Treat Rep 61: 237.

3. Weibel E M. 1979. Stereological methods. Vol 1, Academic Press, New York.

Prostate Cancer, Part A: Research, Endocrine
Treatment, and Histopathology, pages 517–528
© 1987 Alan R. Liss, Inc.

THE PROGNOSTIC VALUE OF PATHOLOGICAL FACTORS IN CARCINOMA OF THE PROSTATE

M. BITTARD, JP. CARBILLET, H. WENZEL, H. BITTARD

Service d'UROLOGIE, Service de PATHOLOGIE
C.H.U. SAINT JACQUES - 25000 BESANCON

INTRODUCTION

It may take a very long time for a carcinoma of the prostate to progress spontaneously.

As a matter of fact, most studies about the impact of various treatments such as chemotherapy, radiation therapy or hormonal treatment show no significant differences in the survival rate of untreated patients and of patients having undergone treatment.

Therefore, we have attempted to define prognostic criteria based on pathological features of the tumour at presentation.

I - MATERIAL AND METHODS

Our study is based on the review of 300 primary adenocarcinomas of the prostate recorded between 1971 and 1977, all of them more than 5 years ago. The patients had undergone hormonal treatment (castration) and sometimes radiation therapy. None had had a total prostatectomy.

In an attempt to obtain a more precise view of the prognosis, we carried out 3 types of study :
- survival rate (KAPLAN MEIER - all deaths)
- contingency between tumor features (X^2 test)
- setting up of a prognostic table (method of the logistic function).

The initial specimens were taken from tumours prior to any treatment, in most cases (277 cases) by means of a needle biopsy, less frequently by means of an endoscopic resection (29 cases) or were discovered on adenomectomy material (44 cases).

II - STUDY OF THE SURVIVAL RATE

Our survival rate curves were drawn according to the KAPLAN MEIER method on the basis of all causes of death and of all types of treatments.

Our aim was to define significant clinical factors or initial pathological features of the tumour, as far as survival of the patient is concerned.

We carried out a comparative study of several groups of patients, according to the feature to be assessed. When the difference in the curves is statistically significant (MANTEL-COX test), we consider the feature assessed as having an influence on survival and a prognostic value.

The findings of this study show that this is the case with 3 clinical factors and 5 anatomopathological factors :

A better prognosis can be expected in the presence of the following factors :

- age $\leqslant$ 73 years,
- A and B stages taken together, as opposed to C and D (definition according to JEWETT determinated in the first consultation of the patients befor treatment) - Fig. 1 - (There is no significant difference between A and B, as far as survival is concerned),
- no metastases in other organs, during the followup,
- the tumours with tissue differentiation against the tumours with little or moderate differentiation,
- the moderately atypical nucleus against the severely atypical nucleus,
- mitotic index $\leqslant$ 4 (the mitotic index is the greatest number of mitosis found in a 400 field - enlargement 40 - ocular 10),
- little fibrous stromal reaction,
- no perineural infiltration.

The findings of this study, expressed in survival cumulative percentage with respect to each feature are found in Table 1 and Table 2.

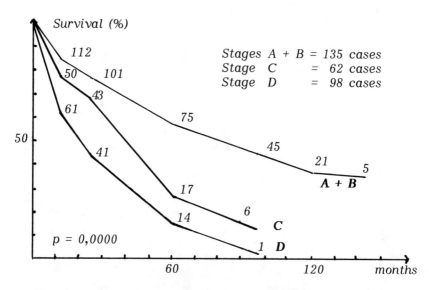

Fig. 1 : Survival curves (KAPLAN MEIER, all deaths), 295
carcinomas of the prostate with respect to the stage

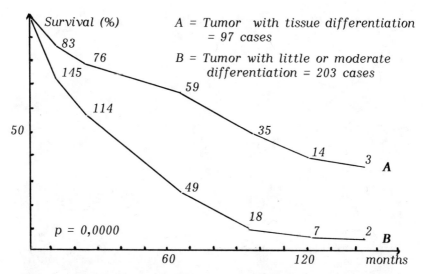

Fig. 2 : Survival curves (KAPLAN MEIER, all deaths), 300
carcinomas of the prostate with respect to tissue
differentiation

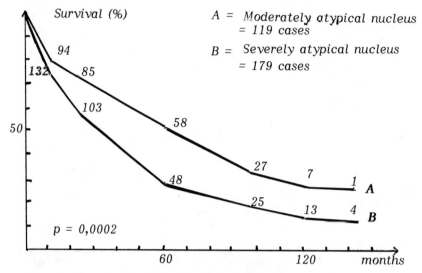

Fig. 3 : Survival curves (KAPLAN MEIER, all deaths), 298 carcinomas of the prostate with respect to atypical nucleus

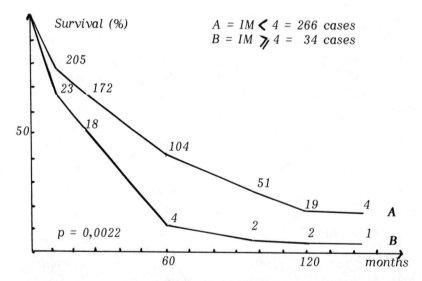

Fig. 4 : Survival curves (KAPLAN MEIER, all deaths), 300 carcinomas of the prostate with respect to the mitotic index

Months	Cases	12	24	60	96	120	144	Surveill. (months)
surviv. rate globale	300	77%	63%	37%	26%	18%	18%	158
Age ⟨73	153	80%	71%	46%	36%	30%	28%	153
Age >73 p = 0,0000	147	73%	58%	29%	12%	6%	6%	158
Stage A±B	135	84%	77%	58%	44%	36%	34%	158
Stage —C	62	79%	69%	28%	15%	–	–	117
Stage —D p = 0,0000	98	62%	43%	15%	2%	–	–	105
Metast. —	146	81%	71%	52%	40%	35%	32%	158
Metast. + p = 0,0000	138	76%	60%	23%	10%	4%	–	133

Table 1 : Cumulative percentage of survival, 300 patients with carcinoma of the prostate, with respect to 3 clinical factors : age, stage, metastases during the followup.

(KAPLAN MEIER, all deaths, average age : 73 years)

Months	Cases	12	24	60	96	120	144	Surveill. (months)
surviv. rate globale	300	77%	63%	37%	26%	18%	18%	158
important *Different.*	97	86%	79%	64%	50%	40%	37%	153
little or moderate p = 0,0000	203	72%	57%	25%	13%	9%	9%	158
moderate atypical nucleus	119	80%	73%	50%	33%	27%	27%	153
important p = 0,0002	179	74%	58%	29%	18%	13%	12%	158
<4 mitotic index	266	78%	66%	41%	27%	20%	19%	153
>4 p = 0,0001	34	68%	53%	12%	6%	6%	6%	158
little stromal reaction	181	81%	66%	46%	33%	25%	23%	153
important p = 0,0001	119	70%	61%	25%	12%	9%	9%	158
− perineural infiltration	159	80%	69%	42%	29%	25%	25%	158
+ p = 0,0097	141	72%	59%	33%	20%	12%	10%	150

Table 2 : Cumulative percentage of survival, 300 patients with respect to 5 anatomopathological factors. (KAPLAN MEIER, all deaths)

III - IS THERE A CORRELATION BETWEEN THE FEATURES (X² TEST) ?

After having determined the 8 progostic criteria, we attempted to find out whether there is any statistical correlation between them.

For that purpose, we used the X^2 comparative method which allows a comparison between the actual and the theoretical distribution of a given feature.

As we compared one feature to all others successively, we were able to show that there are several forms of contingency between those features (given p $<$ 0.05). The findings of the X^2 test are summarized on Table 3.

This tables show that 2 among these features have very little contingency with all others :
- age (no related to each of all other variables),
- mitotic index (related to 3 out of 7 features).

We may conclude that both features are discriminating as far as prognosis is concerned.

All other features are significantly correlated :

- stage, fibrous stromal reaction and perineural infiltration are each tied to 5 out of 7 features,
- more or less atypical nucleus, tissue differentiation and the presence of metastases, tied to 6 out 7 features.

We may conclude that these 6 features are, to a certain extent, interchangeable as far as their prognostic value is concerned.

	Stage	Age	Metast.	Differ. tissue	Atyp. nucleus	Mitotic index	Stromal reaction
Age	O						
Metast.	+++	O					
Differ. tissue	+++	O	+++				
Atyp. nucleus	+++	O	+++	+++			
Mitotic index	O	O	+	++	+		
Strom. react.	++	O	++	+++	++	O	
Infilt. perin.	+++	O	++	+++	+++	O	+++

Table 3 : The X^2 comparative method and 8 features

+++ : very significant correlation (p = 0,0001)
++ : quite significant correlation (p = 0,01)
+   : significant correlation (0,01 $<$ p $<$ 0,05)
O   : no correlation (p $>$ 0,05)

IV - SETTING UP OF A PROGNOSIS TABLE (METHOD OF THE LOGISTIC FUNCTION)

In order to set up a precise and simple prognosis table, to be used by anyone immediately after obtaining the histological data, we have tried to select the smallest number of features providing maximal information about the prognosis.

We selected the step by step logistic regression method, available in the PLR or BMDP (programmes of the information and biomathematics department, Massachussets, USA).

This method allowed to determine the 4 features with the most significant prognostic value :

- stage
- degree of tissue dedifferentiation
- mitotic index
- age

Finally, the logistic function allowed a 5 years survival prognosis of the patients, on the basis of the various possible combinations (Tables 4-5-6). Depending on the case, the percentages obtained vary between 4 % and 79 %.

The concepts of stage and tissue dedifferentiation are familiar in the literature (GLEASON). It did not come as a surprise to find out that they are of the utmost importance   interms of   the findings provided by the logistic function.

On the other hand, the mitotic index is a less known criteria. In prostatic malignancy, it is generally low but when it happens to be high, it has its very own impact on the survival rate. This was another finding of the correlation study.

As for the age factor, we are not surprised about its influence either. We had divided our patients into two groups, under and over the average age of 73 and our survival rates curves considered all causes of death, including age.

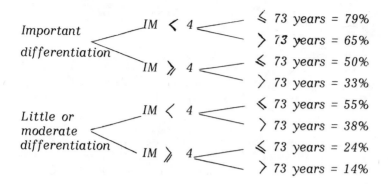

Table 4 : The five years survival rate
including stage A and B

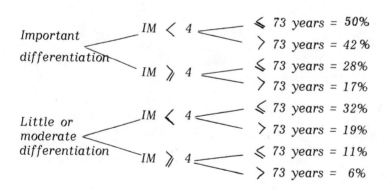

Table 5 : The five years survival rate
including stage C

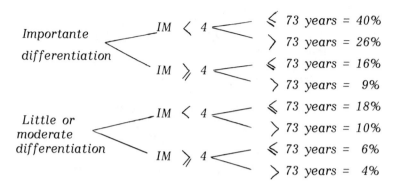

Table 6 : The five years survival rate
including stage D

CONCLUSIONS

This study allowed to determine 4 main factors influencing prognosis of prostatic carcinoma and to set up a precise evolution of a 5 years survival : 4% to 79%.

Age is an important factor which has to be taken into consideration as far as survival is concerned, despite of the fact that there is no relationship between age and the essential malignancy of the tumour.

Clinical factors, the presence of metastases for example are correctly expressed in the stage.

As for the pathological factors, the contingency between them all is extremely significant and a poor differentiation of the tumour alone is an information of the greatest importance with respect to its prognostic value.

Finally, mitotic index is a factor in its own right with little contingency. Its impact on the prognosis is extremely important and is able to modify the 5 years survival chances by 10 to 15%.

REFERENCES

1 - GLEASON DF, MELLINGEN GT and VACURG :
Prediction of progronisis for pronostic adenocarcinoma
by combined histological grading and clinical stating.
Minneapolis, J Urol, 1974, 111, 58.

2 - JEWETT HJ : The prostate. UCNA, 1974, 2, 1, 105-124.

3 - KAPLAN EL and MEIER P : Non parametric estimation
from incomplete observations.
J Am Stat Ass, 1958, 53, 456-481.

4 - MOSTOFI FK : Grading of prostate carcinoma.
Cancer Chemother Rep, 1975, 59, 111-117.

5 - BELIN Thierry.
Contribution à l'étude des facteurs pronostiques
du cancer de la prostate. (A propos de 300 dossiers
informatisés).
Thèse Médecine, Besançon, 85-056, 135 pages.

Prostate Cancer, Part A: Research, Endocrine
Treatment, and Histopathology, pages 529–531
© 1987 Alan R. Liss, Inc.

A.P.U.D. TYPE ENDOCRINE TUMOUR OF THE PROSTATE. INCIDENCE AND PROGNOSIS IN ASSOCIATION WITH ADENOCARCINOMA

M.C. Dauge*, V. Delmas **
* Service d'Anatomie Pathologique, ** Service
d'Urologie, Hôpital Bichat, Paris, France

The review of 100 cases of prostatic adenocarcinoma revealed, after GRIMELIUS' staining, a variable contingent of endocrine-paracrine cells. A.P.U.D. type cells were observed within a typical adenocarcinoma in 31 % of cases. The proportion of these cells in the neoplastic tissue is also variable :
- in 19 cases, there were only a few scattered cells (< 1 %),
- in 7 cases, there were between 1 and 2 % of A.P.U.D. cells,
- in 3 cases, this contingent exceeded 10 % of the neoplastic cells (Fig. 1)
- in 2 cases, the whole tumour presented endocrine features

In these last cases (> 10 % of A.P.U.D. cells), the adeno- carcinomas were generally poorly differentiated, trabecular and, in one case polyadenoidal. These tumours can be considered to be predominantly endocrine tumours sometimes associated with areas of typical adenocarcinoma.

In the 19 cases of rare and dispersed cells, the adenocarcinoma was well differentiated. However, the correlation between the presence of endocrine cells and the degree of differentiation of the adenocarcinoma is not constant, as undifferentiated adenocarcinomas may not present any endocrine cells.

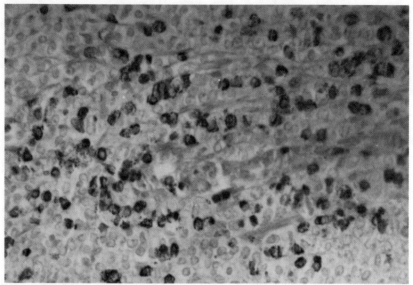

Fig.1: ×325, Grimelius stain. Trabecular carcinoma with numerous argyrophilic cells

It should be noted that the tumours in which the endocrine contingent was greater than 2 % were hormone resistant (oestrogen therapy, pulpectomy, anti-androgen). Chemotherapy was administered in one case and a temporary remission (6 months) was obtained.

The prognosis (Table 1) of endocrine tumours is worse the larger the A.P.U.D. contingent :
- a maximum of 16 months when the percentage of cells was greater than 10 %,
- more than 2 years when this percentage was less than 2 %.

When metastases were biopsied, they showed the endocrine features (carcinoid), which is a sign of rapid progression. Their appearance is independent of the proportion of these cells in the initial tumour : in one of our cases, there were only 1 % of A.P.U.D. cells on the prostatic resection specimen, while the metastases consisted solely of the endocrine contingent (the patient died after 16 months).

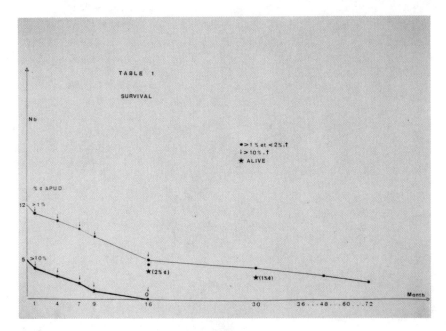

Table 1
Survival graph according to APUD cells' rate

IN CONCLUSION
The identification of endocrine cells by means of GRIMELIUS' stain and their quantitative evaluation within differentiated or undifferentiated prostatic adenocarcinoma therefore has a prognostic and therapeutic significance. In the present state of knowledge, these endocrine cells are of the paracrine type and stimulate the adjacent prostatic cells. Their presence therefore indicates a more agressive tumour.

Prostate Cancer, Part A: Research, Endocrine
Treatment, and Histopathology, pages 533–537
© 1987 Alan R. Liss, Inc.

ARE NUCLEAR SHAPE FACTORS GOOD PREDICTORS OF THE DISEASE
COURSE IN PATIENTS WITH CARCINOMA OF THE PROSTATE

T. Eichenberger, M.J. Mihatsch, M. Oberholzer,
R. Gschwind und G. Rutishauser

Division of Urology (T.E.,G.R), Department of
Pathology (M.J.M.,M.O.) and Department of Scien-
tific Photography, Institute of Physical Chemistry
(R.G.), University of Basel, Switzerland

INTRODUCTION

More sophisticated therapeutic strategies de-
mand higher diagnostic security in morphology
for factors relevant for prognosis. A possible
method to achieve this goal is morphometry- analyses of nuclear shape and size. The major
advantages of morphometry are a high degree of
objectivity of evaluation and reproducibility
(Baak and Oort, 1983).

The prognosis of the carcinoma of the prostate
depends upon age, stage, tumor morphology
including histologic tumor type and grade of
differentiation.

The diagnostic security (reproducibility) for
the above parameters is: age 100%, stage 70%,
histologic tumor type 60% and grade of differentiation 50% (Mihatsch et al., 1983).

Despite these low figures, it would be wrong to
assume that tumor morphology is not important
for prediction of the disease course.

Using both factors age and stage, a correct prediction of the disease course can be achieved in
75% of the cases. However, in a given age group
with a defined stage, tumor morphology allows a
correct prediction in 78% of the cases (Mihatsch
et al., 1983).

These findings formed the basis for our morphometric evaluation. The aim was to increase the
predictibility with that method.

MATERIAL AND METHOD

A tumor area with the least degree of differentiation was selected in HE stained sections. Nuclear shape of 100 nuclei was digitized using a
graphic tablet at a final magnification of 1000 x.
The data were stored on a PC and processed on a
Univac Computer. 12 different nuclear shape factors (roundness factor, ellipsoid factors and
concavity factors) as well as nuclear size were
calculated including mean, SD and relative SD.
Discriminant analysis (BMDP-Program) was used to
select the major factors to differentiate between
groups of patients with a good and a poor prognosis.

Bioptic material from the following patient
groups was investigated.

1. 14 punch biopsies from patients with a mean age
   of 67 years, tumor stage T3. 8 patients had a
   good prognosis and 6 a poor prognosis i.e.
   death from tumor within 5 years after biopsy.

2. 28 prostatectomies from patients with a mean age
   of 66 years, tumor stage T2 and T3, 21 patients
   had a good prognosis, 7 a poor prognosis, i.e.,
   rapid local or systemic progression of disease
   within 3 years after operation.

3. 28 transurethral resection specimens, the mean
   age of the patients was 74 years, tumor stage
   T0; 15 patients had a good prognosis, 13 a
   poor prognosis i.e. rapid local or systemic

tumor progression during a mean duration of
follow-up of 5 years.

RESULTS

In the punch biopsy material, a correlation between prognosis and two morphometric parameters
namely two ellipsoid factors (ELMOI,PDAF) was
found. With these two factors it was possible to
classify all patients correctly into the two
prognostic groups.

In the prostatectomy material a correlation was
found with nuclear size. With nuclear size alone
it was possible to classify 75% of the patients
correctly in the two prognostic groups. The
ellipsoid factors did not increase the predictibility.

In the TUR resection specimens a battery of different factors including ellipsoid (ELMOI, ELFITT,
PDAF), concavity (PCAF, PARIS) and roundness factors correlated with the prognostic groups. 93%
of the cases were correctly classified into the
two prognostic groups.

It must be concluded that in the 3 analyses,
different morphometric parameters are predictive.

In the next step of the analysis we have used the
discriminant function, e.g., of the biopsy material,
to classify the prostatectomy material into the
prognostic groups. The two ellipsoid factors
having a highly predictive value in the biopsy
material gave very poor results within the prostatectomy group. All patients with poor prognosis
were not correctly classified. Accordingly we
have analyzed all possible combinations. The results were good in the group of patients with good
prognosis (80-100%, m 95%),very poor (0-68%, m 20%)
in the group of patients with poor prognosis.

SUMMARY AND DISCUSSION

The following statements can be made:

1. in retrospective analyses morphometric parameters allow a correct assign nt to prognostic groups in more than 75% of the cases. Similar results were obtained by other investigators (Diamond, et al., 1982, Epstein, et al., 1984).

2. in prospective analyses morphometric parameters gave only correct prediction on average in about 70% of the cases, but especially poor was the prediction in patients with poor prognosis.

3. The results of the morphometric analyses are not yet better than the results of standard semiquantitative evaluation. Further studies have to define whether the differences are due to

   a) the heterogeneity of the tumor material, i.e. biopsies, prostatectomies and resection specimens,

   b) the time of fixation i.e. does the nuclear shape change during fixation

In conclusion, morphometry analysis cannot yet be used for daily diagnostic practice and prediction of prognosis.

REFERENCES

Baak JPA and Oort J (1983). Morphometry in diagnostic pathology. Springer Verlag, Berlin Heidelberg New York p2-46.

Mihatsch MJ, Ohnacker H, Oberholzer M, Spichtin HP Eichenberger T,Perret E and Torhorst J (1983). Wie zuverlässig ist die Karzinomdiagnose in der Nadelbiopsie aus der Prostata ? Urologe (A)22: 202-207.

Mihatsch MJ, Rist M, Ohnacker H, Oberholzer M, Spichtin HP, Schmassmann A, Perret A, Torhorst J and Rutishauser G (1983). Das Prostatakarzinom. Z. Urol u. Nephrol 76: 281-297.

Diamond DA, Berry SJ and Umbricht C (1982). Computerized image analysis of nuclear shape as a prognostic factor for prostatic cancer. Prostate 3: 321-332.

Epstein JI, Berry SJ and Eggleston JC (1984). Nuclear roundness factor. A predictor of progression in untreated stage A2 prostate cancer. Cancer 54: 1666-1671.

Prostate Cancer, Part A: Research, Endocrine
Treatment, and Histopathology, pages 539–543
© 1987 Alan R. Liss, Inc.

IS CYTOLOGY A DEFINITIVE DIAGNOSTIC PROCEDURE OF PROSTATIC CANCER ?

A. Steg, P. Attignac, P. Evrard, S. Desligneres
Department of Urology
Hôpital Cochin, 75014 - FRANCE

Fine needle aspiration biopsy (FNAB) is now extensively used as a method of establishing diagnosis of prostatic carcinoma. The advantages of this procedure are obvious : simplicity (out-patient procedure), accuracy (the Franzen needle is easily guided to the suspicious zone), very low complication rate and low cost.

The cytological classification we use in our laboratory is shown in Table I.

Table I. FNA : Cytological classification

I	Normal
II	Negative for malignant cells
III	Atypical
III+	Suspicion for malignancy
IV	Positive for malignant cells
V	Majority of cells positive for malignancy

The purpose of this paper is to report the results of two studies which may help to appreciate the diagnostic value of the procedure.

I) In a first retrospective study, we have analyzed the records of 105 patients in whom carcinoma of prostate has been histologically proven by TURP, and who before operation have undergone fine needle aspiration biopsy.

As seen in Table 2, there were 3 negative results and 9 inadequate cytological samples.

Table 2. 105 cases of prostatic carcinoma. Histologically
documented by T.U.R.

F.N.A. positive	93
F.N.A. negative	3
F.N.A. material inadequate for diagnosis	9

However, one should remember that in all these patients, FNAB has been performed once only just before operation. It is likely that should an aspiration biopsy have been repeated, the number of positive results whould have been higher.

Anyway the fact remains: false negative results exist, which may be explained by failure of technique or insufficient experience of the cytologist. In the literature, the false negative rate varies from 1% to 12% (1-5). For that reason, it must be underlined that *negative fine needle aspiration biopsy cannot rule out cancer.*

II) In a second study, we have analyzed 10 cases in whom prostatic adeno-carcinoma was diagnosed by positive cytology and specific treatment was initiated although histologic examination after TURP was negative for malignancy.

These 10 so called "false positive" cases are figured on Table 3. As seen, in all cases but two, the diagnosis was subsequently confirmed either by histology (case n°2, 3, 4, 5) or by evolution of the disease (case n°1, 8, 9, 10). Only in 2 patients does the diagnosis remain unconfirmed. One patient (case n°7) died a few months after TUR. The death being non related to cancer. The 2nd patient, a 83 year old patient with a typical stony hard prostatic right lobe had undergone 3 FNAB: 2 were classified III+, and 1 classified IV.

He was treated by bilateral orchiectomy in 1980. In July 1984, he has told us by letter that he is doing perfectly well but being 87 and living far from Paris he was not able to come to control (case n°6).

One may conclude that among our 10 patients there is no true false positive case. Considering our experience with these 10 patients, and also the fact that in the literature we did not find any clearly demonstrated false positive results, we should without hesitancy have concluded that a positive FNAB is a reliable procedure and allows to initiate treatment based on this method alone. However our conviction is somewhat weakened by the following case:

Obs. n°11: a 60 year old patient complained with pollakiuria and dysuria. At rectal examination, a little fine area was found in the right

Table 3 - Positive cytology (F.N.A.)/Negative histology (T.U.R.)
(10 cases)

CASE	AGE	CLINICAL STAGE	TREATMENT	EVOLUTION
1 - B.P. 1978	77	C	Orchiectomy	appearance of bone metastases in scan. Dead (1 year after T.U.R.)
2 - D.J. 1982	70	D (prostatic nodule diffuse metastases on bone scan.)	Orchiectomy	local progression of the disease (4 years later second T.U.R. : adeno-carcinoma)
3 - P.H. 1982	89	C	Orchiectomy	dead autopsy : prostatic carcinoma
4 - A.J. 1983	68	B1	no	3 years later second T.U.R. : adenocarcinoma
5 - B.A. 1983	77	C	Orchiectomy	18 months later second T.U.R. : adenocarcinoma
6 - D.M. 1981	83	B1	Orchiectomy	alive N.E.D.(?) : letter
7 - M.J. 1981	76	B2	Orchiectomy	rapid death. Non related to cancer
8 - P.M. 1982	63	B2	Orchiectomy	definite regression of tumor alive N.E.D.
9 - J.J. 1982	67	B1	External beam radiotherapy	definite regression of tumor alive N.E.D.
10 - B.A. 1983	79	C	Orchiectomy	definite regression of tumor alive N.E.D.

lobe of the prostate near the apex which appeared to be heterogeneous at sonography. TURP was performed in September 1983: 22 g of prostatic tissue was removed which at pathology appeared as *benign prostatic dystrophy*.

In spite of the operation, symptoms remained unchanged and at rectal examination, the same firm area persisted. 2 FNAB were performed in November 1983 and June 1984 which demonstrated: "a group of cells typical for malignancy". As at staging there was no extension, radical suprapubic prostatectomy was performed in March 1984.

Pathology demonstrated adenomyoma of prostate, with some cells showing slight atypia, without any visible malignant growth (complete examination of prostate). No cancer was found !!

The follow-up is now 2 years and the patient is doing well NED. This case seems to be the first one published in which a positive cytologic results was unconfirmed by complete step-sectioning of a surgically removed gland.

We have no explanation for this observation. Was a little carcinomatous prostatic area left in place during surgery ? Or was it been unrecognized by histology in spite of complete step-sectioning ? Or is it the first case of *true false positive result* ? We cannot conclude positively.

The slides were read again by 3 Cytologists. For 2, the cells were considered as malignant (stage IV) and for I they were "suspicious for malignancy" (III+).

Anyway, this case undoubtedly makes our appreciation of FNAB more reserved and careful. Finally FNAB appears as a very interesting diagnostic procedure but in order to avoid the only major risk which is a false positive result we consider as does Chokak (2) that a FNAB positive for malignancy can only be considered as definite if two conditions are fulfilled:

1°) the malignant cells have to be very numerous,

2°) the malignant cells have to be poorly differenciated and if these 2 conditions are fulfilled we think that FNAB allows staging work-up and treatment. If not, histological control is required.

REFERENCES

1 - Ballentine Carter H., Riehle R.A., Koizumi J.H., Amberson J., Darzalott Vaugham E., Jr. - Fine needle aspiration of the abnormal prostate : a cytohistological correlation. J. Urol. 135:294, 1986.

2 - Chodak G.W., Steinberg G.D., Bibbo M., Wied G., Strauss F.S., Vogelzand J., Shoenberg H.W. - The role of transrectal aspiration biopsy in the diagnosis of prostatic cancer. J. Urol. 135:299, 1986.

3 - Epstein N.A. - Prostatic biopsy : a morphologic correlation of aspiration cytology with needle biopsy histology. Cancer 38:2078, 1976.

4 - Murphy G.P. - The diagnosis of prostatic cancer. Cancer 37:589, 1976.

5 - Zattoni F., Pagano F., Rebuffi A., Constantin G. - Transrectal thin needle aspiration biopsy of prostate : four years experience. Urology 23:69, 1983.

Prostate Cancer, Part A: Research, Endocrine
Treatment, and Histopathology, page 545
© 1987 Alan R. Liss, Inc.

PROSTATIC CYTOLOGY: PERSONAL EXPERIENCE

Zattoni F., Costantin G.

Istituto di Urologia, Università di Padova
Centro Tumori, Servizio di Citologia II, Ospedale civile, Padova

SUMMARY

The clinical significance and diagnostic possibilities
of prostatic cytology are confirmed in the present report.

From 1979 to 1985, 2749 transrectal aspiration biopsies have been performed on 1934 patients at the Urologic
Clinic of Padua University. Diagnostic accurancy of prostatic transrectal aspiration biopsy was achieved in 96% of
the cases. Correlation between cytologic and histologic gra
ding in our series was 85.8 per cent. Cytological findings
and morphological changes due to Hormone and Radio-treat
ments have been proved to be a good parameter in order to
evaluate the effects of the therapy.

A good correlation between morphological changes and
clinical course has been demonstrated in 133 patients with
prostatic carcinoma treated by conservative treatments.

Cytologic examination is a simple method, quickly
carried out repeatable for several times and of high diagno
stic value. Moreover this method associated with the other
traditional parameters is indicated in the follow-up of
treated carcinomas.

Prostate Cancer, Part A: Research, Endocrine
Treatment, and Histopathology, pages 547–550
© 1987 Alan R. Liss, Inc.

ROLE OF CYTOLOGY IN THE FOLLOW-UP OF PROSTATE CANCER

L. Andersson, P.O. Hedlund, D. Das, P. Esposti
and T. Löwhagen
Departments of Urology, Cytology and Medical
Oncology, Karolinska sjukhuset, Stockholm,
Sweden

In recent years it has become widely accepted that
cytologic evaluation of prostate smears is a reliable and
reproducible method to verify the diagnosis of prostate
cancer and to ascertain the malignancy grade, provided we
have an adequate expertise in cytology available. It is
still a matter of debate whether cytology is useful even in
the follow-up of patients who are subjected to various modalities of conservative treatment, such as androgen deprivation or radiation therapy.

Since Franzén and co-workers introduced the transrectal fine needle biopsy technique in 1960 we have used
this technique as a routine procedure in the work up of
prostate cancer patients. Aspiration biopsy is also done as
part of our follow-up procedure.

In cases where there have been clinical evidence of
tumour regression such as disappearance of palpable tumour
mass, relief of obstruction etc there were usually observed
some cytomorphologic phenomena of a characteristic nature,
indicating cell injury or cell death.

Signs of cell injury are vacuolization of the cytoplasm
and "hazyness" of the cell structures, both in the nucleus
and the cytoplasm. The nuclear borders are diffuse. Large
nuclei with vacuoles indicate cell death. Nuclear pyknosis
and karyorrhexis are classical signs of cell death.

Squamous cell metaplasia is seen frequently following
estrogen treatment. There is disagreement whether the squa-

mous metaplasia affects the tumour cells or the normal
prostate epithelium. Presumably both kind of cells can undergo metaplasia. When squamous cells are scattered within
a cluster of cancer cells it is probable that they originate from tumour cells. Some of the squamous cells contain
glycogen.

Squamous cell metaplasia may be observed even after
orchidectomy although to a much lesser degree than following estrogenic hormone. Shrinkage of the nuclei and pyknosis
are more common indications of tumour cell degeneration
following orchidectomy.

Following radiation therapy there may occur some pe-
culiar alterations of the tumour cells with "ballooning"
of the nuclei and with very large nucleoli.

In those cases where the treatment induced no alteration of the cytomorphologic pattern there usually occurred
a progression of the disease.

In a number of patients there was a temporary cytologic improvement followed by a subsequent occurrence of
more active-looking tumour cells in the smears but with no
clinical evidence of tumour progression. In several of these
cases it became obvious a few months later that the disease
was in a progressive state with enlargement of the primary
tumour and appearance of metastatic lesions. On the other
hand, we have observed cases where the cytomorphologic
pattern indicated active tumour disease but where even a
prolonged follow-up failed to indicate tumour progression.

With the aim to evaluate the reliability of cytology
in the follow-up of prostate cancer patients we have done
a more systematic analysis of prostate smears with the
Franzén technique in series of 59 patients who were given
estrogenic treatment, either in the form of i.m. polyestra-
diol phosphate, 80 mg once per month, + oral ethinylestradiol, 150 μg per day, or oral estramustine phosphate,
560-840 mg per day.

The age of the patients at the initiation of therapy
was 48-82 years (m = 68 years) and the follow-up periods
6-12 months (m = 48 months).

The palpatory control was performed by one and the

same urologist and the cytologic evaluation by one and the
same cytologist.

The palpatory findings were classified as no tumour
palpable, unclear finding or suspicion of remaining tumour,
and a clearly palpable tumour infiltrate.

The cytologic evaluation was divided into four patterns.
1. No tumour cells in the smear. Ordinary or atrophic glandular cells $\pm$ metaplastic squamous cells.
2. Atrophic or degenerated tumour cells $\pm$ metaplastic squamous cells.
3. A few groups of well preserved malignant cells amongst
predominantly atrophic tumour cells or normal cells $\pm$ metaplastic squamous cells.
4. Predominantly well preserved malignant cells (of equal
or altered differentiation compared with the initial smear)
$\pm$ metaplastic squamous cells.

The patterns 1 and 2 were considered indications of a
good response to the treatment, whereas the patterns 3 and
4 were regarded to indicate treatment failure.

The correlation between the palpatory and the cytologic findings is seen in Table 1. Remission of the disease,
at least as far as the local tumour was concerned, as well
as treatment failure was fairly well reflected in the cytologic pattern of the smears. The value of cytology in the
patients with non-conclusive palpatory finding can only be
judged when there appears additional indication of progression and regression of the disease.

Table 1. Correlation between palpatory and cytologic evidence of remission

Palpation	n*	Cytologic pattern	
		1-2	3-4
No tumour	89	88%	12%
Doubtful	178	71%	29%
Tumour	39	13%	87%

* number of observations

In 19 patients both methods indicated tumour remission
throughout the observation period. In 7 cases progression

of the tumour was detected with palpation and cytology on the same occasion. In 22 cases there was cytologic evidence that the tumour had escaped from remission but no tumour infiltrate was palpated. After an interval of 2-24 months (m = 8 months) there was even palpatory evidence of progression. The opposite occurred in 7 patients - tumour infiltrate was palpated but cytology verified the progression 4-40 months (m = 12 months) later. In the remaining 4 cases there was suspicion as to progression but neither palpation nor cytology was conclusive.

Squamous cell metaplasia was seen in all the patient categories but significantly less in those cases where there was no evidence of remission, whether by palpation or cytology. The occurence of squamous cell metaplasia was found of little help to evaluate the response to treatment.

It is evident that rectal palpation has not a very high accuracy in the estimation of the size and shape of the tumour infiltrate in the prostate. To compensate for this we had one and the same observer, with long experience (P.O.H.) to examine all the patients. We do not have access to transrectal ultrasonotomography.

In the present series cytology and prostate palpation correlated well in those cases where there was a clear response or non-response to the treatment. In more than one third of the patients cytology signaled tumour progression earlier than palpation. We therefore consider cytology to be helpful in the follow-up of prostate cancer. It should not be the only investigation method but be correlated with other clinical parameters. The occurrence of well preserved tumour cells in the smears should be considered an indicator that the tumour disease is not under control, and the search for additional criteria should be intensified.

REFERENCE

Franzén S, Giertz G, Zajicek J (1960). Cytological diagnosis of prostatic tumours by transrectal aspiration biopsy: A preliminary report. Br J Urol, Vol 32, No 2:193.

Prostate Cancer, Part A: Research, Endocrine
Treatment, and Histopathology, pages 551–558
© 1987 Alan R. Liss, Inc.

AN EVALUATION OF FIVE TESTS TO DIAGNOSE PROSTATE CANCER

Patrick Guinan, Paul Ray, Rashid Bhatti and
Marvin Rubenstein

Divisions of Urology of the University of
Illinois and Cook County Hospitals Chicago,
Illinois 60612

ABSTRACT

In an effort to determine which of five tests was the
most efficient in the diagnosis of prostate cancer, 280
male patients were screened employing aspiration cytology,
transrectal ultrasound, acid phosphatase, prostate specific
antigen, and the digital rectal examination. The digital
rectal examination was the most efficient (75%) and in
order of decreasing accuracy were prostate specific antigen
(74%), prostatic ultrasound (71%), acid phosphatase (66%),
and finally aspiration cytology (63%).

In an era when what are more expensive and more technology are assumed to be better, what is simple and traditional is ignored. From an evaluation of these patients it
appears that the digital rectal examination still retains
its diagnostic efficiency. Finally, in this age of escala-
ting medical costs and physician accountability for these
expenses, you can't beat the cost – benefit ratio for the
old fashioned rectal exam.

INTRODUCTION

The digital rectal examination has traditionally been
the best technique to diagnose prostate cancer. Recently,
reports have suggested that aspiration cytology (Kline,
1982) and transrectal ultrasound (Pontes, 1984) can more
accurately detect prostatic malignancies than traditional
techniques. Modern technology has provided the physician
with more expensive and sophisticated diagnostic techniques

to diagnose prostate cancer. But are they better? We recently evaluated 280 consecutive male patients to determine
whether the newer diagnostic modalities of aspiration cytology and transrectal ultrasound were more accurate than
the time-honored digital rectal examination. In addition,
we included the standard prostate cancer marker, acid phosphatase, as well as the newer prostate specific antigen
test.

METHODS AND MATERIALS

    Patients. Two hundred and eighty male patients ad-
mitted to the Urology Service of Cook County Hospital were
evaluated. All patients had urologic complaints but were
not known to have cancer of the prostate (CAP). The mean
age of the patients was 68.1 years. All patients had a
transrectal biopsy and 77 (28%) had a histologic diagnosis
of adenocarcinoma of the prostate.

    Aspiration Cytology. Employing Esposti's method,
(Esposti, 1966) aspirations were taken from the prostate,
Papanicolaou stained and examined microscopically.

    Transrectal Prostatic Ultrasound. The Bruel and Kjaer
3604 ultrasound with a 3.5 m Hz radial scanning transducer
was utilized. A condom was placed over the transducer and
after the unit was inserted into the rectum the condom was
filled with water to allow an adequate interface for scanning. The scans were recorded on Polaroid film and read independently by three staff urologists with experience in
interpreting ultrasonic images. Unsatisfactory scans were
read as an incorrect diagnosis.

    Acid Phosphatase. Determinations of serum acid phos-
phatase were performed with thymolphthalein phosphate substrate, according to the method of Roy et al (Roy, 1971).
Acid phosphatase levels were expressed in Worthington units,
and the normal range was 0.2 to 0.6 units.

    Prostate Specific Antigen. Prostate specific antigen
determinations were performed employing the Hybritec TAN-
DEM- R PSA kit (Killian, 1986). The upper limit of normal
was the mean plus one standard deviation.

    Digital Rectal Examination. Digital rectal examina-
tions were performed by board-certified urologists or senior

residents with five years experience in urology; this was
done after blood samples had been drawn for tests of acid
phosphatase and leukocyte-adherence inhibition but before
the cytologic tests were begun. When the examiners recorded
their diagnostic impression, they did not know the results
of any of the other tests. The diagnostic criteria for examination of the prostate conformed with the guidelines
given by Carlton (Carlton, 1978); these guidelines are simple yet complete. A diagnosis of absence of malignant tumor
was made on the basis of the palpation of the smooth and
uniform prostate; the prostate could be larger than the
normal "chestnut" size although its configuration would have
to be relatively symmetrical. A diagnosis of possible presence of carcinoma was made if the prostate contained areas
of induration or nodular irregularities, which could be
small or could involve extensive areas of stone-hard projections with lateral fixation. The results were recorded
in the patient's medical record as well as on data collec-
tion sheets.

Statistical Analysis. Our analysis was based on the
predictive-value theory of test accuracy as reflected in
Bayes' (Bayes, 1763) theorem and as further defined by
Galen and Gambino (Galen, 1975).

Sensitivity was determined as the percentage of positive tests in patients who had prostate cancer, and specificity as the percentage of negative tests in patients who
did not have prostate cancer. The predictive value of a
positive test was defined as the percentage of patients who
had a positive test and prostate cancer, and the predictive
value of a negative test as the percentage of patients who
had a negative test and did not have prostate cancer.

Efficiency was defined as the percentage of patients
who were correctly classified, and was determined according
to the formula $(pa + [1 - p] b) \times 100$, where "a" represents
sensitivity, "b" specificity, and "p" prevalence (the percentage of patients who had prostate cancer in the population studied).

RESULTS

Aspiration Cytology. Of the 163 patients who had an
aspiration cytology 44 had a histologic diagnosis of CAP
and 129 had a diagnosis of BPH (TABLE 1). Of the 34 CAP

TABLE 1

DIAGNOSTIC TESTS FOR PROSTATE CANCER

DIAGNOSIS	TEST RESULT	ASPIR- ATION	ULTRA- SOUND	ACID PHOSPHATASE	PROSTATE SPECIFIC ANTIGEN	RECTAL EXAM
Benign Prostatic Hypertrophy	True Negative	93	38	127	45	143
	False Positive	36	15	55	15	45
	Total	129	53	182	60	188
Prostate Cancer	True Positive	20	22	42	31	51
	False Negative	14	9	23	11	19
	Total	34	31	65	42	70
	Total Examined	163	84	247	102	258

patients 20 were correctly diagnosed and 93 of the 129 BPH patients were correctly diagnosed for an efficiency rate of 63% (TABLE 2).

Transrectal Ultrasound. Of the 84 patients who had transrectal ultrasound examinations 31 had a histological diagnosis of CAP and 53 had a diagnosis of BPH. Of the 31 CAP patients, 22 were correctly diagnosed, and of the 53 BPH patients 38 were correctly diagnosed for an efficiency rate of 71%.

Acid Phosphatase. Of the 247 patients who had an acid phosphatase determination, 65 had a histologic diagnosis of CAP and 182 had a diagnosis of BPH. Of the 65 CAP patients, 42 were correctly diagnosed, and of 182 BPH patients 127 were correctly diagnosed for an efficiency rate of 66%.

Prostate Specific Antigen. Of the 102 patients who had a prostate specific antigen determination performed, 42 had a histologic diagnosis of CAP and 60 had a diagnosis of BPH. Of the 42 patients with CAP 31 were correctly diagnosed and 45 of the 60 BPH patients were correctly diagnosed for an efficiency rate of 74%.

Digital Rectal Examination. Of the 258 patients who had a digital rectal examination, 70 had a histologic diagnosis of CAP and 188 had a diagnosis of benign prostatic hypertherapy (BPH). Of the 70 CAP patients 51 were correctly diagnosed for an efficiency rate of 75%.

DISCUSSION

Prostate cancer is the second leading cause of male cancer deaths in the United States accounting for 26,100 estimated fatalities in 1986 (Silverberg, 1986). There will be 90,000 new cases of this disease in 1986 and its incidence is half again more common in the black male. Prostate cancer is curable if diagnosed while localized; however only 10-15% is detected while still confined to within the prostate capsule. Until 1936 the only test to detect prostate cancer was the rectal examination. In that year Gutman described the first marker for any human cancer, acid phosphatase (Gutman, 1936). There have been numerous modifications of the serum acid phosphatase test and more recently there has been the development of an antigenically more specific marker, the prostate specific antigen test.

TABLE 2

	#PATIENTS	EFFICIENCY SENSIVITITY	SPECIFICITY	EFFICIENCY
Aspiration Cytology	163	59	72	63%
Prostate Ultrasound	84	71	72	71%
Prostate Specific Antigen	102	74	75	74%
Acid Phosphatase	247	65	69	66%
Digital Rectal Examination	258	73	77	75%

Two non-serum diagnostic modalities: aspiration cytology and transrectal ultrasound, have been reported to be
accurate in detecting prostate cancer. Aspiration cytology
of the prostate, while first reported by Esposti in 1956,
has only recently become popular in the United States. Its
advantage over core biopsy is simplicity and a low incidence
of sepsis. Prostatic ultrasound is expensive and a scanning
unit can cost $30,000 to $50,000.

In on-going efforts to find better methods to diagnose
prostate cancer we evaluated 280 consecutive male patients,
who also had a histologically confirmed diagnosis by core
biopsy, with one or all tests: aspiration cytology, transrectal ultrasound, acid phosphatase, prostate specific antigen and the digital rectal examination. Statistical analysis revealed that the rectal examination was the most
efficient.

Unfortunately modern medicine has become enamored with
technology (which is usually expensive) and has become less
reliant upon, and proficient with, the old fashioned history
and physical examination (which may be more diagnostic).

Moreover, with the rectal examination the practitioner
can also evaluate the rectum for rectal cancer and the stool
for the presence of gastrointestinal bleeding. In addition,
the anus can be evaluated for hemorrhoids and anal disease
as well as sphincter tone.

The digital rectal examination has been overshadowed
by more glamorous technologic and expensive tests. But
since the rectal exam is cost efficient and no less diag-
nostically accurate, it behooves all practitioners to routinely perform this test on all of their patients.

REFERENCES

Bayes T (1763). An essay toward solving a problem in the
    doctrine of chance. Philos Trans R Soc Lond Biol 53:370-418.
Carlton CE Jr (1978). Initial evaluation: including history
    physical examination, and urinalysis. In Harrison JH
    Gittes RF Perlmutter AD Stamey TA Walsh PC (eds): Camp-
    bell's Urology Vol 1 Philadelphia: WB Saunders 203-221.
Esposti PL (1966). Cytologic diagnosis of prostatic tumors
    with the aid of transrectal aspiration biopsy: a critical
    review of 1,110 cases and a report of morphologic and cy-

tochemical studies. Acta Cytol 10:182-186.

Galen RS Gambino SR (1975). Beyond normality: The predictive value and efficiency of medical diagnoses, New York:
John Wiley.

Gutman EB Sproul EE and Gutman AB (1936). Increased phosphatase activity of bone at site of osteoblastic metastases secondary to carcinoma of prostate gland. Am J Cancer
28:485-495.

Killian et al (1986). Relative reliability of five serially
measured markers for prognosis of progression in prostate
cancer. JNCI February 76:179-185.

Kline TS Kohler F˜Kelsey DM (1982). Cytology (ABC) its
use in diagnosis of lesions of the prostate gland. Arch
Pathol Lab Med 106:136-139.

Pontes JE Ohe H Watanabe H Murphy G (1984). Transrectal
ultrasonography of the prostate. Cancer 53:1369-1372.

Roy AV Brower ME Hayden JE (1971). A new acid phosphatase
substrate with greater prostatic specificity. Clin Chem
17:653.

Silverberg E (1986). Cancer statistics. Ca 36:9-25.

Prostate Cancer, Part A: Research, Endocrine Treatment, and Histopathology, pages 559–568
© 1987 Alan R. Liss, Inc.

EXPERIMENTAL INDUCTION OF ATYPICAL HYPERPLASIA IN RAT VENTRAL PROSTATE

Armand Abramovici, Ciro Servadio,
Josef Shmuely, Uriel Sandbank
Laboratory of Development Pathology, J.Casper Inst.
of Pathology and Department of Urology, Beilinson
Medical Center, Petah Tikva, Tel Aviv University
Sackler School of Medicine, Israel

INTRODUCTION

The search for an animal model especially among rodents, for the study of prostatic growth abnormalities is hampered by the relatively high resistance of old rodents to develop spontaneously hyperplastic (Franks,1967) or neoplastic changes (Shain et al,1975; Noble, 1980).

The experimental induction of neoplastic lesions in animals were obtained after prolonged treatment with androgens (Grayhack, 1965; Walvoored et al,1976; Jacobi et al,1978; De Klerck et al, 1979; Moore et al,1979; Noble, 1980; Karr et al,1984), methylcholantrene (Scott and Angbrey,1978), and nitrosamines (Pour, 1981). In all these reports the pathological lesions of the prostate were found to be quite identical to the human entity (Scott and Angbrey,1978; De Klerck et al, 1979).

In a previous study we demonstrated that a daily topical application of citral (Abramovici et al,1985) on back skin of adolescent male rats initially induces benign prostatic hyperplasia (BPH), changes observed already 10 days after citral administration. A longer period of treatment (30 days) significantly enhanced the acinar hyperplasia of ventral prostates, whereas the stroma remained more resistent (Servadio et al, 1986). Characteristic BPH lesions involving both prostatic compartments were found after 3 months of treatment (Abramovici et al,1985).

The citral (3,7 dimethyl-2,6 octadienal) is a constituent of natural essential oils extracted from various plants, mainly citrus fruits. Nowadays, it is mostly synthesized on an industrial scale,being widely used in cosmetics cleaning products and food industry because of its pleasant lemon scent (Bedoukian,1965; Opdyke,1979).

Citral also posses a hyperplastic effect on sebaceous glands of the dorsal skin as well as induces epidermal hyperkeratosis on the application site (Abramovici et al, 1983). Since it is known that testosterone is involved on growth modulation of both prostate (Lasnitzki, 1955;Isaacs and Coffey,1981) and sebaceous glands(Ebling, 1957;Strauss and Pochi, 1963), we assumed that the citral effect on these structures may be a testosterone dependent phenomenon. Moreover, citral administration following bilateral orchidectomy did not prevent the prostate involution process (Servadio et al,1986).

The question arises whether the citral effect might be influenced by the testosterone levels in plasma at the time of treatment or determined by its own absorption rate through the hyperkeratotic skin lesions (Abramovici et al,1983) following permanent application of citral. Preliminary study (unpublished data) showed that the total testosterone levels in the plasma of young male rats (42 days old) have a circadian rhythm which gradually decreases with age and disappears among retired breeder rats (1 yr.old). The highest testosterone levels were found in the morning, attaining a nadir in the evening. Therefore, we decided to change the time sequence frequency and the location of the citral application, namely giving every four days pulse instead of a daily one, and smearing the citral at a different location each time. This change in the experimental schedule induced relevant histological lesions of atypical acinar hyperplasia of the ventral prostate, instead of BPH as obtained by a daily citral treatment in a constant skin area.

MATERIAL and METHODS

Thirty-five young male Wistar rats (6 wks.old,150gr.B.W.) were maintained in a climatized environment with a 12 hr. light/dark cycle. Standard Purina chow pellets and water were supplied ad libidum.

The citral (Fluka,Buchs, Switzerland) was dissolved in 70% ethanol solution and administered at a dose of 185 mg/kg body weight according to the experimental group as follows:

a) daily smearing at 8 am on the same area of the shaved back skin.

b) smearing once in a four days at 12 am each time on different areas of the shaved back skin.

c) untreated animals as controls.

The animals were sacrificed at 30 days from the initiation of the experiment.

The prostate glands were excised, freshly weighed, fixed thereafter in Stieve's fluid overnight at room temperature (Lillie,1965), and embedded in paraffin wax. Sections 5 um thick were routinely proceeded and stained with Harris haematoxilin-eosin method for histological examination. The statistical analysis of prostate weight was done using the Student t-test.

RESULTS

The ventral prostates of both experimental groups and control rats were macroscopically alike. However,the daily treated animals – group a – had a heavier prostate (875 ± 12mg.) than those treated once in four days – group b – (800 ± 11mg.) and control rats (820 ± 15mg.). The difference in the prostatic wet weight between groups a and b was found to be statistically significant at a confidence limit of 0.05 p 0.01.

The histology of normal rat ventral prostate is characterized by random distribution of equal size acini containing a conspicuous eosinophilic material and surrounded by a very delicate fibro-vascular stroma (Fig.1). The low columnal epithelial cell lining appeared uniform and devoid of papillary projections (Fig.2), their nuclei placed at the basal pole of the cell.

The prostate of citral daily treated rats (group a) showed typical lobular hyperplasia characterized by varying degrees

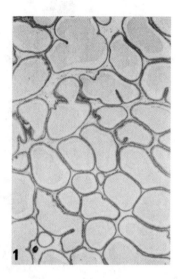 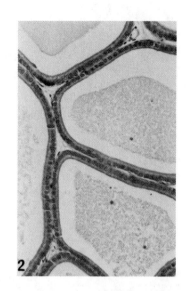

Figure 1. Normal prostate,
equal size acini contain-
ing eosinophilic homo-
genuous material   x28

Figure 2. Uniform acini with
low columnar epithelial
cells lining and minimal
interaciniar stroma   x150

of acinar proliferation (Fig.3). The acini showed a hetero-
genicity in size and shape, large or small round acini intermingled with tortuous and irregular ones. They were densely
packed and presented intraluminal small papillary projections
(Fig.4). High columnal epithelial cells containing large intracellular apical clear cytoplasm and nuclei of round to ovoid
shape, were found together with the slight loss of polarity
in cell arrangement (Fig.4). A slight increase of fibrovascular stroma was noted and the basal membrane was found normal.

At low power magnification the ventral prostate of rats
treated once every four days (group b) at noon,showed at first
glance similar morphological pictures as the group-a treated
rats. However,the acini were apparently less crowded and contained a reduced amount of light eosinophilic secretory ma-

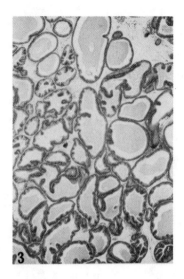

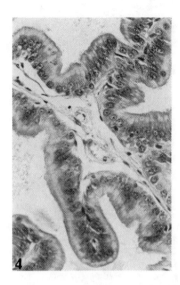

Figure 3 Daily treatment:
varying degree of aciniar
hyperplasia   x 25

Figure 4 Intraluminal papillary projections of high
columnal epithelium with
apical clear cytoplasm.
x250

terial (Fig.5). Examination at a higher magnification, revealed definite histopathological changes of atypical hyperplasia.
Abundant intraluminal papillary projections at different ex-
tends were observed attaining a cribriform pattern in some areas
(Fig.6). Foci of epithelial "pilling up" and unisokaryosis,
together with a net loss of nuclear polarity were also seen(Fig.
7). Relatively few mitotic figures were noted. In few acini,
budding of small groups of irregular small epithelial cells
crossing the basal membrane of the acini were seen(Fig.8).
These cell groups budding seemed to be strictly limited to the
bursting site and did not extend further.

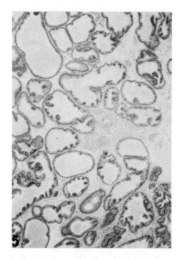

Figure 5   Every 4 days treatment: similar changes as
in Fig. 4   x25

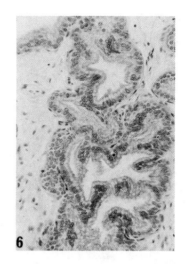

Figure 6   Abundant intraluminal papillary projections
and a cribiform acinus
                              x150

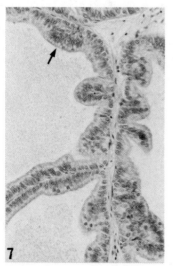

Figure 7   Foci of epithelial
pilling up (arrow), uni-
sokaryosis and loss of
nuclear polarity   x150

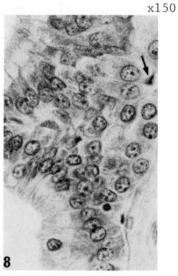

Figure 8   Budding of epithelial cells crossing
the basal membrane. Mi-
totic figure present
(arrow)   x600

DISCUSSION

Atypical hyperplasia of human prostate (AHP) was first described by McNeal(1965) as an abnormal cellular and glandular proliferation and has been considered as a precancerous state. This entity was long time disputed and not unanimously accepted as a diagnostic entity by most of the pathologists (Gleason, 1985). Efforts for a more comprehensive analysis of the morphological criteria defining the atypical hyperplasia lesions were continued and nowadays its biological behaviour is considered as a precursor of prostatic neoplasia (Gleason, 1985; McNeal & Bastwick, 1986).

Our previous studies revealed that daily citral administration induced BPH lesions in rats and do correspond morphologically to the human counterpart excepts of the delay in stromal participation at the early stages (Abramovici et al 1985; Servadio et al, 1986).

Changing the schedule time of citral administration while relating it to the circadian rhythm of testosterone concentration in rat plasma, as well as, the site of smearing, induced an atypical hyperplasia,quite identical to that described in human prostates (Gleason, 1985; McNeal & Bastwick, 1986). We prefered to use the term of atypical hyperplasia (Gleason, 1985) rather than intraductal dysplasia proposed by McNeal & Bastwick (1986), since morphogenetically, the cytological features seemed to be derived from the BPH pattern, also induced by citral in different experimental conditions (Abramovici et al, 1985; Servadio et al, 1986). Moreover, our findings did not seem to be limited to the intraductal compartment, but a tentative for extra-acinar budding of epithelial cells was observed.

Noteworthy that the variability in size and shape of prostatic acini and the presence of some cribriform structures, are also in favour of an atypical hyperplastic process. The presence of pilling-up foci in the acini, as characterized by multilayering of the nuclei, might reflect an accelerate local proliferation. Such a process will promote the loss of nuclear polarity, and also an exacerbation of the papillary intraluminal projection with cribriform pattern formation, as observed in this study.

The significant difference in the prostate weight found between the experimental groups, might be explained by the reduction in the amount of prostatic secretion encountered among AHP acini and also to their relatively less crowdedness as compared to the BPH acini.

The exact mechanism of action of citral upon the adolescent rat prostate is as yet unknown. The fact that citral might affect other tissues known to be monitored by sex hormones such as rat ovary (Toaff et al, 1979) and sebaceous glands (Abramovici et al, 1983) suggest an interreaction between citral and the sex hormones at the level of these target organs. Also to remind that citral administration could not prevent the prostate involution process in bilateral orchidectomized rats(Servadio et al, 1986).

Paradoxically, the atypical hyperplastic changes were obtained by relatively lower amounts of citral administered once in a four day pulses, while a daily smearing induced only typical BPH lesions. Such an increase of citral efficiency might partially be explained by the fact that it was administered each time on a different skin area, thus avoiding the hyperkeratotic skin lesions induced by daily smearing on the same area(Abramovici et al,1983) and subsequently to an improvement of its absorbtion rate. Moreover, the administration schedule of citral at noon when plasma testosterone levels are much lower than during the morning might also play an important role on the promotion of atypical hyperplasia by citral.

The relatively short induction time of such lesions among adolescent rats are definitely not connected with the senescence process, but they are rather dependent on the androgens homeostasis and/or circadian rhythm interphases. The present findings represent a first attempt to study the evolution of prostatic acinar transformation from benign to a typical hyperplasia by modulating the amount and the time of citral administration.

In conclusion this animal model opens a new and unique opportunity to study the prostatic growth pathophysiology and its possible interconnections with the neoplastic growth process.

REFERENCES

Abramovici A, Servadio C, Sandbank U (1985) Benign hyperplasia of ventral prostate in rats induced by a monoterpene. Prostate 7:389-394.

Abramovici A, Wolf R, Sandbank M (1983). Sebaceous glands changes following topical application of citral. Acta Dermatol Venerol (Stockh) 63:428-432.

Bedaukian PZ (1965). "Perfumery and flavoring synthetics". Amsterdam Elsevier Publishing Comp. 2nd edition, pp.99-111.

De Klerk DP, Coffey DS, Ewing LL, McDermott IR, Reiner WG, Robinson CH, Scott WW, Strandberg JD, Talalay P, Walsh PC, Wheaton LG, Zirkin BR (1979). Comparison of spontaneous and experimentally induced canine prostatic hyperplasia. J Clin Invest 64:842-849.

Ebling FJ (1957). The action of testosterone in the sebaceous glands and epidermis in castrated and hypophysectomized male rats. J Endocrinol 15:297-306.

Franks ML (1967). Normal, pathological anatomy and histology of the genital tracts of rats and mice. In Cotchin E, Roe FJC (eds)"Pathology of laboratory rats and mice" Oxford Blackwell Scientific Publ. pp.469-499.

Gleason DF (1985). Atypical hyperplasia, benign hyperplasia and well differentiated adenocarcinoma of the prostate. Amer J Surg Pathol 9 Suppl:53-67.

Grayhack JT (1965). Effect of testosterone-estradiol administration on citric acid and fructose content of the rat prostate. Endocrinology 72:1068-1074.

Isaacs JT, Coffey DS (1981). Changes in dihydrotestosterone metabolism associated with the development of canine benign prostatic hypertrophy. Endocrinology 108:445-453.

Jacobi GH, Moore RJ, Wilson JD (1978). Studies on the mechanism of 3 androstanediol induced growth of the dog prostate. Endocrinology 102:1748-1755.

Karr JP, Kim U, Resko JA, Schneider S, Chai LS, Murphy GP, Sandbery AA (1984). Induction of benign prostatic hypertrophy in baboons. Invest Urol 23:276-289.

Lasnitzki I (1955). The effect of testosterone propionate on organ cultures of mouse prostate. J Endocrinol 12:236-240.

Lillie BD (1965). "Histopathologic technic and practical histochemistry" 3rd edition New York McGraw-Hill Book Comp. pp.48-49.

McNeal JE (1965). Morphogenesis of prostatic carcinoma. Cancer 18:1659-1666.

McNeal JE, Bastwick DG (1986). Intraductal dysplasia: A premalignant lesion of the prostate. Hum Pathol 17:64-71.

Moore RJ, Gazak JM, Quebbeman JF, Wilson JD (1979). Concentration of dihydrostestosterone and 3 androstanediol in naturally occurring and androgen induced prostatic hyperplasia in the dog. J Clin Invest 64:1003-1010.

Noble RL (1980). Production of Nb rat carcinoma of the dorsal prostate and response of estrogen dependent transplant to sex hormones and tamoxifen. Cancer Res 40:3547-3550.

Opdyke DLJ (1979). Citral. Food Cosmet Toxicol 17:259-266.

Pour PM (1981). A new prostatic cancer model: systemic induction of prostatic cancer in rats by a mitrosamine. Cancer Lett. 13:303-308.

Scott R, Angbrey E (1978). Methylcholantrene and cadmium induced changes in rat prostate. Brit J Urol 50:25-28.

Servadio C, Abramovici A, Sandbank U, Savion M, Rosen M (1986). Early stages of the pathogenesis of rat ventral prostate hyperplasia induced by citral. Eur Urol (in press).

Shain SA, McCullough B, Segaloff A (1975).Spontaneous adenocarcinoma of the ventral prostate of aged AXC rats. J Nat Cancer Inst 55:181-190.

Strauss JS, Pochi PE (1963). The human sebaceous gland: Its regulation by steroidal hormones and its use as an organ for assaying androgenicity in vivo. Recent Prog Horm Res 19:385-444.

Toaf ME, Abramovici A, Sporn J, Liban E (1979). Selective oocyte degeneration and impaired fertility in rats treated with aliphatic monoterpene, citral. J Reprod Fertil 55:347-352.

Walvoord DJ, Resnick MI, Grayhack JT (1976). Effect of testosterone, dihydrotestosterone, estradiol, and prolactin on the weight and citric acid content of the lateral lobe of the rat prostate. Invest Urol 14:60-65.

Prostate Cancer, Part A: Research, Endocrine
Treatment, and Histopathology, pages 569–571
© 1987 Alan R. Liss, Inc.

SCLEROTIC BONE METASTASES OF PROSTATIC ORIGIN AND
OSTEOMALACIA. IMPORTANCE OF A HISTOMORPHOMETRY STUDY.

Franck Bürki, Jean-Michel Coindre and Louis
Mauriac
Department of Medicine (F.B. , L.M) and
Department of Pathology (J.M.C), Fondation
Bergonié, 180, rue de Saint-Genès, 33076,
Bordeaux Cédex, France.

INTRODUCTION

Bone metastases from prostatic carcinoma are usually
sclerotic and sometimes extensive. Patients must produce
large amounts of bone tissue and the resulting, markedly
increased requirement for calcium and phosphorus often
leads to hypocalcemia and hypophosphoremia. Osteomalacia
(OM) is rarely reported, but its incidence is certainly
underestimated because clinical and radiological signs of
such osteopathy are systematically attributed to bone
metastases. In such a situation, only histomorphometry on
undecalcified bone biopsy specimens with measurement of
the calcification rate makes diagnosis of osteomalacia
possible .

PATIENTS AND METHODS

Patients

Eighteen patients, 62 to 82 years old, with confirmed
sclerotic bone metastases from prostatic carcinoma, were
investigated. These patients were under estrogen therapy.
They all experienced bone pain resistant to estrogen and
analgesic treatment.

Methods

- Pelvis, ribs, dorso-lumbar spine, femur X-rays and
bone scan were performed.
- Serum calcium, phosphate, alkaline phosphatases, and
urinary calcium excretion were determined.

    - Bone biopsy:
    . After double labelling of the calcification front with tetracycline
    . Embedding in methacrylate without prior decalcification
    . Histomorphometric study.

RESULTS (Tables 1 and 2)

    . Histomorphometry showed that 3 patients had osteomalacia (OM +)
    . These patients differed from the others in that the pain they experienced in their bones was stronger, more diffuse and often more permanent.
    . All three had a fracture of the femoral neck.
    . Osteomalacia was cured by doses of vitamin D and calcium in one patient. The other two died too quickly for vitamino-calcic treatment to be administered.

Table 1 : HISTOMORPHOMETRIC DATA (Group 1 = OM + ; Group 2 = OM -)

	TBV (%)	RS (%)	OV (%)	OS (%)	TIO	CR(μm/day)
All patients (18)	48.5±22.0	8.7±4.7	13.5±15.2	50.6±22.4	22.1±15.0	0.66±0.29
Group 1 (OM+) (3)	59.4± 0.17	5.5±2.6	43.8± 8.9	84.3± 2.4	51.8± 9.9	(0.20
Group 2 (OM-) (15)	45.6±23.4	8.2±4.6	7.0± 3.7	43.4±17.3	15.6± 3.7	0.79±0.15
Normal values	17.8± 4.9	3.6±1.1	2.7± 1.7	15.5± 8.2	17.6± 4.8	0.72±0.12

TBV = trabecular bone volume RS = resorption surfaces
OV = osteoid volume OS = osteoid surfaces
CR = calcification rate TIO = thickness index of the osteoid seams

Difference between groups 1 and 2 is significant for all data (p < 0.01) except for TBV (N.S.).

Table 2 : BIOCHEMICAL DATA (Group 1 = OM + ; Group 2 = OM -)

	Serum calcium (mmol/1)	Serum phosphorus (mmol/1)	Serum alkaline phosphatase (IU/1)	Urinary calcium (mmol/24 h)
All patients (18)	2.11±0.16	0.93±0.18	1 471± 966	1.39±0.86
Group 1 (OM+)(3)	1.93±0.25	0.66±0.17 *	1 231± 472	1.46±1.16
Group 2 (OM-)(15)	2.14±0.11	0.97±0.14	1 522±1 048	1.37±0.84
Normal values	2.35±0.25	1.10±0.30	135± 65	5.60±1.87

(* Difference between group 1 and group 2 = $p < 0.05$).

DISCUSSION

. Phosphocalcic metabolism anomalies in bone prostate cancer metastases have been known for a long time. Histologic proof of osteomalacia has been reported more recently in a few cases and in limited series.

. The clinical symptoms of osteomalacia are somewhat similar to pain related to bone metastases. Apart from phosphatemia, biology is of no use to the clinician for diagnosis. In such circumstances, only bone histomorphometry makes possible the diagnosis of osteomalacia in patients presenting intractable pain.

. Causes of osteomalacia in prostatic cancer are :
- an increased need for calcium owing to sclerotic diffuse metastasis,
- vitamin D deficiency owing to aging,
- estrogenotherapy which inhibits bone resorption when used at low doses.

CONCLUSION

1. Osteomalacia is not rare in patients with bone metastases of prostatic origin.

2. In such patients, osteomalacia can be reliably diagnosed only by bone histomorphometry.

3. This examination may be used in patients undergoing hormonal therapy and suffering from diffuse skeletal pain or bone fragility, and from hypocalcemia or phosphatemia.

4. This type of osteomalacia can be cured by treatment with vitamin D and calcium.

Index

573